Cultures of Intoxication

Fiona Hutton
Editor

Cultures of Intoxication

Key Issues and Debates

palgrave
macmillan

Editor
Fiona Hutton
Victoria University
Wellington, New Zealand

ISBN 978-3-030-35283-7 ISBN 978-3-030-35284-4 (eBook)
https://doi.org/10.1007/978-3-030-35284-4

Cover illustration: Phanie / Alamy Stock Photo

This Palgrave Macmillan imprint is published by the registered company Springer Nature Switzerland AG.
The registered company address is: Gewerbestrasse 11, 6330 Cham, Switzerland

This book is dedicated to Wendy Chambers, a woman who was known (on occasion!) to enjoy being intoxicated. I enjoyed our many intoxications, and I miss you.

Acknowledgements

The idea for this book came about over many conversations and ponderings about the notion of intoxication—what it means, what it feels like, how is it different for different people, and does it change over time? These are just a few of the questions I have considered on plane and train journeys, at conferences ('The Dangerous Consumptions Colloquium' crowd needs a special mention here), whilst observing the effects of intoxication in myself and others as well as through asking people about a variety of intoxications over several research projects. Helping these ponderings were a number of academics and researchers whose work I found interesting and inspiring, so I decided to ask them to collaborate on this book with me—I was delighted when they said 'yes'. So many thanks to all the authors who have contributed their chapters to this edited collection—you have all been wonderful, and (mostly!) on time. Your thoughts, contributions and hard work have been much appreciated.

Thanks also go to Josie from Palgrave, who prompted me to start the process of getting this book together, and to Liam and his colleagues who took over and had the unenviable task of trying to get me to be organised and efficient in terms of deadlines.

There are many people who contributed to this book in numerous ways, but special thanks go to Archie and Grace, who were fantastic, understanding when mum was 'always working' and amusing themselves without getting into too much trouble. Special thanks also go to Steve—

this book would not have been written without your sacrifices, and I couldn't have done this without your incredible support as well as your continual encouragement to keep at it. My friends and colleagues at the Institute of Criminology and beyond also need a special mention: Helen, Jo, Sian, Paul, Karen, Desna, Lizzy, Antonia, Sarah, Jan, Lynzi, Trevor, Sally and Jordan in particular—thank you for your words of encouragement, cups of tea and chocolate. Lastly, to my parents Val and David, thank you for your endless love and encouragement over many years of ponderings and for not minding my own (often spectacular!) intoxications.

Contents

Notes on Contributors

Tammy Ayres is Lecturer in Criminology at the University of Leicester. Ayres has been undertaking research within the field of drugs for almost two decades, with extensive experience of investigating vulnerable populations, particularly problematic drug users, prisoners, people with mental ill health and trauma both in the community and in prisons. She is co-chair for the British Society of Criminology's Critical Criminology Network and a member of the Deviant Leisure Research Group and the Extreme Anthropology Network.

Angus Bancroft is Lecturer in Sociology at the University of Edinburgh. He researches illicit digital markets, intoxication experiences and cultures, and the relationship between deprivation and drug problems.

Adrian Barton is Senior Lecturer in Criminology working at the University of St Mark and St John. His research has been focused on the interface of criminal justice policy and practice and its relationship with health and welfare provision. Barton's work has been published widely in those areas including journal articles, books and commissioned research reports. He has conducted research into both licit and illicit drug use and is working with offenders within prisons, looking at how social interventions may impact on their substance use.

Nicolas Droste has accumulated ten years of research experience in the fields of alcohol and other drug (AOD) use in nightlife and emergency service contexts. He has been involved in multiple collaborative projects evaluating and refining youth outreach services, and is an author on approximately 60 papers in the fields of AOD use/misuse and emergency mental health/AOD services. In 2012 he was awarded an Australian Research Council (ARC) PhD scholarship to undertake a study of combined alcohol and energy drink use based in Geelong, Australia, which was completed in March 2016. Droste researches alcohol-related violence and injuries in emergency department settings.

Sarah Herbert (Ngāti Kahu ki Whangaroa) is a lecturer at Te Kupenga Hauora Māori, the University of Auckland, New Zealand (NZ). She completed her PhD (Critical health psychology), in 2017, from Massey University in New Zealand, which explored the social contexts of (older) Māori alcohol use. Broadly, her interests lie in the field of Māori health advancement and achieving health equity for Māori. Her expertise is in qualitative research and her research interests include Māori alcohol use, social justice and critical policy analysis including responsiveness to Māori and Te Tiriti o Waitangi.

Fiona Hutton is an associate professor at the Institute of Criminology at Victoria University, New Zealand. She has taught and researched in the areas of criminology, specifically criminological theory, youth crime and cultures, drug policy, harm reduction, alcohol and other drugs for the past 20 years. Her research work has been published extensively in New Zealand and international journals. She is the author of *Risky Pleasures? Club Cultures and Feminine Identities* (2006). Her research projects include exploring the ways drug use and drug users are demonised and stigmatised through a variety of media and other discourses; critically exploring the concept of intoxication, and how the intoxication practices of diverse groups are experienced and responded to; and a qualitative project examining people's experiences of receiving a drug-related conviction.

Helen Keane is a professor in the School of Sociology at the Australian National University in Canberra, Australia. Her primary research focuses on drug use, including pharmaceutical, recreational and illicit substances (and the relationships between these categories and forms of use). Her work on these topics has been published widely in journals such as *Social Science & Medicine*, *International Journal of Drug Policy* and *Feminist Theory*. She has a particular interest in concepts of addiction and critical addiction studies. She is the co-author of *Habits: Remaking Addiction* (Palgrave Macmillan, 2014) with Suzanne Fraser and David Moore. This book builds on her earlier work *What's Wrong with Addiction?* (2002).

Kate Kersey is a lecturer in Auckland University of Technology (AUT) University and has a background in public health, health policy and regulation, and health law. She is enrolled at Victoria University of Wellington, New Zealand, as a PhD student. Her research aims to explore how midlife women make sense of their and others' alcohol use and how social, economic and cultural contexts play a role in this sense-making, in order to inform appropriate cohort-specific policy responses.

Toby Lea is a Humboldt Foundation Research Fellow at the German Institute for Addiction and Prevention Research, Cologne, Germany, and an adjunct lecturer in the Centre for Social Research in Health, the University of New South Wales (UNSW) Sydney, Australia. He is an applied social health researcher focused on the use of psychedelics as novel therapies for mental health, and substance use and harm reduction among sexual and gender minority people.

Antonia Lyons is Professor of Health Psychology and head of school in the School of Health at Victoria University of Wellington, New Zealand. Her research has focused on the social, cultural and mediated contexts of behaviours related to health and well-being outcomes. She is co-editor for *Qualitative Research in Psychology*, associate editor for *Psychology and Health* and is also co-editor (with Prof. Kerry Chamberlain) of the book series *Critical Approaches to Health*.

Tim McCreanor is a senior Pākehā social scientist at Social and Health Outcomes Research and Evaluation (SHORE) & Whariki Research Centre, College of Health, Massey University in Auckland. Key interests are public health, health disparities, racism, marginalisation, Te Tiriti o Waitangi and decolonisation in Aotearoa New Zealand. The marketing of alcohol to young people has also been a specific focus with a particular orientation to understanding and critiquing the use of social media in this domain. His main approaches are qualitative with innovative techniques such as photovoice, go-along video interviewing, sitting alongside critical discursive work and thematic analyses based on conventional audio interviews and focus groups.

Peter Miller is Professor of Violence Prevention and Addiction Studies at the School of Psychology, Deakin University. He is the Director of the Deakin University Centre for Drug use, Addictive and Anti-social behaviour Research (CEDAAR: www.deakin.edu.au/cedaar). His research interests include alcohol and drug-related violence, predictors of violence (including family and domestic violence) and corporate political activity of alcohol and dangerous consumptions industries. He is running major studies assessing the impact of restricted trading hours in Queensland and testing the impact of last drinks data collected in emergency departments to identify and intervene with problem venues across Australia.

David Moore is a professor in the Drugs, Gender and Sexuality (DruGS) Program at the Australian Research Centre in Sex, Health and Society at La Trobe University, and an adjunct professor at the National Drug Research Institute at Curtin University. His current research explores how gender influences the use of performance and image-enhancing drugs, and research and policy on alcohol-related violence. Moore has written extensively on youth, gender, alcohol and other drug use, addiction concepts and policy, including *The Lads in Action: Social Process in an Urban Youth Subculture* and (with Suzanne Fraser and Helen Keane) *Habits: Remaking Addiction*.

Dean Murphy is a senior research associate in the Department of Gender and Cultural Studies at the University of Sydney. His book, *Gay Men Pursuing Parenthood Through Surrogacy: Reconfiguring Kinship*, was published in 2015. His writings in the areas of kinship, sexuality and gender; drug-consumption practices; HIV biomedical prevention technologies; and understandings of health risks have been published.

Amy Peacock is a senior research fellow and a National Health and Medical Research Council (NHMRC) Early Career Fellow at the National Drug and Alcohol Research Centre, University of New South Wales, and a conjoint fellow in the School of Medicine, University of Tasmania. She graduated with a PhD in Psychology in 2014 from the University of Tasmania. Her programme of research focuses on quantifying problematic alcohol and illicit drug use and harms in Australia and globally. She uses various methods for this, including systematic reviews, linkage of routinely collected administrative data, prospective cohort studies and cross-sectional surveys.

Amy Pennay is an NHMRC Early Career Fellow at the Centre for Alcohol Policy Research (CAPR), La Trobe University. Her PhD explored the social, cultural and economic contexts of alcohol and 'party drug' use among young people patronising the night-time economy. Pennay has worked in alcohol and drug research for more than ten years across a diverse range of methodologies including both qualitative and quantitative studies. Her recent work at CAPR has included studies on the use and effects of alcohol combined with stimulants (including energy drinks) among young adults, alcohol practices among same-sex-attracted women and studies of drinking cultures.

Kiran Pienaar is a research fellow in the Department of Sociology, School of Social Sciences, Monash University. Her research interests include the body in society, gender and sexuality, and science and technology studies. Her work has been published in the areas of drugs, addiction and the self; gender and the body; and health and disease, and her first book is titled *Politics in the Making of HIV/AIDS in South Africa* (2016).

Kane Race is Professor of Gender and Cultural Studies at the University of Sydney. His works on HIV prevention, sexuality, drug use, biomedicine, care practices and digital culture have been published widely. He is the author of *Pleasure Consuming Medicine: The Queer Politics of Drugs* (2009), *Plastic Water: The Social and Material Life of Bottled Water* (co-authored with Gay Hawkins and Emily Potter, 2015) and *The Gay Science: Intimate Experiments with the Problem of HIV* (2018).

Robin Room is a sociologist who has directed alcohol and drug research centres in the United States, Canada, Sweden and Australia. He is a professor at the Centre for Alcohol Policy Research at La Trobe University in Melbourne, as well as at Stockholm University, and has advised the World Health Organization on alcohol issues for more than 40 years. His research is on social, cultural and epidemiological studies of alcohol, drugs and gambling behaviour and problems; on social responses to such problems; and on effects of policies and regulation.

Andy Ruddock is Lecturer in Communications and Media Studies at Monash University, Melbourne. He has authored four books on the social impact of the media. Ruddock's fifth monograph, *Cultivation Theory and Digital Media*, applies George Gerbner's work on media violence to topics including Trumpism, rampage murders, reality TV, right-wing extremism and digital activism. Over 40 book chapters and articles of his on topics including violence, political celebrity, pornography, alcohol marketing and the military applications of social media have been published.

Stuart Taylor is Senior Lecturer in Criminal Justice at Liverpool John Moores University, UK. Prior to entering academia, Taylor worked for the National Probation Service, latterly specialising in substance use. His main research interests focus on drug use and drug policy with a particular interest in the sociolegal construction of drugs and the role and place of substance use in contemporary society. Recent studies have considered the role of cannabis use and cultivation on a community level and the inferences of using a private drug testing kit amongst a collective of ecstasy users.

List of Tables

1

Introduction

Fiona Hutton

The Importance of Intoxication

As is often noted by scholars writing about intoxication, historically, there is no recorded fully formed society that has existed without using psychoactive substances[1]—intoxication through a variety of means is a universal human theme (Walton, 2001, p. 2), and has a central role in diverse societies. In early societies intoxication and the use of psychoactive substances were seen as ways to commune with the gods through carefully constructed rituals, although later, intoxication came to be viewed as interfering with divine communion and was viewed instead as immoral, sinful and with disapproval (Walton, 2001). Intoxicants are often disapproved of when they are perceived as related to rebelliousness, disorder and immorality, and there have been strenuous attempts over the centuries to curtail the use of intoxicants, and the unfortunate, but pervasive punitive approach of prohibition (despite welcome challenges to

F. Hutton (✉)
School of Social and Cultural Studies, Institute of Criminology,
Victoria University, Wellington, New Zealand
e-mail: fiona.hutton@vuw.ac.nz

F. Hutton (ed.), *Cultures of Intoxication*,
https://doi.org/10.1007/978-3-030-35284-4_1

this in recent years). These efforts, to curtail the use of psychoactive substances, have largely failed because the demand for intoxicants has endured over Millenia. Intoxication, therefore, is embedded in our social worlds, and even though intoxicants and their users may be disapproved of and legislated against, this does not mean that the demand for altered states of consciousness has ceased to exist. Intoxication is so embedded in human societies that Siegel (2005, p. 10) refers to it as the 'fourth drive', as much a feature of human existence, as other biological drives such as hunger, sex and thirst, and describes Homo sapiens as the 'king (*and queen?*) of intoxication' (Siegel, 2005, p. 10, emphasis added). Perhaps the attraction of intoxication is that it makes us feel different in comparison to our normal, everyday selves. Whether substances are used to soothe the pains of illness or trauma or simply to have fun and socialise, it is what intoxicants do and the effects they have that are often sought out by diverse groups across equally diverse societies: the enjoyment of experiencing an alternative feeling of self.

However, although intoxication is a feature of almost all societies globally, referred to by Herring, Regan, Weinberg, and Withington (2013, p. 1) as a *modern obsession*, people often have a troubled relationship with experiences of intoxication. Addictions to a variety of substances, both legal and illegal, cause harms to users, their families and communities, and dependent use can lead to problematic use of some substances by some users. These kinds of troubled intoxications are often what are represented in media and public discourse, representations often light on fact and heavy on fiction, giving a skewed notion of problematic relationships with intoxication (Alexandrescu, 2019; Ayres & Taylor, Chap. 11 this volume; Ayres & Jewkes, 2012). This leaves many struggling to see intoxication in anything but a negative light. The pleasures and benefits of intoxications are often seen as impermissible in this kind of climate and are side-lined in public and policy discourse around the use of psychoactive substances—almost as if there was something immoral in itself about referring to the pleasures of intoxication (Ettorre, 2015; O'Malley & Valverde, 2004). This aversion to pleasure is also puzzling, as the vast majority of global populations engage in intoxication, often on a daily basis, from minor intoxications via nicotine and caffeine, to more 'spectacular' intoxications via illegal drugs and alcohol.

Intoxication: Towards a Definition

'Intoxication', for the purposes of this edited collection, is viewed as a set of social and cultural practices, norms and values. Douglas (1987, p. 4) argued in relation to alcohol consumption that it is a *highly patterned learned comportment which varies from one culture to another*, so the debates presented here explore these settings and contexts in relation to diverse 'intoxications', and the ways in which individuals *manage, maintain or change the experience of the self in the world* (Bancroft, 2009, p. 5).

However, trying to define 'intoxication' is deceptively simple. A broad all-encompassing definition such as that used by Becker (1967, p. 164) viewing intoxication as 'the aim of artificially inducing a change in one's consciousness' is useful as it covers intoxication by any means, both legal and illegal. Bancroft (2009, p. 15) similarly views intoxication as related to the ways in which individuals mange experiences in relation to their social worlds, affected by a variety of forces that shape human behaviour such as culture, habit and emotion. Although useful and important, what these kinds of definitions often struggle with are the complexities in defining what and what should not be counted as 'intoxication'. For example, after drinking a cup of tea or coffee, the 'user' could be construed as 'intoxicated', but is this what intoxication is or how it should be defined? Perhaps instead a narrow definition could be used in which the intoxicated person is displaying visible signs of being intoxicated, such as excitement, slurred speech and so on. However, this type of definition also encounters problems as visible signs of intoxication occur often when a person has *over* consumed or is viewed as *overly* intoxicated such as staggering after drinking too much alcohol. Also, in terms of intoxication via substances like nicotine, as Keane in Chap. 3 notes, these micro-intoxications serve to provide excitement of sorts and breaks in routines from otherwise mundane working and leisure lives. This leads to the observation that intoxication itself is not necessarily visible, although it is often the *visible* signs of intoxication that are socially and culturally censored and disapproved of. Furthermore, some substances such as methamphetamine, heroin or crack cocaine, for example, can be viewed as *symbolically or dangerously intoxicating*. The use of these substances is universally censored whether the person using them is visibly intoxicated or not, and people who use them are viewed as *symbolically or dangerously intoxicated* simply by being associated with such illegal substances.

Bearing these complexities of definition in mind, intoxication in this introductory discussion refers to using legal or illegal drugs to alter one's state of consciousness, whether visible to others or not, in order to change the way that the person interacts with the world. The notion of intoxication, thus, has some kind of *purpose*, whether to ease pain and trauma, to have fun, to socialise, to rebel, to express anger, to fit in, to chill out, to work long hours, relax or simply to provide a break in a mundane routine, as with the micro-intoxications related to smoking tobacco or drinking tea or coffee. However, it is also acknowledged that visible signs of intoxication are often what causes social and cultural anxieties around particular groups, and that this is important when considering issues like femininity, masculinity, ethnicity and sexuality in relation to intoxication. Women, for example, are often viewed as *dangerously or symbolically intoxicated* through associations with a variety of substances, and it is these associations that affect social anxieties about women's intoxication.

The Purpose of This Book

Academic writing about intoxication, whether related to alcohol or other drugs has a long history with many important and key debates explored and discussed (e.g. See Bancroft, 2009; Herring et al., 2013; Siegel, 2005; Walton, 2001). That the common human desire to become intoxicated, recognised across thousands of years, is often ignored or side-lined in debates about 'drugs' and illicit drugs in particular has led scholars in this area to argue that societies have a muddled and contradictory relationship with intoxication (Bancroft, 2009, p. 6). Intoxication practices are subject to the contradictory measures of surveillance, control, legislation, encouragement, as well as moral approval or disapproval.

Against the backdrop of existing research, this book seeks to consider the global discourses and debates about 'intoxication', and to engage in critical academic discussion around practices of 'intoxication'. The way that intoxication has been engaged with over the centuries has affected how particular groups are perceived and responded to, resulting in punitive responses such as drug prohibition and harsh treatment of those who are seen to transgress societal norms and values. Therefore, this collection seeks to unsettle the dominant discourses about intoxication and to consider this concept in new, critical ways. Intoxication is also defined here in its broadest sense, from 'energy drinks' and other legal drugs, to recreational use of ecstasy and cocaine, to injecting and problematic drug use. By recognising that intoxication can be achieved through a variety of means through both legal or illegal drugs, the aim is to consider the diversity involved in and related to intoxication.

This collection also seeks to build on previous work such as that of Bancroft (2009) and Douglas (1987) to consider intoxication in relation to difference in contemporary society. For example, in exploring the ways that intoxication is related to masculinities and femininities, ethnicity and sexuality, and to consider how intoxication is *brought into being* (Du Rose, 2015) for these diverse social groups. In asking authors to grapple with the concept of 'intoxication', this book offers new and critical ways of exploring the use of drugs in society, contributing to the existing debates on this topic, rather than privileging a particular way or ways of exploring 'intoxication'.

Much of the literature about intoxication is focused on alcohol, and it is research around alcohol as an intoxicant, which has driven much of the theorising about contemporary 'cultures of intoxication' embedded in neo-liberal societies that emphasise consumption. As such, the literature often leans towards Westernised cultures such as those in the UK, US, Australia and Aotearoa, New Zealand, societies that have well-developed, consumer-orientated, night-time economies (NTE). Although in exploring the issues related to alcohol intoxication, researchers have often noted the exclusion of particular populations who are marginalised, precisely because they either do not fit with dominant constructions of the 'ideal' patron in the NTE or are unable to compete in this consumption focused arena of intoxication.

Research in the same Westernised nations has also demonstrated a clear change in drinking practices, particularly in the NTE (McEwan, Campbell, Lyons, & Swain, 2013; Measham & Brain, 2005). These changes have been influenced by factors such as the deregulation of the alcohol industry with many countries liberalising their liquor laws and regulations around sale and supply from approximately the late 1980s,[2] as well as by increasingly sophisticated marketing strategies, particularly via social media platforms (Carah, 2017; McCreanor et al., 2013; Nicholls, 2012). Contemporary research on social media and intoxication, with a focus on alcohol, has noted the relationships between the construction of identities, social media and intoxication. Young people enact their drinking identities online in ways that previous generations did not have to negotiate. However, online identities are still constrained by patriarchal notions of femininity and dominant ideas about ethnicity, class and sexuality when engaging with social networking sites (SNS) (De Ridder & Van Bauwel, 2013; Dobson, 2014; Hutton, Griffin, Lyons, Niland, & McCreanor, 2016).

The focus on young people's conspicuous public consumption of alcohol and the rise of 'binge drinking'[3] both in academic research and media sensationalism has drawn attention to changes in the relationship between intoxication and alcohol. Intoxications via illicit drugs, such as ecstasy, have also been explored with research focusing on femininities (Hutton, 2006; Measham, 2002; Pini, 2001), masculinities (Malbon, 1998), as well as the meanings that these kinds of intoxications have for those engaged in dance and clubbing scenes (Duff, 2008). Research about illicit drug use in clubbing contexts also noted how the development of the NTE meant an explosion in spaces for consumption of intoxicants both legal and illegal. The concept of polydrug use becomes salient here with the blurring of boundaries between spaces for consumption of alcohol and spaces for consumption of illicit drugs such as ecstasy. Cocaine and alcohol use in the UK context, in bars with late licences and dance floors, were argued to be the drugs of choice for the rave generation that 'grew up' (Hutton, 2006), intensifying the relationships between alcohol and other drugs and the search for altered states of being.

The 1990s also saw the development of the 'normalisation' thesis in relation to illicit drugs such as cannabis (Parker, Williams, & Aldridge, 2002). Intoxication via some illicit drugs was argued to have become normalised in contemporary British society, driven by 'rave' culture (as it was termed in the 1980s) and the deregulation of the NTE (Hadfield, 2006, 2009). However, despite developments in the NTE of westernised nations, and the arguments for the normalisation of the use of some drugs, other kinds of drug users persist as the excluded others on the margins of society. People who inject drugs (PWID), street drinkers and people whose drug use causes them, their families and communities harm remain outside of debates about intoxication. Injecting drug use, addiction and those who engage in 'risky' drug-using practices are viewed as 'other' and as abject. Several authors in this collection draw attention to the importance of intersectional approaches to intoxication and the debates surrounding class, ethnicity, sexuality, alongside a multitude of social and cultural factors that are entangled in the practices of, and responses to, intoxication, and the diversity of intoxicated bodies.

The debates presented in this book aim to build on this body of work about intoxication, its complexity and diversity. The chapters also aim, where appropriate, to broaden out the debates about intoxication to include illicit drugs, and intoxicants like 'energy drinks', rather than confining the discussion solely to alcohol. Although this is not to critique authors (including myself) who have taken this approach, nor to denigrate the value of such work, rather the aim here is to recognise the importance of viewing 'intoxication' from multiple, diverse perspectives.

The Structure of This Book

The development of drinking and drug cultures over the last 30 years or so has brought the notion of intoxication itself to the fore and prompted a number of questions: what *is* intoxication?; *what* does it mean for those who engage in it?; *how* is intoxication experienced by diverse groups? It is these kinds of important questions that the authors contributing to this book explore and discuss.

The book is broadly split into four parts; 'drugs' and intoxication; intoxication and diversity; representations of intoxication; and responses to intoxication. Part I, Chaps. 2, 3, 4, 5 and 6, explore the issues associated with different 'drugs', ranging from alcohol, tobacco and illicit drugs, to 'energy drinks' and new psychoactive substances (NPS). Lyons and Kersey in Chap. 2 begin by highlighting that historically, alcohol is socially and culturally embedded in many societies, but that it also has a long history of regulation. They draw attention to the complexity of intoxication, its meanings in a range of different contexts, as well as noting the tensions in debates about alcohol use. A public health approach focuses on harm, risk and dependency while research based in the social sciences focuses on the meanings of alcohol consumption for consumers, as well as changes in the social, cultural and historical environments for alcohol consumption and intoxication. Their chapter also notes key debates surrounding gender, femininities and masculinities, citing the importance of intersectionality and approaches that take into account the diversity of intoxication practices.

In Chap. 3, Keane argues that nicotine is not usually a drug that is associated with the concept of intoxication. However, she takes an inclusive approach to the concept of intoxication and notes the more subtle, micro-intoxications that occur through nicotine use, as well as the changing contexts in which nicotine is and has been used. This chapter about smoking moves debates about intoxication away from alcohol towards considering this concept in light of the use of other drugs in society, and the pleasures and benefits small intoxications have for people who engage in them.

Bancroft in Chap. 4 also broadens out the debate in considering illicit drugs in relation to intoxication. In a novel discussion, Bancroft argues that the use of illicit drugs is related to drugs as cultural algorithms and that intoxication and desire are embedded in these algorithms. Power and the symbolic order are also key debates in his discussion, in terms of the economic power and cultural status of producers and consumers of illicit drugs.

Hutton and Droste, Pennay, Peacock and Miller continue this theme of broadening out the debates surrounding intoxication, considering it in relation to 'new' psychoactive substances (NPS) and 'energy drinks'. Hutton's discussion in Chap. 5 highlights that drug-using repertoires have expanded in recent years to include intoxication via new psychoactive substances (NPS). Also discussed is that the market for NPS such as BZP (benzylpiperazine)-based party pills (BZP-PPs), mephedrone (Meow) and synthetic cannabis (Spice) has developed rapidly over the last decade or so, alongside legislation attempting to control the harms related to the use of these 'new' substances. Definitions of NPS and the history of their use in

New Zealand is explored, alongside global debates about stigma, disadvantage and NPS use. There have been shifts in the use of NPS, synthetic cannabis in particular, towards more marginalised users, which are significant in terms of responses to NPS and how they are represented in media and public discourse.

Droste et al. in Chap. 6 discuss 'energy drinks' or more correctly 'alcohol mixed with energy drinks' (AmED), to explore the research related to this novel beverage category. AmED use is discussed within a framework of social identity, environmental contexts and a functional approach to understanding the 'culture' of AmED intoxication. Much of the research relating to AmED notes that consumers positively identify as high-risk drinkers, and that despite some negative physiological side effects, AmED use is viewed positively with importance placed on the desired effects, such as extending the effects of intoxication on a night out.

Part II of the book, Chaps. 7, 8, 9 and 10 shifts the focus towards some of the issues related to intoxication and diversity, examining key debates around sexualities, ethnicities, masculinities and femininities. Pienaar, Murphy, Race and Lea, in Chap. 7, present the results of research that draws on qualitative interviews from an Australian study of drug practices among gender and sexual minorities. They consider how LGBTQ consumers pursue particular drug effects to transform or enhance their experience of gender and/or sexuality. Their analysis notes that for LGBTQ consumers, intoxication materialises in relation to sex, desire and play, and that in sexual contexts it enhances pleasure, enables disinhibition and facilitates endurance. Furthermore, in the context of gender variance, intoxication often has therapeutic benefits such as facilitating free gender expression and promoting healing from trauma and gender dysphoria.

Intersectionality and intoxication are further explored by Herbert and McCreanor in Chap. 8. Ethnicity and indigenous alcohol use are discussed in relation to Māori, the indigenous people of Aotearoa, New Zealand, and the problematising of indigenous alcohol use is challenged. In taking a historical view of the development of alcohol intoxication, they argue that biased legislation in colonial times stigmatised indigenous drinking practices and fostered the idea that indigenous drinking was problematic. Biases in the reporting of indigenous peoples' alcohol use are argued to have led to misconceptions that indigenous people misuse alcohol simply because they do not conform to western ideas of acceptable alcohol use. The health disparities in terms of alcohol-related harms between Māori and non-Māori are also noted in this chapter alongside Herbert's work exploring the meanings of alcohol consumption among older Māori. This chapter demonstrates that more nuanced understandings of Māori and other indigenous intoxication practices are needed if health and harm disparities are to be effectively addressed.

In Chap. 9, Hutton focuses on the theoretical developments in debates about intoxication and femininities. The focus is on how women negotiate the tensions and inconsistencies in enactments of intoxication. The discussion explores how women engage with the NTE, the arguments surrounding hypersexual femininities, post-feminism, intersectionality and the narrow categories that women's intoxications are placed within. Some of the ways that women negotiate the risks and pleasures of intoxication are noted and in order to broaden out the debate, intoxication through alcohol and illicit drugs is considered, emphasising the diversity of both femininity and intoxication. The idea that some women are viewed as *symbolically and dangerously intoxicated* is also considered alongside the stigma that affects, in particular, women who inject drugs (WWID).

Moore in Chap. 10 takes a similar theory-focused approach to masculinities and intoxication, viewing them as co-constituted and contingent on the collective activity of diverse human and non-human elements. In considering these debates, Moore draws on feminist theory, feminist science studies and science and technology studies, as well as empirical work that utilises these approaches. He explores literature from both masculinity and drug studies in order to consider how to move forward from social constructionist debates about masculinities, towards an approach that recognises how masculinity and femininity are co-constituted. This approach is then discussed in light of drug effects and intoxication, with the idea that drug effects emerge, and are co-constructed by the complexities of elements assembled in consumption networks or events.

Part III of the book moves into considering representations of intoxication and how a variety of intoxication practices are presented via news media (Ayres and Taylor) and the social media site Tumblr (Ruddock).

Ayres and Taylor in Chap. 11 explore the socio-cultural framing of intoxication via the lens of news media and argue that the moral good of capitalist consumer society is entwined with who consumes what, how they consume it and the results of such consumption. Their chapter problematises the neo-liberal capitalist notion of 'choice' and questions the extent of choice for some groups in society: those whose intoxications evoke concern and focuses on the media emphasised object—*the intoxicated. The intoxicated* are situated as the symbolic 'other', the existence of whom emphasises the contradictions inherent in consumer capitalism—we must consume but only in a 'civilised' and non-risky way.

Representations of intoxication are also explored by Ruddock. However, his chapter (Chap. 12) focuses on cultural artefacts and what they can reveal about intoxication, rather than intoxication practices themselves. His innovative discussion explores the use of a particular image of a meth pipe from a popular television series 'Breaking Bad' on a blog site that, in part, discusses the pleasures of methamphetamine use: a taboo subject given the heavy stigmatisation of this particular drug. Ruddock argues that posting this meth smoking device is part of a larger timeline of media narration of 'deviance' and highlights the ambiguity of representations of drugs in media forms. Social media are positioned as allowing ways of representing intoxication which are not possible in other arenas. The ideas of Becker and Gerbner are also explored in this chapter in relation to the cultural meaning making of drug use and intoxication, as is the idea that social media are integral to telling contemporary stories of intoxication.

The final part of the book explores some of the responses to intoxication with Room in Chap. 13 arguing that intoxication is often not accepted by the majority in contemporary society, and that intoxication varies in its extent and manifestation, dependent on the socio-cultural expectations about the meanings attached to intoxication. These issues are important in considering social and legal responses to intoxication, not least because intoxication tends to be heavily moralised and often subject to legal prohibitions. Room's chapter explores these social and cultural boundaries related to intoxication as well as variations in the acceptability of drinking to intoxication across a wide variety of countries. A number of societal responses to and social handlings of intoxication are also explored, with Room noting that discouragement of intoxication has had limited success with effective policies resisted by political elites and alcohol industry interests.

Furthering the debate about responses to intoxication, Barton in Chap. 14 explores the debates surrounding harm reduction, arguing that definitions of harm reduction are often problematic, focused solely on illicit drugs. He usefully points out that all drugs, legal and illegal, have the capacity to cause harm, and that responses should be based on more than simply requiring abstinence from particular substances, as well as that harms from alcohol and other drug use are moral judgements related to markers of identity such as class, sexuality, gender and ethnicity. Barton uses Barad's (2003) work on materiality to underpin the discussion in his chapter, namely that reactions to intoxication are based on the morality of the user rather than the substance itself. The history of harm reduction as an approach to drug-related harms is described, such as the development of syringe exchange programmes in the 1980s. Barton also presents a critical discussion of the political reluctance to acknowledge harm reduction related to drug use and intoxication more broadly, which often hampers attempts to initiate effective harm reduction strategies.

Notes

1. The only exception to this is the Inuit (Eskimos) who were unable to grow anything in the harsh conditions under which they live, although European explorers introduced this society to alcohol (Walton, 2001, p. 2).
2. For example, in New Zealand, the 1989 Sale of Liquor Act relaxed the licensing application process leading to the increased availability of alcohol (See Hutton, 2009).
3. 'Binge drinking' is a term that refers to drinking an often large amount of alcohol in one sitting to reach a particular level of intoxication. The term is often seen as problematic as it means different things in different social, cultural and historical contexts. Furthermore, unit-based definitions of binge drinking often vary and can result in discrepancies in levels of binge drinking, resulting in inaccuracies in measuring binge drinking among particular populations.

References

Alexandrescu, L. (2019). Streets of the 'spice zombies': Dependence and poverty stigma in times of austerity. *Crime, Media, Culture*. https://doi.org/10.1177/1741659019835274

Ayres, T., & Jewkes, Y. (2012). The haunting spectacle of crystal meth: A media-created mythology? *Crime Media Culture, 8*, 315–332.

Bancroft, A. (2009). *Drugs, intoxication and society*. Cambridge: Polity Press.

Barad, K. (2003). Posthumanist performativity: Toward an understanding of how matter comes to matter. *Signs: Journal of Women in Culture and Society, 28*(3), 801–831.

Becker, H. (1967). History culture and subjective experience: An exploration of the social bases of drug induced experiences. *Journal of Health and Social Behaviour, 8*(3), 163–176.

Carah, N. (2017). Alcohol corporations and marketing in social media. In A. Lyons, T. McCreanor, I. Goodwin, & H. Moewaka Barnes (Eds.), *Youth drinking cultures in a digital world: Alcohol, social media and cultures of intoxication* (pp. 115–131). London: Routledge.

De Ridder, S., & Van Bauwel, S. (2013). Commenting on pictures: Teens negotiating gender and sexualities on social networking sites. *Sexualities, 16*(5), 565–586.

Dobson, A. S. (2014). "Sexy" and "Laddish" girls: Unpacking complicity between two cultural imag(inations)es of young femininity. *Feminist Media Studies, 14*(2), 253–269.

Douglas, M. (1987). *Constructive drinking: Perspectives on drink from anthropology*. London: Routledge.

Du Rose, N. (2015). *The governance of female drug users: Women's experiences of drug policy*. Bristol: Bristol University Press.

Duff, C. (2008). The pleasure in context. *International Journal of Drug Policy, 19*(5), 384–392.

Ettorre, E. (2015). Embodied deviance, gender and epistemologies of ignorance: Re-visioning drug use in a neurochemical, unjust world. *Substance Use and Misuse, 50*(6), 794–805.

Hadfield, P. (2006). *Bar wars: Contesting the night in contemporary British cities*. Oxford: Oxford University Press.

Hadfield, P. (2009). *Nightlife and crime: Social order and governance in international perspective*. Oxford: Oxford University Press.

Herring, J., Regan, C., Weinberg, D., & Withington, P. (Eds.). (2013). *Intoxication and society: Problematic pleasures of drugs and alcohol*. Houndmills, Basingstoke, Hampshire: Palgrave Macmillan.

Hutton, F. (2006). *Risky pleasures? Club cultures and feminine identities*. Aldershot: Ashgate Publishing Limited.

Hutton, F. (2009). New Zealand. In P. Hadfield (Ed.), *Nightlife and crime: Social order and governance in international perspective*. Oxford University Press.

Hutton, F., Griffin, C., Lyons, A., Niland, P., & McCreanor, T. (2016). "Tragic girls" and "crack whores": Alcohol, femininity and Facebook. *Feminism & Psychology, 26*(1), 73–93.

Malbon, B. (1998). Clubbing consumption and identity and the spatial practices of every-nightlife. In T. Skelton & G. Valentine (Eds.), *Cool places: Geographies of youth cultures*. London: Routledge.

McCreanor, T., Lyons, A., Griffin, C., Goodwin, I., Moewaka Barnes, H., & Hutton, F. (2013). Youth drinking cultures, social networking and alcohol marketing: Implications for public health. *Critical Public Health, 23*(1), 110–120.

McEwan, B., Campbell, M., Lyons, A., & Swain, D. (2013). *Pleasure profit and pain: Alcohol in New Zealand and the contemporary culture of intoxication*. Hamilton, New Zealand: University of Waikato.

Measham, F. (2002). "Doing gender"—"Doing drugs": Conceptualizing the gendering of drugs cultures. *Contemporary Drug Problems, 29*(2), 335–373.

Measham, F., & Brain, K. (2005). 'Binge' drinking, British alcohol policy and the new culture of intoxication. *Crime Media Culture: An International Journal, 1*(3), 262–283.

Nicholls, J. (2012). Everyday, everywhere: Alcohol marketing and social media – Current trends. *Alcohol and Alcoholism, 47*(4), 486–493.

O'Malley, P., & Valverde, M. (2004). Pleasure, freedom and drugs: The uses of 'Pleasure' in liberal governance of drug and alcohol consumption. *Sociology, 38*, 25–42.

Parker, H., Williams, L., & Aldridge, J. (2002). The normalisation of 'sensible' recreational drug use: Further evidence from the North West England longitudinal study. *Sociology, 36*, 941–964.

Pini, M. (2001). *Club cultures and female subjectivity: The move from home to house*. Palgrave Macmillan.

Siegel, R. (2005). *Intoxication: The universal drive for mind-altering substances*. Vermont: Park Street Press.

Walton, S. (2001). *Out of it: A cultural history of intoxication*. London: Hamish Hamilton.

Part I

'Drugs' and Intoxication

2

Alcohol and Intoxication

Antonia Lyons and Kate Kersey

Introduction

Alcohol is one of the oldest and most widely used psychoactive substances (O'Brien, 2018). Recent archaeological evidence suggests that alcohol was consumed in great quantities by large groups of people as far back as the Stone Age. In 2018, a vast festival site was discovered in southern Turkey where, over 10,000 years ago, "men and women came to feast and to drink beer by the trough-load" (McKie, 2018). Throughout history, alcohol has been a legal drug in many parts of the world, and it continues to be socially and culturally embedded in many societies. In most Western countries, the use of alcohol has been socially acceptable and permitted for

A. Lyons (✉) • K. Kersey
School of Health, Victoria University of Wellington,
Wellington, New Zealand
e-mail: antonia.lyons@vuw.ac.nz; kate.kersey@vuw.ac.nz

F. Hutton (ed.), *Cultures of Intoxication*,
https://doi.org/10.1007/978-3-030-35284-4_2

certain groups (e.g. middle- and upper-class White men), but it also has a long history of government regulation restricting consumption for other groups (e.g. women, specific ethnic groups) and intoxicated and drunken behaviour (Measham, 2011). Other countries continue to ban alcohol consumption entirely, largely because of religious and cultural factors (e.g. Muslim countries; Manthey et al., 2019; The Social Issues Research Centre, 1998).

In recent decades, there has been concern about a 'culture of intoxication' involving "culturally embedded celebrations of alcohol and intoxication, firmly enmeshed in the social life of many countries" (Hutton, 2016, p. 136). Although many adults within Western societies consume alcohol, there are wide differences in the ways in which they drink, the types of alcoholic beverages they drink, where they drink, when they drink, who they drink with, why they drink and their intentions around intoxication. Given this diversity, meanings of alcohol consumption, as well as experiences of intoxication, vary widely across different local, national and international contexts, as well as by different age groups, gender identities, social classes, sexualities, geographic regions and other identity vectors. Yet, despite these vast differences across diverse settings and groups of people, there is a shared desire to ingest alcohol as a substance to alter one's state of consciousness.

In this chapter, we outline what intoxication is and how it has been understood both generally and within the alcohol field. We then consider the broader political, economic, regulatory and social shifts that have occurred in Western societies in recent years, and their implications for alcohol consumption, drinking cultures and drinking practices, particularly those involving drinking to intoxication. Within this contextual framing, we go on to describe the different approaches taken to the study of alcohol and intoxication, and the ways in which it has been regulated. In the final sections of the chapter, we explore how meanings and experiences of alcohol consumption and intoxication vary widely across different social groups and sectors of society.

What Is Alcohol Intoxication?

Experiences of alcohol intoxication can range from the calming effect of a glass of wine in the liminal space between work and home, to the increase in sociability when drinking with friends, and to drinking that causes loss of control of bodily functions and physical actions, including vomiting, unconsciousness, violence or unwanted violent or sexual behaviour. Everyday terms in English convey the varying levels of intoxicated states, such as 'tipsy', 'blotto' and 'dead drunk' (Measham, 2011). Additionally, differing embodied states, or changes in consciousness, may be specifically sought out as a by-product of drinking. These varied experiences and aims of drinking make it difficult to ascribe one meaning to the concept of intoxication (Hunt & Antin, 2019).

The term 'intoxication' has generally been used to refer to stronger behavioural responses to alcohol consumption. Synonyms include 'drunkenness', 'inebriation' and 'insobriety' (Collins English Thesaurus, n.d.). A recent British Broadcasting Corporation (BBC) article claiming that there are 3000 words for being drunk in the English language highlighted some of the more colourful descriptors such as 'bladdered', 'wasted' and 'tanked' (Dent, 2017). Researchers in this area also use terms and concepts that emphasise the intentional processes of reaching a state of 'intoxication' through heavy drinking, such as "extreme drinking", "binge drinking", "calculated hedonism", "determined drunkenness" and "heavy episodic drinking" (Measham, 2011, p. 121).

Alcohol, and specifically the chemical ethanol, has physiological effects. Ethanol is absorbed through the gastrointestinal tract and, put simply, influences neurotransmitters and hormones, including those in the adrenal cortex (Stockley & Saunders, 2011). Intoxication is described as acute alcohol consumption that disturbs a number of normal, physical, mechanical and biochemical functions (Stockley & Saunders, 2011, p. 17). These 'symptoms' of consumption depend on the amount consumed, and range from disinhibition, talkativeness and flushed skin to the stronger effects of slurring of speech, blackouts and unconsciousness (Stockley & Saunders, 2011). Speed of consumption, sex, genetics, weight, food consumption and tolerance (inherited or developed) are all factors that influence the impact of alcohol on a person's motor and cognitive functioning (Grant & MacAvoy, 2011).

Nevertheless, experiences of consumption and resulting behaviour are not a straightforward biological calculation, with researchers commenting that "the existence of a predictable dose-response relationship is most likely a convenient fiction" (Grant & MacAvoy, 2011, p. 4). In fact, how alcohol is experienced and who will be 'drunk' is dependent on a complex interaction between expectancies around its use, and the social and cultural context in which it is consumed. State of mind at the time of consumption, together with learnt behaviours and social and cultural expectancies of the effects of alcohol, contributes to the experience of intoxication, level of impairment and how people behave during and after alcohol consumption (Grant & MacAvoy, 2011; Hart & Ksir, 2011; Stockley & Saunders, 2011). The importance of cultural, economic and social contexts of drinking for experiences of intoxication is shown in the "certain uniformity of drunken behaviour within most cultures and subcultures" (Grant & MacAvoy, 2011, p. 4). It follows that the responses people exhibit, such as happiness, sociability, aggressiveness, extraversion, relaxation or anxiety, are learnt and socialised, shaped by cultural norms and expectations around alcohol use (Grant & MacAvoy, 2011).

Changing Patterns of Alcohol Consumption and Intoxication Within Late Modernity

Increases in consumption and changes in patterns of drinking have occurred in Western societies in the past three decades alongside significant societal shifts, including the pursuit of neoliberal state governance arrangements and changing social positions for women (McEwan, Campbell, Lyons, & Swain, 2013; Mercille, 2016). Neoliberal ideals prioritising individual choice and limiting government involvement in market economies have led to the deregulation of the alcohol industry and permissive social and policy conditions around its promotion and sale (Babor et al., 2010; Goodwin & Griffin, 2017; Mercille, 2016). By utilising 'unfettered' marketing and promotion efforts, increasingly globalised alcohol companies are able to shape positive social and cultural norms around alcohol and its use in social settings, creating an encouraging climate for alcohol use (Casswell, 2012). Marketing in countries experiencing economic transitions, economic growth and greater disposable income, such as India and China, highlights the ever-continuing pursuit of growth by the alcohol sector (Casswell, 2012). It is predicted that the number of overall heavy episodic drinkers will increase from 20% to 23% by 2030, with the upward trend forecast to be most significant in the Western Pacific and South-East Asia regions (Manthey et al., 2019).

Recent efforts to increase sales in Western countries have seen the redesign and development of products and commercial spaces to attract younger people and women, groups viewed as key emerging markets (McCreanor, Barnes, Kaiwai, Borell, & Gregory, 2008; McEwan et al., 2013). Alcohol companies use sophisticated marketing techniques to link products and ways of drinking with processes of identity creation, making the meanings of alcohol increasingly relevant to targeted cohorts (Lyons, McCreanor, Goodwin, & Moewaka Barnes, 2017; McCreanor, Greenaway, Moewaka Barnes, Borell, & Gregory, 2005). Products and their associated branding have been developed to appeal to emerging markets, such as the development of sweeter (and cheaper) premixed drinks for women and younger drinkers and craft beer for middle-class drinkers. With consumption choices becoming an increasingly important signal of identity (McCreanor et al., 2005), selection of alcohol beverage and place of location have become 'symbolically marked' (Brierley-Jones et al., 2014). For men, this is apparent in attempts to associate brands with sporting teams and other aspects of traditional masculinity (Hall & Kappel, 2018), while for women it is evident in the 'pinking' of products, and the creation of diet, 'mommy' and sophisticated feminine drinks (European Centre of Monitoring Alcohol Marketing, 2008). Alcohol is also marketed as relevant for all aspects of everyday life, including for relaxation, as a reward, for socialising and for celebrating events and achievements (Babor, Robaina, Noel, & Ritson, 2017; European Centre of Monitoring Alcohol Marketing, 2008). Companies also employ social media platforms to undertake highly effective alcohol marketing to targeted youth cohorts in a virtually unregulated domain (Lyons et al., 2017; McCreanor et al., 2013), including using often undisclosed relationships with Instagram personalities to promote their products (VicHealth, 2019).

Countries that strongly embraced neoliberal philosophies involving pursuing profit and growth (such as Ireland and Aotearoa [New Zealand]) have witnessed an expansion in off-licences selling alcohol as well as the sale of alcohol in supermarkets (Casswell, 2012; Mercille, 2016). Furthermore, relaxed alcohol licencing in bars and restaurants (including "bring your own") enabled the development of "purpose built 'urban playscapes'" (Chatterton and Hollands, cited in McCreanor et al., 2008, p. 939). Here, night-time leisure opportunities are provided via cafes and bars selling alcohol to a wide clientele, particularly women and those in the 18–30 age group (Bailey, 2012; Hutton, Wright, & Saunders, 2013; McEwan et al., 2013; Measham, 2004).

The development of the night-time economy, longer opening hours for establishments and increased retail availability of alcohol resulting from weak regulation have encouraged heavy drinking (Goodwin & Griffin, 2017; Mercille, 2016), and normalised intoxication in public spaces (Pennay & Measham, 2016). In this "social context of late modernity of neoliberalism", commentators have described "a shift into a 'new alcohol order'" (Brain, 2000, cited in Hutton & Wright, 2014, p. 102), with young people increasingly socialised into excessive drinking underpinned and promoted by corporate alcohol (Goodwin & Griffin, 2017). Functioning as a space for young people to spend their clearly demarcated leisure time (Measham, 2011), the night-time economy has become "a largely unregulated zone of quasi-liminality awash on a sea of alcohol" (Hobbs, Lister, Hadfield, Winlow, & Hall, 2000, p. 710). Here, displays of 'determined drunkenness' are seen as an understandable pursuit of leisure and pleasure in the course of socialising and celebrating by groups such as university students or young professionals (Hutton, 2016; McEwan et al., 2013; Measham & Brain, 2005). Factors such as the ability to preload with cheap drinks before a night out, higher potency of drinks, more frequent mixing of drinks and the increased popularity of shots have all enabled heavy drinking practices to thrive (Measham, 2011).

Approaches to Alcohol and Intoxication

Hunt and Antin (2019) identify two main disciplinary approaches to the study and regulation of intoxication and drunkenness. Public health research and policy has been primarily concerned with the harms that result from certain types of alcohol use. Within this field, intoxication has been linked with heavy alcohol use and drunkenness and conceptualised predominantly as physically harmful, as well as socially and morally problematic (Grant & MacAvoy, 2011; Hunt & Antin, 2019). Research within this approach has traditionally been underpinned by a strong focus on alcoholism, dependence and toxicity (Hunt & Barker, 2001). Outcomes have focused on measuring harms, such as alcohol-related deaths, injury, self-inflicted injury, alcoholism/dependence, poisoning, crime and assault, drink driving, risky sexual behaviour and foetal alcohol spectrum disorder (see Huckle, Yeh, Lin, & Jensen, 2013; Loring, 2014). More recently, there has been a focus on the longer-term health outcomes of different levels of alcohol consumption, including cancer and other diseases, with recent research concluding that there are *no* safe drinking levels (Connor, 2017; GBD 2016 Alcohol Collaborators, 2018; Slade et al., 2016).

The other dominant approach to the study of alcohol and intoxication has come from researchers who have taken a broader view, seeking to understand the historical development and contemporary understandings of alcohol's role, meaning and function within societies, cultures and subcultures. This social science-oriented approach does consider harms but also focuses on gaining insight into the symbiotic relationship between alcohol use and the social and cultural environment, where alcohol is understood as integral to the constitution of much social and cultural life (Grant & MacAvoy, 2011). For example, as noted above, this research considers the influence of culture-specific norms around alcohol use in religious, celebratory and social settings in establishing a country's drinking levels and patterns (Gordon, Heim, & MacAskill, 2012; The Social Issues Research Centre, 1998). Researchers ask questions that explore what people are seeking when using alcohol to change their consciousness (O'Brien, 2018), and the individual and collective meanings of drinking and drinking to get drunk (Grant & MacAvoy, 2011; see also Hutton, 2016).

There are tensions between these two dominant approaches, with one focused primarily on harm and negative outcomes and the other focused more on insight and understanding, including people's perceptions, motivations and meanings. Public health discourse constructs intoxication primarily as a harm that results from risky ways of drinking alcohol (Keane, 2009), and much of the research funding for alcohol is linked to developing ways to reduce harmful use. Yet, intoxication is frequently constructed by drinkers as "a positive and enhanced state: a form of bodily pleasure" (Keane, 2009, p. 135) that provides benefits such as relaxation and sociability. Research shows that seeking intoxication and drunkenness is for many a deliberate act, a way to pursue pleasure and, in some cases, a transcendence of everyday life and social norms (Measham, 2006, 2011; Measham & Brain, 2005). Much academic research on alcohol (and other drugs) has neglected the study of pleasure and enjoyment from intoxication, particularly bodily pleasure (Bunton & Coveney, 2011). Yet, greater insight into cultures of drinking, particularly cultures of intoxication and hedonistic consumption, will enhance public health understandings of the risks and pleasures of alcohol.

Restricting and Regulating Alcohol Consumption

Regulation of alcohol and attempts to minimise its harms have occurred for centuries. Regulation has ranged from the extremes of prohibition in the USA in the early twentieth century to bans on alcohol sales to certain groups of people. For example, in colonial Aotearoa New Zealand in the late 1800s, it was illegal for women and Māori to consume alcohol (Hutton, 2009). Generally, regulatory responses are presupposed on definitions of 'harmful' consumption, where health, social and economic problems occur from heavy drinking or toxicity (see the World Health Organization's [WHO's] 2010 *Global Strategy to Reduce Harmful Use of Alcohol*, discussed in Bacchi, 2015). For most countries, this includes regulations selected from the "WHO's so-called best-buys": taxation, pricing limits, age restrictions and restrictions on the sale and marketing of alcohol (Manthey et al., 2019, p. 8). Most countries have age restrictions for purchasing alcohol (reflecting higher rates of reported harm to adolescents whose cognitive and emotional functioning is still developing [Stockley & Saunders, 2011]), and laws preventing drink driving. Public drunkenness is a criminal offence in some parts of the world, while undesirable behaviours arising from alcohol use, such as assault, are usually dealt with under the relevant provisions of the criminal law in many places.

In addition to these direct restrictions, limiting alcohol availability or accessibility is the main mechanism for addressing problematic drinking. These regulatory approaches have been critiqued as assuming that alcohol use leading to a high level of intoxication is caused by a lack of individual willpower which can be addressed by restricting access or raising prices, ignoring pleasure and sociability as rational reasons for consumption (Bacchi, 2015). Additionally, while there is evidence that increasing price decreases alcohol-related harm in developed and developing countries, there is evidence that the real price of alcohol has been decreasing over time due to liberalised environments (Babor et al., 2010).

Many countries also include restrictions on advertising or marketing of alcohol in traditional media, although broader marketing initiatives such as sponsorship are often not captured (Babor et al., 2010). The use of new and social media for marketing and promotion also occurs in a largely unregulated environment, primarily due to such developments occurring at a time of neoliberal ideology favouring free-market approaches (Casswell, 2012). As an alternative to legislative restrictions, many countries rely on alcohol companies adopting voluntary codes of conduct such as the Code for Advertising and Promotion of Alcohol in New Zealand (Advertising Standards Authority, n.d.) and, in the UK, the UK Code of Broadcast Advertising (Advertising Standards Authority and Committee of Advertising Practice, n.d.-a) and the UK Code of Non-broadcast Advertising and Direct and Promotional Marketing (Advertising Standards Authority and Committee of Advertising Practice, n.d.-b). Despite findings of breaches of codes, there exists doubt as to the efficacy of industry-based efforts to encourage good practice, and these are more likely used as a mechanism by alcohol companies to reduce regulatory scrutiny (Babor et al., 2010; Casswell, 2012).

Other than the regulatory measures above, governmental responses to binge drinking, associated disruptive behaviour and the longer-term health harms of alcohol (including cancer as noted earlier) have been based on guidelines for 'safe' drinking levels. Such responses often recommend maximum units of alcohol to be consumed in any one drinking episode (Goodwin & Griffin, 2017). In Aotearoa New Zealand, it is recommended that women drink no more than two standard drinks a day (and no more than four standard drinks on any occasion) and men drink no more than three standard drinks a day (and no more than five on any single occasion) (Ministry of Health, 2019). In the UK, the latest guidelines simply state that no more than 14 units should be consumed per week, preferably spread across this time (UK Chief Medical Officers, 2016). However, there are difficulties with such unit-based recommendations as they do not always converge with people's own understandings of their drinking (Emslie & Macdonald, 2017). Amounts consumed by those who label themselves 'moderate drinkers' vary greatly, showing little association with government unit recommendations (Green, Polen, Janoff, Castleton, & Perrin, 2007). Rather, individual ideas of heavy and moderate drinking, and the experience of drunkenness itself, are highly subjective (Measham, 2011). Many people make decisions about their consumption levels as they are drinking based on their feelings of being drunk, the extent to which they experience negative consequences and whether they perceive themselves to be dependent on alcohol (Lyons, Emslie, & Hunt, 2014). There is thus a gap between public health messages and personal experiences, particularly among people who actively pursue intoxication and drunkenness as a pleasurable leisure activity (Keane, 2009; Measham, 2011).

The 'recommended' units of consumption approach is in line with many health promotion policies by neoliberal governments where responsibility is devolved to individuals to manage their health risks and choose healthy lifestyles (Ayo, 2012). Government policy discourses and regulatory controls tend to hold a strong line that drinking alcohol is an individual choice and that 'moderate' drinkers—those who can 'handle' their drinking—should not be unfairly penalised (Ayo, 2012; Room, 2011), while problematising alcoholics and publicly disruptive heavy drinkers.

Those labelled as 'alcoholics' are generally considered to have a disease and little agency over their drinking, requiring medical intervention to cease or reduce consumption. In contrast, people who choose to consume alcohol to get drunk as a leisure activity are perceived negatively (Measham, 2011); their public drunken behaviour (particularly vomiting, unconsciousness or violence) attracts a higher level of social opprobrium. Unlike tobacco laws which responded to increasing evidence of disease, alcohol policies in most Western countries remain premised on the basis of "deserving and responsible citizens … earn[ing] an *environment* where alcohol is easily accessible" (Goodwin & Griffin, 2017, p. 21).

Some researchers have critiqued how harm is defined in alcohol policies, examining whose behaviour is being labelled as problematic and the consequences that flow from such constructions (e.g. Keane, 2009). Identifying certain groups or individuals as having 'problematic' alcohol consumption may exacerbate unhealthy behaviour or cause harm through negative or disproportionate social or legal responses, a legacy of which exists today for many ethnic and minority groups such as Māori in New Zealand (Bacchi, 2015; Hutton, 2009). Locating 'the problem' and the responsibility for harm with certain groups or individuals, while at the same time construing others as engaging in 'socially acceptable' alcohol use (e.g. drinking heavily but at home with friends over a meal), may prevent an acknowledgement that society encourages and promotes unhealthy drinking practices across groups. The support of drinking by deregulation of the alcohol industry, increased availability and accessibility of alcohol and the growth of the night-time economy all sit in direct contrast with a public health approach seeking to address intoxicated behaviour and reduce overall consumption levels.

Diversity in Meanings and Experiences of Intoxication

Meanings and functions of alcohol consumption vary across the localised social and cultural environment in which it takes place, including by socio-economic status, age, sexuality and gender groups (Day, 2012; Lyons et al., 2017; McCreanor et al., 2016). These factors combine to shape how individuals experience alcohol consumption, the meanings they attach to drinking and how they negotiate those meanings (Hunt & Antin, 2019). In the remainder of this chapter, we explore some of the key social vectors of people's lives and their role in the experiences, understandings and meanings of alcohol and intoxication. Reflecting the research in this field, we focus initially on masculinities and femininities in relation to alcohol and intoxication, before considering how these intersect with other identities and groups. With millennials more likely to consider themselves multiracial and to "adopt unconventional gender identities" (Johfre & Saperstein, 2019), exploring intersectional identities and drinking practices is increasingly important.

Masculinities, Femininities and Intoxication

Drinking alcohol, particularly beer, and drinking in public have traditionally been practices engaged in by men and linked to enacting masculine identities (Lemle & Mishkind, 1989). Drinking to intoxication has been a way for men to demonstrate hegemonic masculinity in Western societies (Peralta, 2007; Willott & Lyons, 2012). Hegemonic masculinity is a dominant position that is constructed in relation to femininities and subordinated masculinities, and that functions to legitimate patriarchal social relations (Connell, 1995; Connell & Messerschmidt, 2005). Drinking heavily has been linked with other traditionally masculine behaviours such as aggressiveness and assertive sexual conduct (Campbell, 2000; Hunt & Antin, 2019; Hutton, 2016). Men have traditionally been expected to consume large quantities of alcohol, but to 'hold' their drink and demonstrate control over their body by not overtly displaying any physical signs of intoxication (such as slurring, stumbling and passing out) (Campbell, 2000; Peralta, 2007; Thurnell-Read, 2013).

However, in more recent times, many young people in Western societies, both men and women, drink intentionally to get drunk and lose control, and alcohol is central to their experiences of enjoyment, pleasure and sociability (e.g. Griffin, Bengry-Howell, Hackley, Mistral, & Szmigin, 2009; Lyons et al., 2014). Their drinking is organised and planned, bounded by times and places (e.g. Friday nights, pubs and bars), undertaken with friends and often described by participants as loads of 'fun'. Some groups of young men explicitly drink to achieve a drunken loss of physical control while socialising together, including during stag nights/weekends (Thurnell-Read, 2011), during rites of passage in the US fraternities (Measham, 2011), and following rugby (or other sports) matches (e.g. Willott & Lyons, 2012). Drinking to intoxication, losing control of one's body, and sometimes one's memory, is described as pleasurable, providing shared experiences that function to solidify friendship bonds (Griffin et al., 2009; Niland, Lyons, Goodwin, & Hutton, 2013).

The changes in Western societies over the last decades (as noted earlier) have shifted some of the traditional links between heavy alcohol consumption and masculinities (Lyons & Willott, 2008). Alcohol is more widely available and accessible, there are many more products on the market, there are a much broader range of places to purchase and consume alcohol, and there has been a convergence between men's and women's drinking (although men still consistently drink more than women) (Slade et al., 2016). These shifts have provided ways for men to consume alcohol differently, and produce alternative masculinities, although in ways that ensure they remain differentiated from femininities and women's consumption (Lyons, 2009; Lyons & Gough, 2017). There are different masculine identities related to different forms of alcohol consumption for (particularly young) men (Mullen, Watson, Swift, & Black, 2007). Products can also differentiate across class identities for men, although in-depth qualitative research demonstrates that men tend to have to justify non-normative drinking choices (Emslie, Hunt, & Lyons, 2013; Willott & Lyons, 2012).

Drinking to intoxication has also been linked to men having the opportunity to transgress idealised and normative forms of masculinity. This includes a desire for a release from the ongoing, everyday imperative to be engaged in controlled, rational, autonomous and independent embodied masculine performances (Lyons & Gough, 2017; Robertson, 2007; Thurnell-Read, 2011, 2013). For example, young men have talked about how they use alcohol, and drunkenness, to engage in non-masculine behaviours such as expressing pain, crying and being emotional, as well as to engage in homosexual behaviours (de Visser & Smith, 2007; Peralta, 2008). These behaviours are also documented and shared on Facebook;

analyses of male students' drinking photos in the UK demonstrated that they overwhelmingly displayed homosocial behaviours, including men touching, kissing and dancing with each other at parties, in pubs and clubs (Scoats, 2015). This suggests that transgressions of heteronormative masculinity while drinking are acceptable—and understandable—outside of the immediate context in which they occur. Among older Scottish men, research has found that their descriptions of drinking in the pub with other men entailed a space for them to talk about their emotions, well-being and mental health (Emslie et al., 2013). The men noted that alcohol was an important aspect of this context, and that it would not be the same with a non-alcoholic drink, suggesting the act of drinking alcohol provided a kind of masculine protection, an allowance for masculine bonding that may not otherwise have been possible (Emslie et al., 2013).

Changes in women's drinking practices in Western societies over recent decades—notably increasing amounts and frequencies of consumption, particularly in young women—have been linked to changes in women's position in society (Lyons & Willott, 2008; Rahav, Wilsnack, Bloomfield, Gmel, & Kuntsche, 2006). Alongside greater economic freedom and pursuing careers, many women have taken up the 'work hard, play hard' lifestyle that has been traditionally linked to men. Heavy drinking for young women may also provide a way of 'letting go' of dominant and expected performances of femininity (Stepney, 2015; Waitt, Jessop, & Gorman-Murray, 2011).

Surrounded by a discourse that celebrates women's social drinking, there remains significant disapproval of women drinking to excess or being out of control due to alcohol consumption (Lennox, Emslie, Sweeting, & Lyons, 2018; Rolfe, Orford, & Dalton, 2009; Room, 2011; Skeggs, 2005). As Hutton, Griffin, Lyons, Niland, and McCreanor (2016) have noted, "a '*drinking* femininity' is acceptable, but a '*drunken* femininity' is not" (p. 85). There has been concern about excessive drinking and 'out-of-control' drunken behaviours of younger women, with 'ladettes' (working-class women in the UK) singled out as particularly problematic (Day, Gough, & McFadden, 2004; Hunt & Antin, 2019). This social anxiety and moral panic around women's drinking and drunkenness (particularly working-class women [Lindsay & Supski, 2017]) and its 'appropriateness' can be traced back to the early twentieth century

(Jackson & Tinkler, 2007), where women's drinking and intoxication was stigmatised, considered unfeminine and non-respectable (Ettore, 2004). Women are also highly judgmental of other women's drinking, with middle-class women condemning of 'unfeminine' drinking behaviours of their working-class counterparts (Lennox et al., 2018). Some commentators suggest that problematising women's heavy drinking occurs because it has the potential to disrupt traditional female gender roles such as carers and mothers (Day et al., 2004). It may also be viewed as an unwanted attempt to appropriate public drinking spaces that have traditionally been male-dominated (Day et al., 2004).

The feminisation of the night-time economy, and the active push by alcohol companies to develop female drinkers as a key market starting in the 1990s, provided women with female-friendly places to drink and (increasingly strong) products to consume (Griffin, Szmigin, Bengry-Howell, Hackley, & Mistral, 2013; Szmigin et al., 2008). Young women became engaged in the routine and oftentimes expected practice of drinking to intoxication, alongside young men (Griffin et al., 2013; Lindsay & Supski, 2017). Feminist researchers sought to explore these behaviours and what meanings they held for those taking part in the culture of intoxication, locating the behaviours "within a wider analysis of the contemporary social and gendered position of young women" (Hunt & Antin, 2019, p. 73). Some of this work usefully linked young women's (heavy) drinking to theorisations of broader neoliberal imperatives for the individual to actively seek continual self-transformation and improvement, performing authentic feminine identities in the night-time economy (Goodwin & Griffin, 2017; Griffin et al., 2013). Research has also demonstrated the inaccuracy of dominant postfeminist discourses in the media that portray the obsolescence of feminism and the achievement of equality between men and women (Gill, 2007). This research highlights the very different meanings attached to men's and women's drinking, with women's drinking viewed more negatively, and continuing gendered double standards in meanings of drunkenness (e.g. de Visser & McDonnell, 2012; Lyons et al., 2016; Lyons & Willott, 2008). This is supported by research from the Stanford Center of Inequality and Poverty which suggests that although gender identities are broadening, gender stereotypes remain entrenched (Johfre & Saperstein, 2019).

Gender Identities and Intersectional Considerations

Much of the research on drinking and intoxication has focused on young, middle-class, White, heterosexual men and women, while those who sit outside these groups remain invisible (Hunt & Antin, 2019). While some work has investigated the importance of social class for women's meanings and experiences of drinking to intoxication in the UK (e.g. see Bailey, Griffin, & Shankar, 2015; Griffin et al., 2013), much less has examined ethnicity, sexuality and non-binary gender identities (although see Emslie, Lennox, & Ireland, 2017; Hunt, Kolind, & Antin, 2018; Hunt, Antin, Sanders, & Sisneros, 2019). According to Hunt and Antin (2019), an intersectional approach that explores experiences and understandings that occur where two or more social identities—age, life stage, ethnicity, social class, sexuality and gender—intersect has been slow to be taken up in alcohol-related research.

Age, life stage and gender have been investigated in terms of differences in consumption levels and patterns of drinking, but less work has interrogated how meanings and understandings of alcohol and drinking vary across the lifespan. Midlife people use alcohol as an escape from everyday gendered routines, as a reward and to celebrate (Emslie, Hunt, & Lyons, 2015). For example, research highlighted that midlife drinkers in Scotland used alcohol to alter their "subjective embodied experience of everyday gendered roles and responsibilities" (Lyons et al., 2014, p. 264). They had their own histories of drinking and described detailed self-knowledge about their bodies while consuming alcohol, knowledge that they used to ensure they consumed alcohol to a point of being 'in the zone'—enjoyably intoxicated, but not too drunk. This experiential embodied knowledge was prioritised over any other kind of knowledge (such as health promotion advice) to regulate their drinking (Lyons et al., 2014). Mothers with young children have also been found to discuss the pleasures of alcohol and how appealing drinking is; they viewed alcohol as a reward for getting through their days, as a way to relax and as a form of 'adult time out' from the demands of mothering. However, given their role as mothers of young children, they both self-monitored and policed other women's drinking to ensure nights involving intoxication were only undertaken when their children were being cared for by someone else (Pedersen, 2019). Thus, the pleasures of alcohol are highly context-dependent; they are "embodied, social and situational" rather than fixed and static (Keane, 2009, p. 141).

Some research has examined alcohol use in gay, lesbian and bisexual people, finding higher rates of use and alcohol-related problems in these groups compared to their heterosexual counterparts (Bloomfield, Wicki, Wilsnack, Hughes, & Gmel, 2011; Hughes, Wilsnack, & Kantor, 2016). Such work positions the drinking of lesbian, gay, bisexual, transgender, queer and intersex (LGBTQI) populations within a problem or pathology frame (Hunt et al., 2019) and locates higher consumption as due to the stress and stigma associated with their lives. This provides little insight into the meanings and pleasures of alcohol use for these groups of people, or the importance of alcohol use for relationships, identities, sexualities and socialising. Recent research highlights how "social and cultural practices of alcohol consumption play a role in the performance of sexual and gender identities" and ideas about masculinity and femininity can be "de-coupled from sex-gendered bodies" (Hunt et al., 2019, p. 383). Safe, comfortable and meaningful spaces in which to socialise and drink have been found to be important for LGBTQI people, particularly spaces where hegemonic masculinity and heteronormativity are absent or less dominant (Adams, Asiasiga, & Neville, 2019; Hunt et al., 2019). Other work also demonstrates that people drink particular drinks to convey or express specific sexual identities and to challenge dominant preconceptions about gender (Emslie et al., 2017).

Conclusion

As a legal drug in most parts of the world, alcohol holds a paradoxical position. Much research, time, effort and money are devoted to focusing on the harms of consumption, particularly intoxication, and finding ways to reduce the risks associated with alcohol. Yet alcohol is a socially valued, heavily marketed and economically significant product (Babor et al., 2010; Keane, 2009). The alcohol industry has strong links with governments and lobbies hard to ensure there are few policy restrictions on the sale and supply of alcohol, particularly those found to be effective in reducing population consumption such as regulations and taxes (Casswell, 2009). This is due in part to the wide acceptance of 'social drinking'. Room (2011) describes the moderate drinker as the "hero of the economic system" (p. 147); this drinker engages in the socio-economic imperative to consume, while also meeting increased expectations of 'sober attention' in the post-industrial world. Creating identities through drinking performances and consuming particular alcohol brands fit neatly with the 'good corporate citizen' of neoliberalism, where successful individuals are those who exercise "consumer-based lifestyle choices" (Goodwin & Griffin, 2017). Alcohol use has been normalised to such an extent in Western societies that adult men and women report social difficulties in reducing or abstaining from alcohol (Research New Zealand, 2018) and feel stigmatised for not drinking alcohol in social situations (Bartram, Eliott, & Crabb, 2017; Hutton, 2016). However, as this chapter highlights, in addition to legitimising socially appropriate drinking, this has likely fuelled 'cultures of intoxication' and created a disjunct between published drinking guidelines and subjective experiences of drinking.

As a psychoactive drug, alcohol is also a product that is used in different ways by different people for different functions, but its effects are overwhelmingly understood as appealing, pleasurable and fun. Certain groups have embraced drunkenness in the pursuit of pleasure, sociability and escape from daily life, as a meaningful and functional aspect of their leisure time (Measham & Brain, 2005), and research highlights the extent to which alcohol's roles and meanings vary across different groups. To gain further insight into the role and meanings of intoxication for people from various backgrounds, classes, gender identities, sexualities, ages and ethnicities, it is essential to theorise beyond binary gender dichotomies and individual markers of identity. As Measham (2011) has neatly stated, how we understand intoxication, and "whether drunkenness is seen as something to strive for or avoid depends, in part, on academics', policy-makers', and drinkers' notions of what drunkenness entails and what they might want to achieve" (p. 147).

References

Adams, J., Asiasiga, L., & Neville, S. (2019). *Drinking cultures of rainbow New Zealanders*. Wellington: Health Promotion Agency.

Advertising Standards Authority. (n.d.). *Code for advertising and promotion of alcohol*. Retrieved July 8, 2019, from https://www.asa.co.nz/codes/codes/code-for-advertising-and-promotion-of-alcohol/

Advertising Standards Authority and Committees of Advertising Practice. (n.d.-a). *The BCAP code: The UK code of broadcast advertising*. Retrieved July 8, 2019, from https://www.asa.org.uk/uploads/assets/uploaded/b6a021eb-2525-40e1-9c44eb6eab1f6797.pdf

Advertising Standards Authority and Committees of Advertising Practice. (n.d.-b). *The CAP code: The UK code of non-broadcast advertising and direct & promotional marketing*. Retrieved July 8, 2019, from https://www.asa.org.uk/uploads/assets/uploaded/ce3923e7-94ff-473b-ad2f85f69ea24dd8.pdf

Ayo, N. (2012). Understanding health promotion in a neoliberal climate and the making of health conscious citizens. *Critical Public Health, 22*(1), 99–105. https://doi.org/10.1080/09581596.2010.520692

Babor, T. F., Caetano, P., Casswell, S., Edwards, G., Giesbrecht, N., Graham, K., … Rossow, I. (2010). *Alcohol: No ordinary commodity: Research and public policy*. Oxford, UK: Oxford University Press.

Babor, T. F., Robaina, K., Noel, J. K., & Ritson, E. B. (2017). Vulnerability to alcohol-related problems: A policy brief with implications for the regulation of alcohol marketing. *Addiction, 112*, 94–101.

Bacchi, C. (2015). Problematizations in alcohol policy: WHO's "alcohol problems". *Contemporary Drug Problems, 42*(2), 130–147. https://doi.org/10.1177/0091450915576116

Bailey, L. (2012). *Young women and the culture of intoxication: Negotiating classed femininities in the postfeminist culture*. PhD, University of Bath, England.

Bailey, L., Griffin, C., & Shankar, A. (2015). 'Not a good look': Impossible dilemmas for young women negotiating the culture of intoxication in the United Kingdom. *Substance Use and Misuse, 50*(6), 747–758.

Bartram, A., Eliott, J., & Crabb, S. (2017). 'Why can't I just not drink?' A qualitative study of adults' social experiences of stopping or reducing alcohol consumption. *Drug and Alcohol Review, 36*(4), 449–455. https://doi.org/10.1111/dar.12461

Bloomfield, K., Wicki, M., Wilsnack, S., Hughes, T., & Gmel, G. (2011). International differences in alcohol use according to sexual orientation.

Substance Abuse, 32(4), 210–219. https://doi.org/10.1080/08897077.2011.598404
Brain, K. J. (2000). *Youth, alcohol and the emergence of the postmodern alcohol order*. Occasional Paper No. 1, Institute of Alcohol Studies, UK.
Brierley-Jones, L., Ling, J., McCabe, K. E., Wilson, G. B., Crosland, A., Kaner, E. F. S., & Haighton, C. A. (2014). Habitus of home and traditional drinking: A qualitative analysis of reported middle-class alcohol use. *Sociology of Health and Illness, 36*(7), 1054–1076. https://doi.org/10.1111/1467-9566.12145
Bunton, R., & Coveney, J. (2011). Drugs' pleasures. *Critical Public Health, 21*(1), 9–23.
Campbell, H. (2000). The glass phallus: Pub(lic) masculinity and drinking in rural New Zealand. *Rural Sociology, 65*(4), 562–581.
Casswell, S. (2009). Alcohol industry and alcohol policy – The challenge ahead. *Addiction, 104*, 3–5. https://doi.org/10.1111/j.1360-0443.2008.02429.x
Casswell, S. (2012). Current status of alcohol marketing policy: An urgent challenge for global governance. *Addiction, 107*(3), 478–485. https://doi.org/10.1111/j.1360-0443.2011.03701.x
Collins English Thesaurus. (n.d.). *Symptoms of 'intoxication'*. Retrieved July 7, 2019, from https://www.collinsdictionary.com/dictionary/english-thesaurus/intoxication#intoxication__1
Connell, R. W. (1995). *Masculinities*. Cambridge, UK: Polity Press.
Connell, R. W., & Messerschmidt, J. W. (2005). Hegemonic masculinity rethinking the concept. *Gender & Society, 19*(6), 829–859.
Connor, J. (2017). Alcohol consumption as a cause of cancer. *Addiction, 112*(2), 222–228.
Day, K. (2012). Social class, socioeconomic status and 'health-risk' behaviours: A critical analysis. In C. Horrocks & S. Johnson (Eds.), *Advances in health psychology: Critical approaches* (pp. 61–73). New York: Palgrave Macmillan.
Day, K., Gough, B., & McFadden, M. (2004). Warning! Alcohol can seriously damage your feminine health. *Feminist Media Studies, 4*(2), 165–183. https://doi.org/10.1080/1468077042000251238
de Visser, R. O., & McDonnell, E. J. (2012). 'That's OK. He's a guy': A mixed-methods study of gender double-standards for alcohol use. *Psychology & Health, 27*(5), 618–639.
de Visser, R. O., & Smith, J. A. (2007). Alcohol consumption and masculine identity among young men. *Psychology and Health, 22*(5), 595–614.
Dent, S. (2017, January 31). *English has 3,000 words for being drunk*. Retrieved May 9, 2019, from http://www.bbc.com/culture/story/20170130-english-has-3000-words-for-being-drunk

Emslie, C., Hunt, K., & Lyons, A. C. (2013). The role of alcohol in forging and maintaining friendships amongst Scottish men in midlife. *Health Psychology, 32*(1), 33–41.

Emslie, C., Hunt, K., & Lyons, A. C. (2015). Transformation and time-out: The role of alcohol in identity construction among Scottish women in mid-life. *International Journal of Drug Policy, 26*(5), 437–445. https://doi.org/10.1016/j.drugpo.2014.12.006

Emslie, C., Lennox, J., & Ireland, L. (2017). The role of alcohol in identity construction among LGBT people: A qualitative study. *Sociology of Health & Illness, 39*(8), 1465–1479.

Emslie, C., & Macdonald, S. (2017). Strong epidemiological evidence that alcohol causes cancer, but how might the public interpret this information? *Addiction, 112*(2), 233–235. https://doi.org/10.1111/add.13687

Ettore, E. M. (2004). Revisioning women and drug use: Gender sensitivity, gendered bodies and reducing harm. *International Journal of Drug Policy, 15*, 327–335.

European Centre of Monitoring Alcohol Marketing. (2008). *Women – The new market.* Retrieved from http://eucam.info/wp-content/uploads/2014/05/women_the_new_market_final.pdf

GBD 2016 Alcohol Collaborators. (2018). Alcohol use and burden for 195 countries and territories, 1990–2016: A systematic analysis for the Global Burden of Disease Study 2016. *The Lancet*. https://doi.org/10.1016/S0140-6736(18)31310-2

Gill, R. (2007). Postfeminist media culture: Elements of a sensibility. *European Journal of Cultural Studies, 10*(2), 147–166.

Goodwin, I., & Griffin, C. (2017). Neoliberalism, alcohol and identity. In A. C. Lyons, T. McCreanor, I. Goodwin, & H. Moewaka Barnes (Eds.), *Youth drinking cultures in a digital world. Alcohol, social media and cultures of intoxication* (pp. 15–30). Oxton, UK: Routledge.

Gordon, R., Heim, D., & MacAskill, S. (2012). Rethinking drinking cultures: A review of drinking cultures and a reconstructed dimensional approach. *Public Health, 126*(1), 3–11.

Grant, M., & MacAvoy, M. (2011). Voices in the debate. In A. Fox & M. MacAvoy (Eds.), *Expressions of drunkenness: (Four hundred rabbits)* (pp. 1–11). New York: Routledge.

Green, C. A., Polen, M. R., Janoff, S. L., Castleton, D. K., & Perrin, N. A. (2007). "Not getting tanked": Definitions of moderate drinking and their health implications. *Drug and Alcohol Dependence, 86*(2–3), 265–273.

Griffin, C., Bengry-Howell, A., Hackley, C., Mistral, W., & Szmigin, I. (2009). 'Every time I do it I absolutely annihilate myself': Loss of (self-)consciousness and loss of memory in young people's drinking narratives. *Sociology, 43*, 457–476.

Griffin, C., Szmigin, I., Bengry-Howell, A., Hackley, C., & Mistral, W. (2013). Inhabiting the contradictions: Hypersexual femininity and the culture of intoxication among young women in the UK. *Feminism and Psychology, 23*(2), 184–206.

Hall, G., & Kappel, R. (2018). Gender, alcohol, and the media: The portrayal of men and women in alcohol commercials. *Sociological Quarterly, 59*(4), 571–583. https://doi.org/10.1080/00380253.2018.1479204

Hart, C. L., & Ksir, C. (2011). *Drugs, society, & human behavior* (14th ed.). New York: McGraw-Hill.

Hobbs, D., Lister, S., Hadfield, P., Winlow, S., & Hall, S. (2000). Receiving shadows: Governance and liminality in the night-time economy. *British Journal of Sociology, 51*(4), 701–717. https://doi.org/10.1080/00071310020015334

Huckle, T., Yeh, L. C., Lin, J., & Jensen, V. (2013). *Trends in alcohol consumption and alcohol-related harms among females in New Zealand*. Wellington, New Zealand: Health Promotion Agency.

Hughes, T. L., Wilsnack, S. C., & Kantor, L. W. (2016). The influence of gender and sexual orientation on alcohol use and alcohol-related problems: Toward a global perspective. *Alcohol Research: Current Reviews, 38*(1), 121–132.

Hunt, G., & Antin, T. (2019). Gender and intoxication: From masculinity to intersectionality. *Drugs: Education, Prevention & Policy, 26*(1), 70–78.

Hunt, G., Antin, T., Sanders, E., & Sisneros, M. (2019). Queer youth, intoxication and queer drinking spaces. *Journal of Youth Studies, 22*(3), 380–400.

Hunt, G., & Barker, J. C. (2001). Socio-cultural anthropology and alcohol and drug research: Towards a unified theory. *Social Science and Medicine, 53*, 165–188. https://doi.org/10.1016/S0277-9536(00)00329-4

Hunt, G., Kolind, T., & Antin, T. (2018). Conceptualizing ethnicity in alcohol and drug research: Epidemiology meets social theory. *Journal of Ethnicity in Substance Abuse, 17*(2), 187–198.

Hutton, F. (2009). New Zealand. In P. Hadfield (Ed.), *Nightlife and crime: Social order and governance in international perspective* (pp. 293–305). Oxford, UK: Oxford University Press.

Hutton, F. (2016). New Zealand students and 'cultures of intoxication'. *Sites: A Journal of Social Anthropology & Cultural Studies, 13*(2), 135–162.

Hutton, F., Griffin, C., Lyons, A. C., Niland, P., & McCreanor, T. (2016). "Tragic girls" and "crack whores": Alcohol, femininity and Facebook. *Feminism & Psychology, 26*(1), 73–93. https://doi.org/10.1177/0959353515618224

Hutton, F., & Wright, S. (2014). 'You don't ditch your girls': Young Māori and Pacific women and the culture of intoxication. *Critical Public Health, 25*(1), 101–119.

Hutton, F., Wright, S., & Saunders, E. (2013). Cultures of intoxication: Young women, alcohol, and harm reduction. *Contemporary Drug Problems, 40*(Winter), 451–480.

Jackson, C., & Tinkler, P. (2007). 'Ladettes' and 'modern girls': 'Troublesome' young femininities. *The Sociological Review, 55*(2), 251–272.

Johfre, S. S., & Saperstein, A. (2019). Racial and gender identities. In Stanford Center on Poverty and Inequality (Ed.), *State of the union: The poverty and inequality report*. Pathways Magazine, special issue.

Keane, H. (2009). Intoxication, harm and pleasure: An analysis of the Australian National Alcohol Strategy. *Critical Public Health, 19*(2), 135–142.

Lemle, R., & Mishkind, M. E. (1989). Alcohol and masculinity. *Journal of Substance Abuse Treatment, 6*(4), 213–222.

Lennox, J., Emslie, C., Sweeting, H., & Lyons, A. C. (2018). The role of alcohol in constructing gender & class identities among young women in the age of social media. *International Journal of Drug Policy, 58*, 13–21.

Lindsay, J., & Supski, S. (2017). Curating identity: Drinking, young women, femininities and social media practices. In A. C. Lyons, T. McCreanor, I. Goodwin, & H. Moewaka Barnes (Eds.), *Youth drinking cultures in a digital world: Alcohol, social media and cultures of intoxication*. Abingdon, UK: Routledge.

Loring, B. (2014). *Alcohol and inequities. Guidance for addressing inequities in alcohol-related harm*. Copenhagen, Denmark: WHO Regional Office for Europe. Retrieved from http://www.euro.who.int/__data/assets/pdf_file/0003/247629/Alcohol-and-Inequities.pdf

Lyons, A. C. (2009). Masculinities, femininities, behaviour and health. *Social and Personality Psychology Compass, 3*(4), 394–412.

Lyons, A. C., Emslie, C., & Hunt, K. (2014). Staying "in the zone" but not passing the "point of no return": Embodiment, gender and drinking in midlife. *Sociology of Health and Illness, 36*(2), 1–14. https://doi.org/10.1111/1467-9566.12103

Lyons, A. C., Goodwin, I., Griffin, C., McCreanor, T., & Moewaka Barnes, H. (2016). Facebook and the fun of drinking photos: Reproducing gendered regimes of power. *Social Media and Society, 2*(4), 1–13. https://doi.org/10.1177/2056305116672888

Lyons, A. C., & Gough, B. (2017). Masculinities, alcohol consumption and social networking. In A. C. Lyons, T. McCreanor, I. Goodwin, & H. Moewaka Barnes (Eds.), *Youth drinking cultures in a digital world: Alcohol, social media and cultures of intoxication*. Abingdon, UK: Routledge.

Lyons, A. C., McCreanor, T., Goodwin, I., & Moewaka Barnes, H. (Eds.). (2017). *Youth drinking cultures in a digital world: Alcohol, social media and cultures of intoxication*. Abingdon, UK: Routledge.

Lyons, A. C., & Willott, S. A. (2008). Alcohol consumption, gender identities and women's changing social positions. *Sex Roles, 59*, 694–712.

Manthey, J., Shield, K. D., Rylett, M., Hasan, O. S. M., Probst, C., & Rehm, J. (2019). Global alcohol exposure between 1990 and 2017 and forecasts until 2030: A modelling study. *The Lancet*. https://doi.org/10.1016/S0140-6736(18)32744-2

McCreanor, T., Barnes, H. M., Kaiwai, H., Borell, S., & Gregory, A. (2008). Creating intoxigenic environments: Marketing alcohol to young people in Aotearoa New Zealand. *Social Science and Medicine, 67*, 938–946. https://doi.org/10.1016/j.socscimed.2008.05.027

McCreanor, T., Greenaway, A., Moewaka Barnes, H., Borell, S., & Gregory, A. (2005). Youth identity formation and contemporary alcohol marketing. *Critical Public Health, 15*(3), 251–262. https://doi.org/10.1080/09581590500372345

McCreanor, T., Lyons, A. C., Griffin, C., Goodwin, I., Moewaka Barnes, H., & Hutton, F. (2013). Youth drinking cultures, social networking and alcohol marketing: Implications for public health. *Critical Public Health, 23*(1), 110–120. https://doi.org/10.1080/09581596.2012.748883

McCreanor, T., Lyons, A. C., Moewaka Barnes, H., Hutton, F., Goodwin, I., & Griffin, C. (2016). 'Drink a 12 box before you go': Pre-loading among young people in Aotearoa New Zealand. *Kotuitui: New Zealand Journal of Social Sciences, 11*(1), 36–46. https://doi.org/10.1080/1177083X.2015.1037314

McEwan, B., Campbell, M., Lyons, A. C., & Swain, D. A. (2013). *Pleasure, profit and pain: Alcohol in New Zealand and the contemporary culture of intoxication*. Hamilton, New Zealand: University of Waikato Faculty of Arts & Social Sciences.

McKie, B. (2018, September 1). 10,000 years of cheers: Why social drinking is an ancient ritual. *The Guardian International Edition*. Retrieved from https://www.theguardian.com/society/2018/sep/01/social-drinking-moderation-health-risks?

Measham, F. (2004). The decline of ecstasy, the rise of 'binge' drinking and the persistence of pleasure. *Probation Journal, 51*(4), 309–326. https://doi.org/10.1177/0264550504048220

Measham, F. (2006). The new policy mix: Alcohol, harm minimisation, and determined drunkenness in contemporary society. *International Journal of Drug Policy, 17*(4), 258–268. https://doi.org/10.1016/j.drugpo.2006.02.013

Measham, F. (2011). Drunkenness – A historical and contemporary cross-cultural perspective: "A voluntary madness". In A. Fox & M. MacAvoy (Eds.), *Expressions of drunkenness: (Four hundred rabbits)* (pp. 121–153). New York: Routledge.

Measham, F., & Brain, K. (2005). 'Binge' drinking, British alcohol policy and the new culture of intoxication. *Crime, Media, Culture, 1*(3), 262–283. https://doi.org/10.1177/1741659005057641

Mercille, J. (2016). Neoliberalism and the alcohol industry in Ireland. *Space & Polity, 20*(1), 59.

Ministry of Health. (2019, January 5). *Alcohol.* Retrieved July 8, 2019, from https://www.health.govt.nz/your-health/healthy-living/addictions/alcohol-and-drug-abuse/alcohol

Mullen, K., Watson, J., Swift, J., & Black, D. (2007). Young men, masculinity and alcohol. *Drugs: Education, Prevention and Policy, 14*(2), 151–165.

Niland, P., Lyons, A. C., Goodwin, I., & Hutton, F. (2013). "Everyone can loosen up and get a bit of a buzz on": Young adults, alcohol and friendship practices. *International Journal of Drug Policy, 24*, 530–537.

O'Brien, J. (2018). *States of intoxication: The place of alcohol in civilisation.* Routledge.

Pedersen, M. (2019). 'Feels a bit naughty when you're a mum': Alcohol use amongst mothers with preschool children. Doctor of Clinical Psychology thesis, Massey University.

Pennay, A. E., & Measham, F. (2016). The normalisation thesis – 20 years later. *Drugs: Education, Prevention and Policy, 23*(3), 187–189. https://doi.org/10.3109/09687637.2016.1173649

Peralta, R. L. (2007). College alcohol use and the embodiment of hegemonic masculinity among European American men. *Sex Roles, 56*, 741–756.

Peralta, R. L. (2008). "Alcohol allows you to not be yourself": Toward a structured understanding of alcohol use and gender difference among gay, lesbian, and heterosexual youth. *Journal of Drug Issues, 38*(2), 373–399.

Rahav, G., Wilsnack, R., Bloomfield, K., Gmel, G., & Kuntsche, S. (2006). The influence of societal level factors on men's and women's alcohol consumption and alcohol problems. *Alcohol and Alcoholism, 41*, 147–155.

Research New Zealand. (2018). *Ready to contemplate? Mid-life adults and their relationship with alcohol*. Wellington, New Zealand: Health Promotion Agency. Retrieved from https://www.hpa.org.nz/sites/default/files/Ready%20to%20contemplate%20-%20midlife%20adults%20and%20their%20relationship%20with%20alcohol.pdf

Robertson, S. (2007). *Understanding men and health: Masculinities, identity and well-being*. McGraw-Hill Education, UK.

Rolfe, A., Orford, J., & Dalton, S. (2009). Women, alcohol and femininity: A discourse analysis of women heavy drinkers' accounts. *Journal of Health Psychology, 14*(2), 326–335. https://doi.org/10.1177/1359105308100217

Room, R. (2011). Addiction and personal responsibility as solutions to the contradictions of neoliberal consumerism. *Critical Public Health, 21*(2), 141–151. https://doi.org/10.1080/09581596.2010.529424

Scoats, R. (2015). Inclusive masculinity and Facebook photographs among early emerging adults at a British university. *Journal of Adolescent Research*, 0743558415607059.

Skeggs, B. (2005). The making of class and gender through visualizing moral subject formation. *Sociology, 39*(5), 965–982.

Slade, T., Chapman, C., Swift, W., Keyes, K., Tonks, Z., & Teesson, M. (2016). Birth cohort trends in the global epidemiology of alcohol use and alcohol-related harms in men and women: Systematic review and metaregression. *BMJ Open, 6*(10), e011827. https://doi.org/10.1136/bmjopen-2016-011827

Stepney, M. (2015). The challenge of hyper-sexual femininity and binge drinking: A feminist psychoanalytic response. *Subjectivity, 8*(1), 57–73.

Stockley, C., & Saunders, J. B. (2011). The biology of intoxication. In A. Fox & M. MacAvoy (Eds.), *Expressions of drunkenness: (Four hundred rabbits)* (pp. 13–52). New York: Routledge. Retrieved from http://ezproxy.aut.ac.nz/login?url=http://search.ebscohost.com/login.aspx?direct=true&db=cat05020a&AN=aut.b11744303&site=eds-live

Szmigin, I., Griffin, C., Mistral, W., Bengry-Howell, A., Weale, L., & Hackley, C. (2008). Re-framing 'binge drinking' as calculated hedonism: Empirical evidence from the UK. *International Journal of Drug Policy, 19*(5), 359–366.

The Social Issues Research Centre. (1998). *Social and cultural aspects of drinking. A report to the European Commission*. Oxford, UK. Retrieved from http://www.sirc.org/publik/drinking6.html

Thurnell-Read, T. (2011). Off the leash and out of control: Masculinities and embodiment in Eastern European stag tourism. *Sociology, 45*(6), 977–991.
Thurnell-Read, T. (2013). 'Yobs' and 'Snobs': Embodying drink and the problematic male drinking body. *Sociological Research Online, 18*(2), 3.
UK Chief Medical Officers. (2016). *UK Chief Medical Officers' low risk drinking guidelines*. Retrieved July 8, 2016, from https://assets.publishing.service.gov.uk/government/uploads/system/uploads/attachment_data/file/545937/UK_CMOs__report.pdf
VicHealth. (2019). *Top spin. Under the influence promotion of alcoholic drinks rife on social media*. Retrieved April 11, 2019, from https://www.vichealth.vic.gov.au/media-and-resources/media-releases/under-the-influence-promotion-of-alcoholic-drinks-rife-on-social-media
Waitt, G., Jessop, L., & Gorman-Murray, A. (2011). 'The guys in there just expect to be laid': Embodied and gendered socio-spatial practices of a 'night out' in Wollongong, Australia. *Gender, Place and Culture, 18*(2), 255–275.
Willott, S., & Lyons, A. C. (2012). Consuming male identities: Masculinities, gender relations and alcohol consumption in Aotearoa New Zealand. *Journal of Community and Applied Social Psychology, 22*, 330–345.

3

Smoking and Intoxication: From Control to the Buzz

Helen Keane

Introduction

Smoking is an idiosyncratic form of drug use, at least in its most familiar contemporary forms. Habitual smokers are highly likely to be dependent on nicotine, and they often struggle to quit even if their desire to do so is strong. However, this potentially lethal dependence is normalised, at least to some extent, with smokers occupying the category of 'addict' only in certain limited contexts. For example, unlike other forms of drug dependence, giving up smoking is generally understood simply as cessation of a behaviour, rather than a deeper process of recovery. Becoming a non-smoker is about relinquishing a daily practice. Although quitting is tough and prone to failure, the formation of a new self, based on fundamental transformation of subjectivity, is not usually viewed as a necessary part of the process.

H. Keane (✉)
School of Sociology, Research School of Social Sciences, Australian National University, Canberra, ACT, Australia
e-mail: helen.keane@anu.edu.au

F. Hutton (ed.), *Cultures of Intoxication*,
https://doi.org/10.1007/978-3-030-35284-4_3

The uniqueness of smoking is also reflected in its marginalisation in the field of drug and alcohol studies. In an analysis of journals published in 2010 and 2011, tobacco researcher John Hughes found that the majority of generic studies of drug and substance use did not include nicotine or smoking, and further, that only a very small number of these mentioned this exclusion. According to Hughes (2012), these results, published in an article titled 'Nicotine Don't Get No Respect', suggest that researchers assume that readers will know that generic terms such as 'substance', 'drug' and 'addiction' refer only to alcohol and illicit drug use.

As Courtwright (2005) has observed, however, the inclusion of smoking and tobacco consumption in the category of drug use has varied historically. In the twenty-first century, the rise of neurochemical models of substance use and dependence has promoted the underlying commonality of all forms of drug use as a 'governing idea' in the field. Nicotine, like other drugs, produces rewarding effects by acting on neurotransmitters in the brain. In addition, smoking often takes place at the same time as other forms of drug consumption, with smoking-drinking a familiar form of co-use or 'package deal' in social situations (Nichter et al., 2010). The particular subjective effects produced by concurrent drinking and smoking and the possibility that the two drugs reinforce and enhance the other's effects have been extensively explored (Piasecki, Wood, Shiffman, Sher, & Heath, 2012; Rose et al., 2004). For example, Piasecki et al. (2011, p. 564) found that 'alcohol use increased appraisals of pleasure from smoking and tobacco use increased reported pleasure from drinking' although these effects were small.

The *DSM-5* category of 'tobacco use disorder' also conforms to a generic approach to substance use problems, as its 11 criteria are fundamentally the same as those for other drug use disorders (American Psychiatric Association, 2013). The awkward fit is apparent though, as the examples used to illustrate the criteria are in several cases unconvincing. For example, chain smoking is interpreted as 'spending excessive time' using the substance, despite the fact that it is usually an activity that occurs at the same time as other activities (including other forms of drug consumption).

Whatever the changes in medical discourse and patterns of co-use, the distinctiveness of smoking as a practice remains obvious in everyday life, in terms of its relationship with other activities and its particular constellation of harms. It is easy to attribute the particular role and meaning of smoking to the properties of nicotine and its apparent lack of obvious intoxicating effects. In medical and public health discourse, intoxication is viewed as a pathological state that is both physically harmful and morally suspect (Hunt & Frank, 2017; Keane, 2009). Drunkenness is the iconic state of pathological intoxication, marked by disinhibition, mood lability, impaired judgement, inappropriate behaviour and other signs of diminished physical or mental control (American Psychiatric Association, 2013, pp. 485, 497). Based on this notion of intoxication as loss of control, the *DSM-5* states that 'nicotine intoxication is very rare', and it does not include intoxication as a tobacco-related disorder (American Psychiatric Association, 2013, p. 572). 'Nicotine intoxication' is addressed in the medical literature, but intoxication from this medicalised perspective refers to poisoning. Accounts of nicotine intoxication in the medical literature describe cases of children ingesting 'vape' juice (the nicotine solution used in e-cigarette vaporisers) or acute illness caused by excessive use of nicotine replacement therapy (NRT) (Gupta, Gandhi, & Manikonda, 2014; Palmer, Buckley, & Faulds, 1992).

However, there is a broader understanding of intoxication, which incorporates less florid changes in consciousness than drunkenness. For example, in his book *Drugs, Intoxication and Society*, Sociologist Angus Bancroft introduces the topic by stating 'Whether smoking cigarettes, drinking alcohol and coffee, or taking illicit drugs, for the majority of society's members, some kind of intoxication is a regular, often daily practice' (2009, p. 5). By expanding the category to include substance-induced changes in the relationship between the self and the world, whatever their intensity, Bancroft (2009) normalises the experience of and the desire for intoxication, broadening out the concept of intoxication as something that can be more subtle than ostentatious and visible alcohol and other drug intoxication.

Another expansive definition of intoxication is the use of substances to alter consciousness (Hunt & Frank, 2017, p. 323). 'Altered consciousness' is usually interpreted to entail the experience of a level of awareness significantly divergent from an ordinary or normal state. However, consciousness can be shifted in relatively mild and transient ways, such as a few minutes daydreaming at one's desk. In a recent report on tobacco, nicotine and e-Cigarettes, the US National Institute of Drug Abuse (NIDA) constructs the intoxicating effects of nicotine as powerfully rewarding despite their brevity and modest scale:

> A transient surge of endorphins in the reward circuits of the brain causes a slight, brief euphoria when nicotine is administered. This surge is much briefer than the "high" associated with other drugs. However, like other drugs of abuse, nicotine increases levels of the neurotransmitter dopamine in these reward circuits, which reinforces the behavior of taking the drug. (NIDA, 2018, p. 7)

The notion of a 'slight' euphoria seems oxymoronic at first glance, but it captures the particular capacity of cigarettes to create a brief opening in the smoker's day, which is a minor, but sustaining, enhancement of routine. This form of slight intoxication is also appealing because of its privacy and internality. The act of smoking may be public and visible, but the alteration of mood is not readily discernible to others, including authority figures such as parents, teachers and employers who may have the individual under surveillance. In earlier work, I have described this as the ability of smoking to make time and space (Keane, 2002).

This chapter examines smoking and nicotine consumption in relationship to this broader understanding of intoxication. Its first aim is to illuminate some of the varied effects of nicotine consumption that tend to be sidelined by the medical and public health focus on nicotine addiction. This will include discussion of different forms of social practice, which incorporate nicotine (ritualised, routine and recreational). Its second aim is to contribute to a more nuanced understanding of intoxication, which can attend to small and brief shifts in mood and perception, thereby resisting the dominant view that intoxication is synonymous with harm and loss of control.

Psychoactive Effects and Social Practices

As already suggested, nicotine is a paradoxical drug when considered in the framework of contemporary medicine. It is viewed as both the most and least addictive substance in the range of substances thought of as 'drugs'. The addictive potential of nicotine is stressed in public health discourse on smoking, which warns young people that 'just one cigarette' can get you hooked (DiFranza, 2008). On the other hand, dependence on nicotine does not usually produce the social harms, downward trajectory and loss of control over one's life that are central to models of addiction both medical and popular. Further, in its support of NRT as a cessation aid, medical and public health discourse emphasises that nicotine is not the substance in cigarettes that produces harm.

The most familiar way of explaining the paradoxes of nicotine is by reference to the particular pharmacology and psychoactive effects of the drug. Medical literature describes 'positive effects on mood and cognitive function', 'learning', 'memory enhancement', 'reduction of anxiety and tension' and 'mild euphoria' (Benowitz, 2008; Bruijnzeel, 2017, p. 661). Nicotine combines effects that are experienced as both relaxing and stimulating, which contribute to its versatility as a drug. The blending of controlled pleasure with increased mental performance and focus is ideal for the enhancement and sustaining of productivity desired in many workplaces and institutions.

The pharmacokinetics of nicotine are also noteworthy. The drug is easily absorbed 'from every site on or in the body, including the lungs, buccal and nasal mucosa, skin and gastrointestinal tract' (Julien, 2013, p. 152). It is quickly and thoroughly distributed throughout the body (p. 153). Its ease and speed of absorption means that its effects are rapid and relatively short lived, especially when smoked. However, as sociological and anthropological research on substance use has demonstrated, pharmacology is not the only driver of drug effects. In Zinberg's (1984) classic formulation, the experience of intoxication depends on the combination of drug, set and setting—the substance, the mindset or individual psychology of the user and the social and physical context of use. In more recent work, researchers have highlighted the dynamic processes and the multiplicity of heterogeneous elements involved in drug events that tend to be obscured by terms such as 'set' and 'setting' (Duff, 2007; Moore, 1993).

In this chapter, I turn to practice theory as an approach to social life, which provides insight into substance use by resisting explanations based on universal drug properties and individual psychology (Blue, Shove, Carmona, & Kelly, 2016; Keane, Weier, Fraser, & Gartner, 2017). Theories of practice, built on the work of Bourdieu and, more recently, Reckwitz (2002), Schatzki (2002) and Shove, Pantzar, and Watson (2012) centre on social practices as the unit of analysis. Recent research has demonstrated the usefulness of considering a range of healthy and unhealthy 'behaviours' as forms of social practice (Keane et al., 2017; Will & Weiner, 2014). In this context, a social practice is understood as a routinised or patterned type of behaviour, which brings together forms of bodily activity, forms of mental activity, objects and their handling, types of knowledge and emotional states. Crucially, social practices cannot be reduced to a single element, but depend for their existence on the inter-relatedness of these multiple elements. In Reckwitz's words:

> A practice is…a routinized way in which bodies are moved, objects are handled, subjects are treated, things are described and the world is understood…A practice is social, as it is a 'type' of behaving and understanding that appears at different locales and at different points of time and is carried out by different body/minds. (2002, p. 250)

As he observes, 'bodily movements, things, practical knowledge and routine' (p. 259) are at the centre of practice theory. However, the symbolic remains important, with Shove et al. (2012) usefully identifying the three key elements of social practice as: materials (objects, consumer goods and infrastructures); competence (including understandings of the situation; practical know-how); and meanings (including embodied understandings of the social significance of the practice and past experiences of participation) (cited in Blue et al., 2016, p. 42). Considering smoking as a social practice enables an analysis which acknowledges the pharmaceutical and physiological aspects of nicotine and the materiality of the cigarette, while also attending to the meanings of the activity.

Examining forms of nicotine consumption as social practices highlights diversity and instability, as practices are distinct from each other and change over time. In this way, the approach of this chapter is distinct from the conventional 'history of smoking' narrative which traces a single path from Indigenous American rituals to twenty-first-century vaping. However, the resilience and tenacity of nicotine consumption remain clear, as the drug is assembled into different practices at different times and places. Another advantage of considering smoking as a social practice is that it draws attention to the relationship between smoking and other practices. Smoking is usually combined with other activities and tasks. As Blue et al. (2016, p. 43) explain, practices often hold together in bundles, they become coordinated and mutually dependent, but they can also split apart and compete for time and space. In addition, practice theory refigures individuals as 'carriers' of practices rather than agents of behaviour. This is a radical departure from conventional approaches to 'health behaviours' such as smoking, which remain focused on the individual as the locus of change (even if 'social determinants' are taken into account) (Cohn, 2014). In terms of intoxication, this approach highlights the different types of intoxicating experience that are produced by different social practices located in different times and spaces, even when the same substance is consumed. Intoxication itself is a fluid and changeable category, or perhaps more accurately, it is a shift in one's relationship to the world, with no fixed meaning or inevitable consequences, either negative or positive.

Nicotine Practices: Routine and Ritual

The smoking of commercially cultivated tobacco is the most common and familiar contemporary nicotine-related social practice. According to historian Jordan Goodman (1993, p. 61), tobacco was a mass-consumed commodity by the middle of the eighteenth century. Pipes, snuff and cigars were the most popular modes of early tobacco consumption in Europe, and users were almost exclusively men. The development of the mass-produced cigarette in the late nineteenth century was a transformative material change, which captured and recruited many new users to the practice of smoking, including women and young people. 'Schoolboys', in particular, were regarded as highly susceptible to the lure of cigarettes and were the object of much early anti-tobacco campaigning.

Compared to other forms of tobacco ingestion in practice at the time, cigarettes were convenient, cheap, neat and accessible. Unlike chewing tobacco or snuff, smoking cigarettes did not involve spitting or sneezing and therefore appeared more refined (Hughes, 2003, p. 89). Unlike pipe smoking, there was little additional paraphernalia involved, and a cigarette could be quickly consumed in a couple of minutes. Part of the material innovation of the cigarette was a shift to a new variety of 'bright' flue-cured tobacco, more acidic and milder than earlier forms and easier to inhale. Thus, the specific practical know-how involved in becoming a cigarette smoker included inhalation and the associated coordination of hand, mouth and breath. Hughes (2003, p. 89) argues that the mildness and 'slightness' of the cigarette were central to the success of cigarette smoking as a practice. Compared to other forms of tobacco use 'it had little immediate effect on the smoker' and was therefore a highly adaptable practice, readily coordinated with and incorporated into rhythms of daily life. The portability and wide availability of cigarettes enabled smoking to become a more mobile practice, bundled together with many other daily practices of transportation, work and leisure. New methods of marketing such as packaging and advertising also boosted the popularity of the practice (Brandt, 2004).

However, an association between smoking and intoxication remained. According to Hughes (2003), prior to the development of cigarettes, tobacco use was frequently compared to drinking alcohol. This was partly because no other model for intoxicating substance use existed for the practice in European cultures and partly because the tobacco of the time was stronger and more likely to produce 'drunkenness' (Hughes, 2003, p. 72). In addition, smoking and drinking were routinely combined in the sociability and recreational consumption of the eighteenth-century alehouse, establishing a long-standing practice of public tobacco and alcohol co-use in which the intoxicating effects of the two drugs combined in an enmeshed experience of relaxation and reward. Analogies between the effects of smoking and other less acceptable forms of drug use continued to be deployed in anti-tobacco discourse in Europe and the United States. US physician and author of the early twentieth-century self-help book *Habits that Handicap* (1915) Charles Towns, argued that the process of smoking was fundamentally the same as drinking alcohol and using drugs:

> The relation of tobacco, especially in the form of cigarettes, and alcohol and opium is a very close one. For years I have been dealing with alcoholism and morphinism, have gone into their every phase and aspect, have kept careful and minute details of between six and seven thousand cases, and I have never seen a case, except occasionally with women, which did not have a history of excessive tobacco. (Towns, 2011, p. 72)

Tobacco smoking is therefore presented as linked to, and encouraging, harmful use of other substances, which prompted moral observations such as that by Towns (2011), as well as campaigns against this social practice. In New Zealand, in the 1800s, social puritans saw smoking as a 'lust of the flesh' and labelled those who smoked 'evildoers' (Eldred-Grigg, 1984, p. 220/221). This same group also believed that tobacco led the smoker to other vices such as 'alcoholism, gambling and fornication' (Eldred-Grigg, 1984, p. 221). Young people became the focus for these concerns as the group regarded as the most vulnerable to 'moral contamination'. A bill was introduced into the New Zealand Parliament in 1900 to outlaw smoking by those under 21. The 1903 Juvenile Smoking Suppression Act prohibited the supply of tobacco in any form to children under the age of 15, while also making it an offence for any juvenile to smoke in a public place.

Despite these kinds of moral campaigns and the existence of social proscriptions associated with smoking, Hughes (2003) argues convincingly that cigarette smoking ultimately took on a meaning of self-restraint and control in the twentieth century because it was *not* like drinking and drug use. Mild and transient in its effects, cigarette smoking was compatible with the demands of modern life. As a practice that was well suited to coordination with and supplementation of other activities and tasks (rather than a leisure activity in itself), smoking was constituted as a modern method of coping with stress, boredom and fatigue. In contrast to the intoxicating practice of alehouse pipe smoking/drinking, twentieth-century cigarette smoking was an 'instrument of self-control', which enabled individuals to maintain normality rather than escape it. It could promote productivity at work by acting as a stimulant and aiding concentration, and enhance sociability through relaxation (Hughes, 2003, p. 91).

Smoking developed into a respectable, routine and domesticated practice of daily life for adults, both men and women, in the mid-twentieth century. Its effects on the nervous system were categorised and experienced as welcome and ordinary sensations described in terms such as calming, refreshing and invigorating. These mild changes in mood and alertness were a world away from the 'mind-altering' and destructive effects of other drugs. In the example of cigarette smoking, we can see that intoxication need not be 'other' to normality. Awareness of the link between smoking and disease has had a dramatic effect on the practice of smoking, in both its material and symbolic elements. As Brandt (2004, p. 390) observes 'from a behavior associated with sociability, leisure, and pleasure, smoking increasingly came to be associated with compulsiveness, dirt, and personal disregard for one's health'. Knowledge about the effects of passive smoking was particularly influential in reshaping the practice as it constituted smoking as bad for everyone, not just harmful to the smoker (Berridge, 1999). The rise of tobacco control as a major area of public health and increasingly stringent government regulation has produced a restricted smoking landscape and denormalised the practice (Bell, McCullough, Salmon, & Bell, 2010). Smoking has become 'unbundled' from most forms of work, as well as being excluded from the public social life of restaurants and bars.

However, it is noteworthy that the classification of smoking as a dangerous form of drug consumption has concentrated on and highlighted the risks of addiction to nicotine rather than any concerns about other psychoactive effects (US Department of Health and Human Services, 1988). Smokers are regarded as anti-social and potentially harmful to others, but this is because of the noxious impact of smoke rather than unruly conduct or reckless behaviour produced by intoxication. The smoking subject is disparaged and devalued not because of their unruliness, but because their smoking introduces an unruly and invasive substance into social space (Dennis, 2011). The 'loss of control' of tobacco addiction is not the same as the 'loss of control' of alcoholism. While this distinction may seem obvious, it is connected to the particular mode of consuming tobacco as a mildly pleasurable and non-intoxicating substance that became dominant in a particular historical era.

In contrast to this constitution of smoking as non-intoxicating and mundane are the sacred and ceremonial uses of tobacco. In many Indigenous American belief systems, tobacco is a sacred plant with supernatural origins and powers, which enable interaction with the spirit world (Alderete, Erickson, Kaplan, & Pérez-Stable, 2010; Boudreau et al., 2016; Goodman, 1993). It is also a medicine, connected to physical and spiritual well-being (National Native Network, n.d.). The restoration of traditional tobacco practices, including the cultivation and use of ceremonial tobacco, is a goal of contemporary movements for sovereignty and health equity (Boudreau et al., 2016).

Tobacco is also a central element of South American shamanism, in which altered consciousness, trance states and hallucinations are linked to the power of the shaman to see and communicate with parallel worlds (Alderete et al., 2010; Wilbert, 1991). In this context, the burning and smoking of tobacco is coordinated with practices of prayer, ceremony, celebration, divination, dancing and healing as a crucial element of transformative collective events.

The species and strains of tobacco cultivated and consumed in America prior to European contact were much stronger than contemporary commercial varieties, and therefore were able to produce intoxicating and hallucinogenic effects more readily (Hughes, 2003). However, this pharmacological characteristic should not be regarded as the single determining element that produced the difference between sacred and secular smoking practices. It is the array of practices and elements assembled in the ritualised and ceremonial consumption of nicotine that produces the particular experiences of participants, not simply the properties of the drug. For example, the convulsions, trembling and vomiting that medical discourse defines as symptoms of nicotine poisoning can be positive manifestations of spiritual power in the context of shamanic use (Wilbert, 1991).

By juxtaposing mundane and sacred practices of smoking and highlighting the distinctiveness of commercial and ceremonial tobacco, it can be seen that intoxication does not emerge from a fixed and inherent capacity of a drug. Rather, psychoactive effects are interpreted, heightened, controlled and mediated by their incorporation in an assemblage of associated objects, activities, knowledge and meanings. As practice theory suggests, the habitual use and enjoyment of nicotine consumption emerges from varied socio-material conditions.

Nicotine Practices: Vaping and the Fun of the Buzz

The e-cigarette or personal vaping device, invented in 2003, is the most recent technological innovation in nicotine consumption. These electronic devices produce inhalable aerosol by heating a liquid, which contains varying amounts of nicotine (or no nicotine). As novel nicotine delivery devices that are much less harmful than conventional cigarettes, their rise in popularity has produced intense debate within public health and tobacco control (Bell & Keane, 2012; Royal College of Physicians, 2016). Central to this debate is their safety and their efficacy as smoking cessation aids. However, the success and spread of vaping as a social practice also demonstrate the persistent appeal of nicotine effects, including intoxication.

Vaping devices have undergone substantial changes in material form since their first appearance. As the market grows, new products emerge and online retailers now sell many different models and components, flavours and strengths of juice and accessories (Zhu et al., 2014). The first models on the market, now known as 'cigalikes', were built to resemble conventional cigarettes. Cigalikes usually consist of a low-capacity disposable or rechargeable battery and replaceable pre-filled cartridge containing the nicotine liquid. So-called second-generation models have now eclipsed cigalikes in popularity, especially among experienced users (Farsalinos, Romagna, Tsiapras, Kyrzopoulos, & Voudris, 2014). Second-generation e-cigarettes are bigger (often resembling a large fountain pen), more powerful and feature a refillable tank and replaceable components (e.g. heating coils and wicks for atomisers). Third-generation models also known as 'mods' have even larger-capacity batteries, replaceable components and variable power settings. These devices are highly customisable and come in a variety of styles, shapes and sizes, allowing enthusiasts to put together their own devices (Wagener et al., 2016).

A subculture of vapers and hobbyists has developed, with a flourishing online presence based on blogs, forums, YouTube channels and other forms of social media. Thus, while vaping could be considered as an evolution of smoking, in which a new technology and new competencies alter a long-standing practice, it now makes sense to consider it as a distinct practice of nicotine consumption. The material capacities of electronic devices versus combustible objects enable the practice of vaping to have a characteristic temporal flexibility, for example. The user can take one hit or can vape continuously over a long period of time (Keane et al., 2017; McQuoid, Keamy-Minor, & Ling, 2018). As McQuoid et al. found in their research with young 'poly-tobacco' users, vaping also enables forms of sociability and connection that are different from the routine gift practices of cigarette smokers (2018). While the mass-produced fungibility of cigarettes (and the fleeting nature of 'a light') allows these items to be exchanged outside of close social circles, sharing a vaping device is a more intimate encounter that can act to both produce and signify closeness between friends, partners and family (McQuoid et al., 2018, p. 9).

In addition, the customisability of device and substance that characterises vaping is a stark contrast to the mass-produced and unmodifiable nature of conventional cigarettes. It makes possible a combination of practical know-how, an exercise of choice and pleasurable consumption. In recent research with Australian vapers, this customisability was valued. One participant commented:

> Vaping worked for me because the devices and e-juices were customisable, I could adjust the output power, I could experiment with several different compatible cartridge types until I found the one that fit me perfectly. I was able to purchase e-juices with different amounts of vegetable glycerine (more glycerine, the more vapour exhaled) and different levels of nicotine in order to find the right amount for my requirements for both throat hit and mental stimulation. (Keane et al., 2017, p. 473)

The success of vaping as a practice is also tied to symbolic elements and a dynamic repertoire of meanings, which are in flux (Lucherini, Rooke, & Amos, 2018). In particular, the meanings of vaping among Millennials have developed through a tight relationship with digital and online platforms. Vaping influencers promote brands and models to followers, linking vaping with particular aesthetic styles. A recent article in *The Guardian* described vaping as 'an alternative scene with its own lingo, tricks and superstars' (Usborne, 2018). In the hands of enthusiast vapers, nicotine consumption is refigured as both recreational and a form of identity work. For the most dedicated, it conforms to the characteristics of 'serious leisure' in which a hobby is pursued in a systematic fashion over time, involving the development of skills, expertise and self-identity as a practitioner (Stebbins, 1982). Indeed, vaping has become a lucrative and rewarding profession for a small number of experts.

However, for everyday vapers, it seems that the highly valued social significance of the practice is its relatively low level of stigma rather than a sense that the practice communicates coolness (Lucherini et al., 2018; McQuoid et al., 2018). The obnoxious performativity of some vapers and the 'douche-y bro' identities associated with this performativity can attract derision (McQuoid et al., 2018, p. 6). Related to the relief from stigma, vapers have also reported that while they remain addicted to nicotine, vaping changes the meaning of their nicotine addiction. They no longer feel imprisoned by a habit that was destroying their health. As one participant in the Australian research mentioned previously said, 'I can now enjoy the pleasant effects of nicotine without the fear that it is killing me'. Another stated, 'I went from hating my nicotine addiction to enjoying it' (Keane et al., 2017, p. 472).

In terms of the 'pleasant effects' of the drug, vaping has produced a new discourse and experience of nicotine intoxication in which the transient euphoria characteristic of the drug is explicitly constituted as a key element of the experience. 'The buzz' and how to achieve a pleasurable 'nicotine high' are discussed on online vaping forums, with comparisons routinely made between the smoking buzz and the vaping buzz. Therefore, in this context, the development of vaping as a practice produces a reinterpretation of smoking in terms of particular psychoactive effects. The following two posts from different users on an online vaping forum in

2017 highlight intoxicating effects, including a 'wobbly feel' that is interpreted positively by the user, although this sensation could equally be classified as a sign of exceeding the moderation advised in the first post:

> Nicotine is fun in the right dose. Too much and you end up nastily sick… Try not inhaling so much, just play with it. Be careful. Moderate. It can be a nice buzz. It's short, though.

> I don't really smoke anymore but every couple of weeks I'll bum a few cigarettes off a friend and really enjoy it. It doesn't take long for me to find it unpleasant also but a little bit in between long breaks is really nice I think. Love that head space and wobbly feel of the first cig in a month or two.

The buzz is also a central feature of a recent and dramatic development in vaping practice, the rise of JUUL 'pod' vaporisers, which have become enormously popular in the United States, especially among teenagers (Willett et al., 2019). JUUL vaporisers, launched in 2015, currently have the largest share of the US e-cigarette market (Huang et al., 2019). JUUL has been intensively marketed on social media, and YouTube videos produced by young users number in the hundreds of thousands (Ramamurthi, Chau, & Jackler, 2018). The use of 'Juuling' as a verb is established in youth culture. The material characteristics of JUUL vaporisers underlie the rapid success of 'Juuling' as a social practice among teenagers. The devices use convenient pre-filled cartridges or 'pods' and can be recharged in less than an hour. They are sleek and compact, they resemble USB sticks, and the vapour they produce is relatively inconspicuous. These features enable clandestine use or 'stealth vaping', where the practice is hidden from others, including parents and teachers (Ramamurthi et al., 2018). Here, the ability to consume illicitly while under surveillance and experience intoxicating effects under the noses of unsuspecting adults links the materiality of the device to a desired image of youthful identity as both transgressive and competent.

In the emergent social practice of juuling, the combination of device, substance, user and meanings is assembled into a distinct nicotine experience. At least as the practice appears on social media, this form of nicotine consumption is constituted and experienced as fun, youthful and cool, with the stealth element adding an element of play and/or pleasurable defiance for some users (Kavuluru, Han, & Hahn, 2018). Central to the fun of Juuling is the nicotine 'buzz', which one adolescent user quoted by *The New York Times* described as feeling 'sober and high at the same time' (Barshad, 2018, n.p.).

Similarly to the spread of tobacco cigarettes in the twentieth century, the success of JUUL is, in part based on a material innovation in nicotine formulation. JUUL pods use organic nicotine salts extracted from tobacco leaves rather than the free-base nicotine used in other vaping juices (Huang et al., 2019). This enables JUUL devices to reproduce the rapid 'hit' of a smoked cigarette, delivering nicotine significantly faster than other e-cigarettes. The aerosol that is produced is also apparently less harsh on the throat than that of other devices (Koval, Willett, & Briggs, 2018). Therefore, JUUL produces a fast, fleeting intoxication effect, which readily combines with the thrill of transgression and group belonging for young users. In this way, it has reintegrated some of the material, performative and symbolic elements found in youth smoking practices of the twentieth century.

Not surprisingly, the popularity of JUUL among teenagers has raised public health, school and parental concerns about a new youth nicotine 'epidemic' (US Department of Health and Human Services, 2019). Media coverage of Juuling has focused on telling unsuspecting parents 'what they need to know' about this risky and alarming new practice (Raising Teens Today, 2018).

The mobilisation of medical authorities, parents and teachers against Juuling could enhance its appeal to teenagers, although as its popularity in youth culture is also vulnerable to rapid decline and extinguishment, due to the temporality of social media–influenced trends. In addition, the accessibility of JUUL and other similar devices is currently undergoing a process of restriction that is also likely to affect the future of the practice amongst teens. The US Food and Drug Administration (FDA) has expressed its intention to increase enforcement of e-cigarette sales to minors and to limit the marketing of sweet and fruity flavours, singling out JUUL as a particular concern (Dyer, 2019). After FDA intervention in 2018, JUUL announced that it would restrict availability of its most popular flavours (such as mango) to online sales (Zaleski, 2018). Thus, while at the time of writing, there is an integration of 'material, image, skill' that makes Juuling recognisable as a social practice, this is provisional, rather than stable, and subject to transformation (Pantzar & Shove, 2010). Future innovations in vaping may or may not include 'the buzz' as a central and emphasised element, but the intoxicating potential of nicotine will remain as a potent source of meaning and pleasure that can add to the ability of a consumption practice to take hold.

Conclusion

Dominant medical models of intoxication present it as a state defined by impairment and loss of control, contrasted to the rationality and restraint of normality. From this perspective, smoking is not intoxicating. Rather, in its currently most familiar forms, the consumption of nicotine has been understood as enhancing self-control, helping users cope with the demands of modern life, while maintaining productivity and civility. While awareness of its health effects and the potency of nicotine have undermined the association of smoking with control, the harm of smoking is associated with addiction rather than intoxication.

However, this chapter has argued that the sensations produced by smoking, its mild and transient pleasures, should be recognised and included in an expanded and de-pathologised framework of intoxication. Altered states of consciousness are not necessarily disruptive and dramatic; they can coexist with normal, daily life and become part of its routines. They can be pleasurable and beneficial without being visible as a loss of control.

By bringing together different social practices of nicotine consumption, including domesticated, ritualised and recreational forms, this chapter has also challenged the notion that the pharmacology of nicotine determines the effects and experiences of both intoxication and the drug. Nicotine is a versatile and adaptable drug, and its use can have a range of functions and take on different meanings. By considering the combinations of materiality, know-how and meaning that make up different nicotine-related habits, activities and events, a social practice approach enables a more expansive understanding of these forms of drug use. The rise of vaping in the twenty-first century has produced new practices and affordances, including a re-emergence of 'the buzz' of nicotine, and its capacity to be consumed and enjoyed as an intoxicating drug.

References

Alderete, E., Erickson, P. I., Kaplan, C. P., & Pérez-Stable, E. J. (2010). Ceremonial tobacco use in the Andes: Implications for smoking prevention among indigenous youth. *Anthropology & Medicine, 17*(1), 27–39. https://doi.org/10.1080/13648471003607607

American Psychiatric Association. (2013). *Diagnostic and statistical manual of mental disorders (DSM-5)*. Washington, DC: American Psychiatric Press.

Bancroft, A. (2009). *Drugs, intoxication and society*. Cambridge: Polity.

Barshad, A. (2018). The JUUL is too cool. *The New York Times*, April 7. Retrieved from https://www.nytimes.com/2018/04/07/style/the-juul-is-too-cool.html

Bell, K., & Keane, H. (2012). Nicotine control: E-cigarettes, smoking and addiction. *International Journal of Drug Policy, 23*(3), 242–247. https://doi.org/10.1016/j.drugpo.2012.01.006

Bell, K., McCullough, L., Salmon, A., & Bell, J. (2010). 'Every space is claimed': Smokers' experiences of tobacco denormalisation. *Sociology of Health & Illness, 32*(6), 914–929. https://doi.org/10.1111/j.1467-9566.2010.01251.x

Benowitz, N. L. (2008). Neurobiology of nicotine addiction: Implications for smoking cessation treatment. *The American Journal of Medicine, 121*(4), S3–S10. https://doi.org/10.1016/j.amjmed.2008.01.015

Berridge, V. (1999). Passive smoking and its prehistory in Britain: Policy speaks to science? *Social Science & Medicine, 49*(9), 1183–1195. https://doi.org/10.1016/S02779536(99)00159-8

Blue, S., Shove, E., Carmona, C., & Kelly, M. P. (2016). Theories of practice and public health: Understanding (un)healthy practices. *Critical Public Health, 26*(1), 36–50. https://doi.org/10.1080/09581596.2014.980396

Boudreau, G., Hernandez, C., Hoffer, D., Preuss, K. S., Tibbetts-Barto, L., Villaluz, N. T., & Scott, S. (2016). Why the world will never be tobacco-free: Reframing "tobacco control" into a traditional tobacco movement. *American Journal of Public Health, 106*(7), 1188–1195. https://doi.org/10.2105/AJPH.2016.303125

Brandt, A. (2004). From nicotine to nicotrol: Addiction, cigarettes and American culture. In S. Tracy & C. Acker (Eds.), *Altering American consciousness* (pp. 383–402). Amherst: University of Massachusetts Press.
Bruijnzeel, A. W. (2017). Reward processing and smoking. *Nicotine & Tobacco Research, 19*(6), 661–662. https://doi.org/10.1093/ntr/ntw303
Cohn, S. (2014). From health behaviours to health practices: An introduction. *Sociology of Health & Illness, 36*(2), 157–162. https://doi.org/10.1111/1467-9566.12140
Courtwright, D. T. (2005). Mr. ATOD's wild ride: What do alcohol, tobacco, and other drugs have in common? *The Social History of Alcohol and Drugs, 20*(1), 105–124. https://doi.org/10.1086/SHAD20010105
Dennis, S. (2011). Smoking causes creative responses: On state antismoking policy and resilient habits. *Critical Public Health, 21*(1), 25–35. https://doi.org/10.1080/09581596.2010.529420
DiFranza, J. R. (2008). Hooked from the first cigarette. *Scientific American, 298*(5), 82–87.
Duff, C. (2007). Towards a theory of drug use contexts: Space, embodiment and practice. *Addiction Research & Theory, 15*(5), 503–519. https://doi.org/10.1080/16066350601165448
Dyer, O. (2019). FDA considers regulatory action as vaping among US teens jumps 78% in a year. *BMJ, 364*, l741. https://doi.org/10.1136/bmj.l741
Eldred-Grigg, S. (1984). *Pleasures of the flesh: Sex & drugs in colonial New Zealand, 1840–1915*. Reed: Wellington, NZ.
Farsalinos, K. E., Romagna, G., Tsiapras, D., Kyrzopoulos, S., & Voudris, V. (2014). Characteristics, perceived side effects and benefits of electronic cigarette use. *International Journal of Environmental Research and Public Health, 11*(4), 4356–4373. https://doi.org/10.3390/ijerph110404356
Goodman, J. (1993). *Tobacco in history: The cultures of dependence*. London: Routledge.
Gupta, S., Gandhi, A., & Manikonda, R. (2014). Accidental nicotine liquid ingestion: Emerging paediatric problem. *Archives of Disease in Childhood, 99*, 1149. https://doi.org/10.1136/archdischild-2014-306750
Huang, J., Duan, Z., Kwok, J., Binns, S., Vera, L. E., Kim, Y., … Emery, S. L. (2019). Vaping versus JUULing: How the extraordinary growth and marketing of JUUL transformed the US retail e-cigarette market. *Tobacco Control, 28*(2), 146–151. https://doi.org/10.1136/tobaccocontrol-2018-054382
Hughes, J. (2003). *Learning to smoke: Tobacco use in the West*. Chicago: Chicago University Press.

Hughes, J. R. (2012). Nicotine don't get no respect: A replication test. *Nicotine & Tobacco Research, 15*(2), 588–590. https://doi.org/10.1093/ntr/nts154
Hunt, G., & Frank, V. (2017). Reflecting on intoxication. In T. Kolind, B. Thom, & G. Hunt (Eds.), *The Sage handbook for drug and alcohol studies* (pp. 322–336). London: Sage.
Julien, R. (2013). *A primer of drug action: A concise nontechnical guide to the actions, uses, and side effects of psychoactive drugs* (Revised and updated ed.). New York: Holt Paperbacks.
Kavuluru, R., Han, S., & Hahn, E. J. (2018). On the popularity of the USB flash drive-shaped electronic cigarette Juul. *Tobacco Control, 28*, 110–112. https://doi.org/10.1136/tobaccocontrol-2018-054259
Keane, H. (2002). Smoking, addiction and the making of time. In J. F. Brodie & M. Redfield (Eds.), *High anxieties: Cultural studies in addiction* (pp. 119–133). Berkeley: University of California Press.
Keane, H. (2009). Intoxication, harm and pleasure: An analysis of the Australian National Alcohol Strategy. *Critical Public Health, 19*(2), 135–142. https://doi.org/10.1080/09581590802350957
Keane, H., Weier, M., Fraser, D., & Gartner, C. (2017). 'Anytime, anywhere': Vaping as social practice. *Critical Public Health, 27*(4), 465–476. https://doi.org/10.1080/09581596.2016.1250867
Koval, R., Willett, J., & Briggs, J. (2018). Potential benefits and risks of high-nicotine e-cigarettes. *JAMA, 320*(14), 1429–1430. https://doi.org/10.1001/jama.2018.12328
Lucherini, M., Rooke, C., & Amos, A. (2018). E-cigarettes, vaping and performativity in the context of tobacco denormalisation. *Sociology of Health & Illness, 40*(6), 1037–1052. https://doi.org/10.1111/1467-9566.12741
McQuoid, J., Keamy-Minor, E., & Ling, P. M. (2018). A practice theory approach to understanding poly-tobacco use in the United States. *Critical Public Health*, 1–16. https://doi.org/10.1080/09581596.2018.1541226
Moore, D. (1993). Beyond Zinberg's 'social setting': A processural view of illicit drug use. *Drug and Alcohol Review, 12*(4), 413–421.
National Institute on Drug Abuse. (2018). *Tobacco, nicotine, and e-cigarettes.* Retrieved from https://www.drugabuse.gov/publications/research-reports/tobacco-nicotine-e-cigarettes
National Native Network. (n.d.). *Traditional tobacco.* Retrieved from http://keepitsacred.itcmi.org/tobacco-and-tradition/traditional-tobacco-use/
Nichter, M., Nichter, M., Carkoglu, A., Lloyd-Richardson, E., & Tobacco Etiology Research Network. (2010). Smoking and drinking among college

students: "It's a package deal". *Drug and Alcohol Dependence, 106*(1), 16–20. https://doi.org/10.1016/j.drugalcdep.2009.07.025

Palmer, K. J., Buckley, M. M., & Faulds, D. (1992). Transdermal nicotine. *Drugs, 44*(3), 498–529. https://doi.org/10.2165/00003495-199244030-00011

Pantzar, M., & Shove, E. (2010). Understanding innovation in practice: A discussion of the production and re-production of Nordic walking. *Technology Analysis & Strategic Management, 22*(4), 447–461. https://doi.org/10.1080/09537321003714402

Piasecki, T. M., Jahng, S., Wood, P. K., Robertson, B. M., Epler, A. J., Cronk, N. J., … Sher, K. J. (2011). The subjective effects of alcohol–tobacco co-use: An ecological momentary assessment investigation. *Journal of Abnormal Psychology, 120*(3), 557. https://doi.org/10.1037/a0023033

Piasecki, T. M., Wood, P. K., Shiffman, S., Sher, K. J., & Heath, A. C. (2012). Responses to alcohol and cigarette use during ecologically assessed drinking episodes. *Psychopharmacology, 223*(3), 331–344. https://doi.org/10.1007/s00213-012-2721-1

Raising Teens Today. (2018). JUUL 101: What every parent should know. *Raising Teens Today*. Retrieved from https://raisingteenstoday.com/juul-101-what-every-parent-should-know/

Ramamurthi, D., Chau, C., & Jackler, R. K. (2018). JUUL and other stealth vaporisers: Hiding the habit from parents and teachers. *Tobacco Control*, [epub ahead of print: 13/3/2019]. https://doi.org/10.1136/tobaccocontrol-2018-054455

Reckwitz, A. (2002). Toward a theory of social practices. *European Journal of Social Theory, 5*(2), 243–263. https://doi.org/10.1177/13684310222225432

Rose, J. E., Brauer, L. H., Behm, F. M., Cramblett, M., Calkins, K., & Lawhon, D. (2004). Psychopharmacological interactions between nicotine and ethanol. *Nicotine & Tobacco Research, 6*(1), 133–144. https://doi.org/10.1080/14622200310001656957

Royal College of Physicians. (2016). *Nicotine without smoke: Tobacco harm reduction*. London: RPC.

Schatzki, T. R. (2002). *The site of the social: A philosophical account of the constitution of social life and change*. University Park, PA: Penn State University Press.

Shove, E., Pantzar, M., & Watson, M. (2012). *The dynamics of social practice: Everyday life and how it changes*. London: Sage.

Stebbins, R. A. (1982). Serious leisure: A conceptual statement. *Pacific Sociological Review, 25*(2), 251–272.

Towns, C. (2011). *Habits that handicap: The menace of opium, alcohol and tobacco, and the remedy*. Urbana: Project Gutenberg. Retrieved from http://www.gutenberg.org/ebooks/35270

US Department of Health and Human Services. (2019). *Surgeon general's advisory on e-cigarette use among youth*. Retrieved from https://e-cigarettes.surgeongeneral.gov/documents/surgeon-generals-advisory-on-e-cigarette-use-among-youth-2018.pdf

US Department of Health and Human Services. (1988). *The health consequences of smoking: Nicotine addiction: A report of the surgeon general*. Rockville: US Department of Health and Human Services.

Usborne, S. (2018, June 9). Squonkers, drippers and cloud chasers: The rise of vape culture. *The Guardian*. Retrieved from https://www.theguardian.com/society/2018/jun/09/vape-culture-squonkers-drippers-cloud-chasers-simon-usborne

Wagener, T., Shaikh, R., Meier, E., Tackett, A., Tahirkheli, N., Leavens, E., & Driskill, L. (2016). Examining the smoking and vaping behaviors and preferences of vape shop customers. *Tobacco Prevention & Cessation, 2*(Supplement, 5), 1–7. https://doi.org/10.18332/tpc/65150

Wilbert, J. (1991). Does pharmacology corroborate the nicotine therapy and practices of South American shamanism? *Journal of Ethnopharmacology, 32*(1–3), 179–186.

Will, C. M., & Weiner, K. (2014). Sustained multiplicity in everyday cholesterol reduction: Repertoires and practices in talk about 'healthy living'. *Sociology of Health & Illness, 36*(2), 291–304. https://doi.org/10.1111/1467-9566.12070

Willett, J. G., Bennett, M., Hair, E. C., Xiao, H., Greenberg, M. S., Harvey, E., … Vallone, D. (2019). Recognition, use and perceptions of JUUL among youth and young adults. *Tobacco Control, 28*(1), 115–116. https://doi.org/10.1136/tobaccocontrol-2018-054273

Zaleski, O. (2018, November 13). Juul suspends sales of most flavoured products. *Time*. Retrieved from http://time.com/5453589/juul-curbing-flavored-nicotine-social-media/

Zhu, S.-H., Sun, J. Y., Bonnevie, E., Cummins, S. E., Gamst, A., Yin, L., & Lee, M. (2014). Four hundred and sixty brands of e-cigarettes and counting: Implications for product regulation. *Tobacco Control, 23*(suppl 3), iii3–iii9. https://doi.org/10.1136/tobaccocontrol-2014-051670

Zinberg, N. E. (1984). *Drug, set, and setting: The basis for controlled intoxicant use*. New Haven: Yale University Press.

4

Illicit Drugs and Intoxication

Angus Bancroft

The Historical Emergence and Evolution of Illicit Intoxication

The illicit is a structural factor which looms large in what Duff (2011, p. 149) called intoxication's *enabling place* and Zinberg (1984) it's setting. The illicit is part of the fabric of intoxication, in prisons, in courtrooms, in pubs, clubs, underpasses, streets and private homes, criminalising some intoxications, legitimising others, and also generating entanglements, subjectivities and experiences (Dennis, 2016). The illicit is present in the difference between prescribed, legitimised diamorphine and illicit heroin, between a clinic and a shooting gallery. The illicit is often presented in binary terms. There are illicit drugs and, then, there is everything else. What there is in practice is an overlapping set of regulations and controls which criminalise some intoxication methods and contexts and legitimate others. Illicit drugs as a category is a historical formation

A. Bancroft (✉)
School of Social and Political Science, University of Edinburgh, Edinburgh, UK
e-mail: angus.bancroft@ed.ac.uk

F. Hutton (ed.), *Cultures of Intoxication*,
https://doi.org/10.1007/978-3-030-35284-4_4

that coalesced from a range of different developments that restricted specific drugs and drug users. Starting in the late nineteenth century and early twentieth century, drugs such as opium, cannabis and cocaine began to be governed by law in response to specific public problems in places such as British controlled India (Mills, 2014).

The emergence of global drug control took shape in the early twentieth century at the prompting of the US government (Bewley-Taylor, 2002). Since then, prohibition has been primarily characterised as a US-led policy. While the history of drug control is often seen as the global centre working outwards, the periphery is producing new innovations in drug control or in decriminalisation. For example, the recent securitisation and punitive repression of opiates by some South East Asian governments is seen by them as central to their modernisation and development, while others lead in harm reduction. Repression of opium trafficking and use is framed in terms of a concern for population disorder, fear of being left behind globally, and also racial-national chauvinism (Windle, 2018). So in contrast to the unifying image present in the regime of global drug control, there is a patchwork of varied legal and socially acceptable status for different drugs (Pardo, 2014). Cannabis is legal in Uruguay and Canada, but possession will incur severe legal and social penalties in Sweden and China. Social acceptability and legal status can be reversed. The continental African drug crop is dominated by khat which is legal in some countries but has a dubious social status throughout the countries where it used. On the other hand, cannabis is illegal throughout the continent, but is ubiquitous and therefore has a quasi-legal status (Carrier & Klantschnig, 2017).

As well as more variety in legal controls of drugs, and the grey zone of quasi-legality, the regulation of illicit drugs is more and more a hybrid between public and private, criminal and regulatory and punitive and reformatory. Schools and employers run drug tests and produce both sanctions and data to be fed into systems governed by other algorithms, combining with biometric and facial tracking and digital fingerprinting. Welfare sanctions can be used to control otherwise licit alcohol use or other aspects of behaviour that, while potentially a problem, are not illegal as such. There is a burgeoning set of regulatory modes governing intoxications that might technically be illicit, but that are not directly criminalised, or those that are licit but are subject to sanctioning outwith the process of law. We can understand this by thinking of the law as culturally formed and also having its own culture, but it is only one part of a broader regime that governs intoxication that includes elements unrelated to criminal justice.

An example is the growth of algorithmic governance. An algorithm is a set of instructions which respond to inputs and reach an outcome. Law itself is algorithmic, a set of conditions and instructions that defines rather than solve problems. Globally, societies are increasingly algorithmic, governed by digital and paper instructions, algorithms that are increasingly opaque, private and impenetrable and capable of encoding bias and dogma as unquestionable (Dourish, 2016). The crucial current development is the extent to which algorithms no longer govern individual selves, but rather people's datafied doppelgangers (Smith, Bennett Moses, & Chan, 2017). In considering how illicit intoxications can be understood in the algorithmic age, this discussion focuses on how many of their cultural functions are embedded in algorithms, in software or hardware. Drugs in a sense are themselves analogue algorithms, a set of chemical instructions for body and self, the hardware and software of intoxication. They operate in the same sense that camera film is an algorithm. The chemistry is set to respond to certain kinds of inputs designed in ways, responding differently to light and shade, skin tones and colours. Drugs have these designed in qualities, designed for particular bodies or averages of bodies, or psyches. Drugs embed expectations about pleasure, pain, risk and enhancement. Like algorithms, they are used to produce, interpret and confirm knowledge. Like algorithms, illicit drugs embed culturally mandated and legitimated desire.

Algorithmic Culture and Intoxication

I want to use the concept of algorithmic culture to understand how culture suffuses society and the illicit, from the digital to the economic, and from the illicit to the 'normal'. The concept of culture in relation to illicit drug use has often been used to talk about subcultures or youth cultures as in popular culture, dance culture, grime culture, or that of non-Western indigenous groups. Culture is in that sense 'doing something' to intoxication, producing it, refining it and confining it. However, there is a growing range of intoxication that is not encultured in this way, as can be seen in the spreading use of smart drugs and the effect of pharmaceuticalisation (Abraham, 2010). Illicit drug use cultures are not bounded by nation or formalised symbolic boundaries, but spread along global routes of commodification, trade and cultural exchange. Globally, societies are moving away from 'illicit' to hybrids of illicit means and legitimised ends. We should understand culture in a similar way, as a hybrid and a hybrid producing force that melds the physical, the social, the cultural and the psychological into one simple package. Intoxication is designed into drugs and drug use places, which increasingly are shared with and draw on licit leisure, treatment and employment patterns. Algorithmic culture is a way of governing this hybrid through a combination of technologies, norms and values, which frequently deny the possibility of a public, democratic regulatory regime.

As with digital algorithms, drugs are complex and not predetermined, and in a similar way, intoxication is produced but not determined by culture. They are intricate, rich lattices of objects, habits and sensory experiences out of and into which humans weave our symbolic, cultural, economic and social lives. They are chemical substances to which the ability to change the relationship between self and environment are attributed. They are powerful mediators of social life (MacAndrew and Edgerton, 1969). Among its algorithmic effects, intoxication changes or stabilises the relationship between world and self (Hunt & Frank, 2016). It does so in ways that are symbolic, cultural, psychological and material (Duff, 2014). Illicit drugs are deeply involved in psychoactive geographies and geographies of harm and suffering (Garmany, 2011).

The Work of Culture in the Context of the Illicit

A common perspective shared by many illicit drug users is the presentation of the drug as an agent: it is doing something to them. The viewpoint is shared both by sympathisers and those with an interest in portraying illicit drugs as alien, disease-like entities. However, drugs have to have work done to them before they can be consumed. Work refers to the activity that surrounds the drug and the user, which makes drug use palatable and desirable. From seeking out the substance, haggling, swapping or just posing at a bar to obtain it, practising holding smoke in one's lungs and injecting, these activities are shared, practical and symbolic. All users engage in these activities, all of them work on themselves and the drug they consume. This aspect of drug use is often submerged because it raises difficult questions about where the blame lies for drug problems. To what extent are drug problem produced by drugs, by users, by dealers and traffickers, by failures in social welfare and healthcare? Users are often blamed for their drug use and any problems associated with that use because they 'work' to use drugs but that is not all they do. Users also work at harm reduction and managing those problems, and may see their drug use as a necessity in managing personal trauma and some of the systemic consequences of social deprivation.

Intoxicants have a quality of in-betweenness. Culture does the work of legitimation and normalisation, and de-legitimation and stigmatisation. It can reconcile the desire for pleasure with the needs to display order and compliance (Pennay, 2012). The illicit context makes some of these functions much more salient. Shared cultural understandings are needed to communicate tainted knowledge and to manage economies of scarcity (Bourgois, 1998). Cultural competence and recognition are important in managing drug supply and consumption where those functions are not served by the formal governance system. Medical and treatment concepts attain coherence and stability through their repeated use and reproducing in knowledge generating systems. Are addiction, recovery, intoxication, pleasure and harm coherent concepts or are they quite contingent? What is their contingency built on? It is helpful to view them as concepts with historical and cultural stability, supported by socially validated systems such as the medical system, the legal system, institutions like psychiatry and addiction treatment, academic disciplines like sociology, pharmacology and so on. They act together to produce a stable ontology, reifying their logics and symbolic structures (Manderson, 1995; Seddon, 2016).

This stability and shared understanding of intoxication as a coherent process is mediated through ritual, a set of defined acts that are functional and meaningful (Collins, 2011). Consumption rituals are powerful signs indicating in/out group membership, and marking social time and space (Gusfield, 1987). The array of practices and knowledge around an intoxicant produce it as an affective object with characteristics that vary by time and place and are not solely dependent on its physical nature (Gomart, 2002). Almost all accounts of intoxication include a ritual aspect (Becker, 1953), but this perhaps reflects a research bias. By its nature, ritual is observable, describable and accountable, and the ethnographic methods used with drug users will tend to focus on ritual. Culture also manifests in cue reactivity, risk management and dose titration. These activities, which are vital to make intoxication effective, are part of embedded algorithms shared by users. They can be seen on internet message boards, discussion forums and in the unspoken learning that takes place when users gather. It is also symbolised in the covert information signalled through apps like Tinder and Grindr which are used for drug distribution (Moyle, Childs, Coomber, & Barratt, 2019).

These rituals also transform. Lévi-Strauss (1969) defined civilisation as the distinction between the raw and the cooked. Drugs are likewise cooked, transformed. The argot of heroin users has 'cooking up' as the process of preparing heroin for consumption. Cooking techniques vary depending on form (Strang, Griffiths, & Gossop, 1997). Brown heroin requires heat and acid, white heroin less heat and no acid. Cooking is, therefore, any transformation: from the preparation of heroin to mixing a cocktail—both are 'cooking' and transformative. 'Cooking' is defined here as the combination of preparation, memory and body work that goes into preparing intoxicants, producing intoxication experiences. Both the drug and the user's body are 'cooked' in this process, transformed and turned into a system for drug consumption. 'Cooking' transforms the user between two states: sobriety and intoxication.

Transition is a common feature of intoxication as transitions exist between multiple states. There are age transitions as part of the life course. The shamanic healing ritual and the rite of passage inducting an adolescent into adulthood. Both push the body of the subject of the ritual to its limits. Fly agaric, tobacco, *Spondylus* shellfish and *ayahusca* and other substances with hallucinogenic potential may be employed (Dobkin de Rios, 2009; Glowacki, 2005). The subject goes through death and rebirth, visits the spirit world and returns with his/her status changed permanently. The process of transforming the self necessitates looking inward while also dissolving the distinction between inward and outward. The value of intoxication is in making the users become more what they are, or should be; or getting away from themselves, or taking themselves out of the self. Transitional rituals are about inducting adolescents into culture, into society. The transformational drinking that goes on in Western adulthood is justified in terms of stripping away socialisation, getting one out of one's 'stuck in a rut' adult habits (Hayward & Hobbs, 2007).

The process of transformation involves evoking multiple cues. Cue reactivity has been examined as an automatic response that is often activated by ritual cues or elements of ritualised practice. Cues are the tastes, sights, interactions and actions that have attached to conditioned associations with drug use in the mind of the user. In the case of largely recreational users and examples of use in recreational contexts, cues are built up as part of the process of drug associated learning. Cue reactivity studies foreground exteroceptive inputs such as images, smells, tastes and textures. Cues can also involve familiar conversational terms, money, paraphernalia and other co-occurring associations (Drummond, 2000). In terms of more problematic use of alcohol and other drugs, users may show both aversive and appetitive responses to the introduction of familiar intoxicant related cues (Rodríguez, Fernández, Cepeda-Benito, & Vila, 2005). Cues are recursive. Users become skilled in generating these kinds of effects along with making the substance itself a usable drug through ritualised practices such as preparation and sharing. Cue reactivity is a process that provides an element of somatic feedback in ritual practice and intoxication. The somatic feedback element is a mediator of sensual practice, exploring the combination of preparation, sequence, setting, expectation and working on the body that produces a desired, or sometimes unwanted, outcome. We also consume each other. In some settings, such as nightclubs, the presence of others is part of the setting to be consumed, intentionally developing a collective emotionality. In the experience economy, these settings are closely managed in order to contribute to a commodified intoxication experience.

In my research with student illicit drug users, rituals focused much more on the preparation of the drug, and skill was demonstrated through confident, competent processing of the drug into a state fit to be consumed (Bancroft, 2019). This ethnographic journal recorded by one participant describes the careful, sensory experience of producing a cannabis joint to be shared:

> My skin tingles a little at the crisp sound of the two cigarette papers I lick and stick together, this is followed by a third paper delicately placed in the middle overlapping the other two. I open the cigarette in my hand with one smooth sweeping lick and empty a good part of its contents into the cradled papers. I unwrap the cellophane from the hard brown block resting next to my papers. The smell of earth and wood is singed with my lighter, crumbled between my fingers spread evenly into the joint. I roll the package between my thumb and forefinger. I start from the middle and gradually work my way to the end applying the suited amount of pressure, satisfied I lick the papers together and place a custom made piece of cardboard 'roach' into one end and twist the other. ('Lara' cited in Bancroft, 2019, p. 140)

The satisfaction described by 'Lara' comes from the delicate and precise preparation. Part of the anticipation, represented by her skin tingling, is heightened in the sensory experiences she describes: the sound of cigarette papers rustling, the texture of hash[1] burnt and crumbled between her fingers and the wholesome smell given off by singeing it. Rituals like that depend on cues for their effect. Rituals carefully parse out and employ cue reactivity.

Ritual is also present at other aspects of the illicit intoxication. The process of policing and punishment is partly ritualised, with police and drug dealers playing their roles, engaging in expected denunciations, appeals to rehabilitation and performances of suffering and penitence. Criminalisation creates material realities of surveillance, opacity and punishment. Prison is a site of drug use and exchange (Fleetwood, 2009), as are illicit consumption sites which involve a material culture of harm and harm reduction (Parkin, 2013). Diagnosis of substance addiction also has its ritual element when it links generalised diagnostic categories of addiction, infection and overdose to the specific case of each user (Rosenberg, 2002). The disease entity of addicted intoxication is made culturally recognisable and inscribed in the body of the user in that moment of clinical diagnosis. Settings like hospitals and rehabs clinics function as reinventive institutions (Scott, 2010). Rather than having the self-mortified, as in the total institutions, the client gives up their pre-institutional self voluntarily.

Most of these activities are or soon will be mediated through algorithms. Lara's representation of her joint rolling prowess, the app where she bought the drug, the process of crime detection and adjudication and medical diagnosis and treatment take place in an algorithmically and culturally informed environment.

Ritualised Intoxication in the 'Machine Zone'

A part of algorithmic culture is the zone aspect, a place which creates separation from everyday rhythms, networks and places. Schüll (2012) identifies 'the machine zone' in her study of gambling machines in Las Vegas. The zone is where the players enjoy total focus as they sit in front of the screen and interact with the machine. They play in front of gaming machines that by proxy deliver jolts of dopamine, and the setting is designed to focus attention through a combination of tactile and sensory design which obliterates the periphery and speeds up play. The machines and the environment are carefully designed to maximise 'Time on Device', their metric of value—a devilish bargain the players willingly sign up for. The player is atomised, focused on the interaction with the machine and sophisticated data input and algorithmically informed design is used to keep them there.

Some kinds of drug use can also be described in this way, as can the sites of licit drug use such as superpubs and some nightclubs that are designed to create a separate zone away from the mundane habits of regular life. That aspects of intoxication reflects its rooting in culture and nature (Dennis & Farrugia, 2017), which gives it its partly involuntary feel. This involuntary element, the sense of being swept along, of having the body respond separately from the mind to stimulant cues, is what makes it so potent. Each form of intoxication is a material culture. Intoxication experiences are systematised and designed into environments. The historically novel binge drinking cultures of the 1990s and early 2000s in the UK were a product of the creation of new alcohol commodities and spaces for consumption (Measham & Brain, 2016). Alcohol companies aligned themselves with local and national governments to drive changes in the law alongside product innovation to permit intense, focused consumption (Measham, 2004). These new modes of intoxication could be understood as a machine zone, a carefully constructed set of places where every aspect of the environment was tailored to maximise alcohol consumption. The sounds, the lighting, the carefully constructed interaction spaces, came together to push that zone of intense alcoholic sociality. That was a machine zone of alcoholic intoxication. Illicit intoxication has been both a rider on those processes and an escape from them.

There are striking similarities between the machine zone and student smart drug users, who report similar focusing effects when taking modafinil. Modafinil was introduced as a treatment for the sleep disorder narcolepsy and is one of a set of smart drugs or study drugs that are popular among university students in North America and Europe. The drugs are taken to improve memory, recall and task salience (Jensen, Forlini, Partridge, & Hall, 2016). Students taking modafinil experience a simplifying, satisfying task salience in which they focus wholly on what is in front of them, whether exam cramming, reading or writing. There is a deep delight in separating oneself so wholly from other stimulation. As with most intoxications, the benefit is also a risk. Gamblers and study drug users forget to eat, drink, interact with friends and have to carefully plan to remind themselves to do these things. Pharmaceutical companies produce a new drug indicated for a specific condition such as anxiety, and immediately seek to expand the zone of its application to other conditions like dieting. Smart drug users are doing much the same and indeed a common illicit use of medical amphetamines is for weight reduction. The illicit can be seen as produced by the licit, for example, in demands to use smart drugs. Uber drivers, medical professionals, Amazon warehouse workers, cam girls, all face working requirements that are often fast paced and require them to be always 'on'. It is uncertain though, as to whether these drugs improve cognitive ability or just keep people on task or awake for longer (Arria et al., 2013; Lucke, Bell, Partridge, & Hall, 2011). The pursuit of machine-like intoxication then reflects how power is distributed in society.

Symbolic Order and Power

The focus on algorithms is often taken to mean that these systems are automated and invisible; however, we should not lose sight of the role of the symbolic and of power in shaping how people respond to illicit intoxications. One function of intoxicants is their role in classification of objects and experiences into a symbolic order that divides the sacred from the profane. They are powerful mediators of social structure. Power and resources come to the fore when managing a marginal existence. In situations of structural violence, adaption and survival are managed and negotiated (Haritavorn, 2014; Netherland & Hansen, 2016).

The information served up to users through digital devices is algorithmically determined, in ways that are not frequently legible. This is something new to us as researchers. We have relied on culture to make behaviours and experiences legible, or impenetrably illegible through mythic statements, origin stories and journey narratives that circulate and are shared in user cultures. One narrative is that of recovery from addiction. Drug users perform legibility, for example, when users proclaim that they are competent subjects because they bleach their injection works (Campbell & Shaw, 2008). Users show to the researcher what they know to be a legible cultural performance directed at outside ethnographers, law enforcement, therapists or public health workers. In doing so, they make themselves partially legible. That action is also a strategic one and may hide other equally significant motives such as using drugs for pleasure which is hidden by the dominant cultural narrative of the desireless addict (Dennis, 2017). Treatment programmes have their own cultural norms and performances which make the user legible and 'worthy', as a drug user who uses without pleasure and wishes to reassert their agency over the drug. Initial studies treated drug users' gratification as unintegrated and antisocial (Robbins, 1969). As with drug buying and the cultural representation of drug consumption, that work is migrating to algorithms and algorithmic processes. In the medical sphere, this presents challenges to expert authority which is increasingly embedded in software and hardware devices. This can be an opportunity to use data generating, connected devices to identify dependent patterns of use, but also can lead to the diffusion and denial of responsibility for treatment.

Cultural Mediation of Knowledge

A crucial part of sharing cultural understandings about intoxication is the value and quality of the drug itself, although the make-up of chemical potency is subjective. This is culturally mediated. We might expect in an informationalised world that knowledge about drug content and formulae is ever more precise. However, research with darknet drug markets has shown the opposite (Bancroft & Scott Reid, 2016). Chemical knowledge about drugs has to be understood in a cultural framework. This is a counterpoint to the idea that society is becoming ever more governed by informationalised algorithms. Even where these are in play, culturally mediated understandings of how to interpret and make use of knowledge about drugs must be employed to make sense of them. Algorithms are entangled with culture.

For example, higher pharmacological strength does not necessarily mean a 'better' or 'stronger' effect for the user. Street heroin is often cut with additives, to enhance the pharmacokinetics and the psychoactive experience, such as caffeine, theophylline and procaine. For that reason, a less chemically pure dose may be experienced as much more effectively 'potent' or desirable. Heroin is engineered for different regional markets and by new players in the market (Furst, 2000), and in relation to experiences of intoxication this quality of embedding culturally shared expectations of what the 'right kind' of heroin is becomes important. There are various other physical features and attributes of the substance (name, brand, colour, texture, taste, viscosity) that may or may not have an effect on the user's experience of intoxication. Each of these supposedly objective, separable physical qualities merge with each other. They are created and modified by various factors. In some cases, in response to clinical need, in others marketing, taxation, regulation and surveillance. This was observed this when analysing how cryptomarket drug vendors showed how their business model produced value (see Bancroft, 2019; Barratt and Aldridge, 2016). Some were keen to demonstrate that their business model had instrumental rational value, in the form of economic profitability and sustainability. In contrast, others sought to show the cultural value to their work. A group of cannabis vendors was especially adamant on this point and sought to differentiate both their operations and their product from commercial operations. This quote captured how the instrumental value of their business model had to be demonstrated by educating others about what made for a 'good' drug:

> There is a persistent myth about the trade which is that your top notch weed is dank, fat, thick smelling crystal covered nugs. It isn't a coincidence. Dealers, big commercial growers, seedbanks and breeders keep this myth alive. Commercial farmers who trade in large volumes. We are more like an artisan collective. Our aim is making the best product not the most money. There is vast and deep gulf between commercial indicas which grow rapidly and sativas. Commercial growers use indica because it will grow quickly and they push that as defining what is high quality. Vendor 'HomieGrown'. (Cited in Bancroft, 2019 p. 95)

In this case, what might be expected to be a prime selling point, the chemical potency of high strength cannabis, is viewed as a cheap trick exploited by commercial growers. The seller wants to establish the cultural, rather than chemical, superiority of his or her product. In that example, we see a conflict about motivation and value and whether commercialised growing of illicit cannabis has a lower status than the more ideologically motivated kind of grower (Ancrum & Treadwell, 2017). This process is about power and status. More culturally validated kinds of cannabis growing might be less commercially profitable but have much better recognition and status within the growing and using communities. Better connected criminal groups can negotiate and operate larger, more profitable enterprises, and command more labour. They grow a more homogenised, often more potent, product. Boutique outfits offer a different kind of intoxicant. Buyers from these sellers demonstrate their resistance to commercialisation of the drug, because they view commercialisation as taking away from the drug's cultural significance and worth so that the intoxication ritual loses its significance and meaning.

Looking for Culture in the Wrong Places

The material culture of intoxication is created within global flows, technoscapes and the residue of past efforts. There is no natural, herbal high here, untroubled by cultural norms, political economies and human meddling. Opium, cannabis and coca are all cultivars, plants bred to enhance their intoxicant qualities. Objects have the power of embodying all kinds of relationships and dispositions, of pleasure, pathology and recovery. They can delimit, though not dictate, the terms of their use. Intoxicants mediate such issues as social class (wine), gender (sugar) and savoir-faire (absinthe). In the rhetoric of intoxication, each quality is constructed in relationship to others such that the sweetness of sugar only exists in relation to the bitterness, acidity, saltiness, sourness and umami of other substances. Material culture reproduces and affirms these social relationships which become, in part, relationships between objects. The complex back-and-forth between the drug, its cultural signification and material context of production and consumption constantly regenerates the materiality of intoxication within an algorithmic culture.

This back-and-forth, culturally mediated process happens with scientific knowledge as well. The category of the illicit has had an impact on scientific knowledge, and, in particular, has tended to reduce knowledge about illicit intoxication to the behaviour selected samples of users in treatment or otherwise performing as chaotic, unstable and un-functional (Decorte, 2011). Academic research has its cultures and priorities, and while research showing controlled illicit drug use is likely much more common than chaotic or addictive use, that does not endear academics to governments (Stevens, 2007). A part of the culture of illicit intoxication is, therefore, the cultures of civil service departments, lecturers and researchers who act as gatekeepers to knowledge about the illicit and who give that knowledge force and structure. While users of different drugs share knowledge, academic tribes are quite culturally homogenous and tightly bounded (Becher & Trowler, 2001). They maintain their shared ideology through rituals of reproduction at conferences, in meetings and in academic journals and through in-group terminology (Collins, 2004). Like drug users, academics share folk tales and war stories. Academics are also made up through algorithms where the power of the performance metric and citations core grows stronger each passing year.

The concept of culture has to be adapted. There has sometimes been a background assumption that much contemporary illicit drug use such as smart drug use and the use of recreational drugs bought over the internet lead to de-cultured drug use, without the rich folklore of the urban righteous dope fiend (Agar, 1971). However, research has tended to focus on the public, the street junkie and the male when looking for culture. There, we look for culture in flamboyant performance. The domestic, the private and the female were missing or subordinate in the history of subcultural research on drug users, until this was recognised in the pioneering work of feminist scholars such as Taylor (1993). Culture is just as much a part of these places however, and in relatively atomised and instrumental uses of drugs. What there is less of is a sense of drug using culture as a separate set of spaces and values with its own demographic, performances and symbols. In that sense, the validation of illicit intoxication culture is going to be needed, an approach that traces it throughout different spaces, both digital and material.

Note

1. Hash, short for hashish, is a solid preparation of cannabis. Burning the hash generates a distinctive smell that indicates its quality and makes it easier to crumble into a joint.

References

Abraham, J. (2010). Pharmaceuticalization of society in context: Theoretical, empirical and health dimensions. *Sociology, 44*(4), 603–622. https://doi.org/10.1177/0038038510369368

Agar, M. H. (1971). Folklore of the heroin addict: Two examples. *The Journal of American Folklore, 84*(332), 175–185. https://doi.org/10.2307/538988

Ancrum, C., & Treadwell, J. (2017). Beyond ghosts, gangs and good sorts: Commercial cannabis cultivation and illicit enterprise in England's disadvantaged inner cities. *Crime, Media, Culture, 13*(1), 69–84. https://doi.org/10.1177/1741659016646414

Arria, A. M., Wilcox, H. C., Caldeira, K. M., Vincent, K. B., Garnier-Dykstra, L. M., & O'Grady, K. E. (2013). Dispelling the myth of "smart drugs": Cannabis and alcohol use problems predict nonmedical use of prescription stimulants for studying. *Addictive Behaviors, 38*(3), 1643–1650. https://doi.org/10.1016/j.addbeh.2012.10.002

Bancroft, A. (2019). *The Darknet and Smarter Crime: Methods for Investigating Criminal Entrepreneurs and the Illicit Drug Economy*. Basingstoke: Palgrave Macmillan.

Bancroft, A., & Scott Reid, P. (2016). Concepts of illicit drug quality among darknet market users: Purity, embodied experience, craft and chemical knowledge. *International Journal of Drug Policy, 35*, 42–49. https://doi.org/10.1016/j.drugpo.2015.11.008

Barratt, M. J., & Aldridge, J. (2016). Everything you always wanted to know about drug cryptomarkets* (*but were afraid to ask). *International Journal of Drug Policy, 35*, 1–6. https://doi.org/10.1016/j.drugpo.2016.07.005

Becher, A., & Trowler, P. R. (2001). *Academic tribes and territories*. McGraw-Hill Education (UK).

Becker, H. S. (1953). Becoming a marihuana user. *American Journal of Sociology, 59*(3), 235–242.

Bewley-Taylor, D. R. (2002). *United States and international drug control, 1909–1997*. A&C Black.

Bourgois, P. (1998). The moral economies of homeless heroin addicts: Confronting ethnography, HIV risk, and everyday violence in San Francisco shooting encampments. *Substance Use & Misuse, 33*(11), 2323–2351. https://doi.org/10.3109/10826089809056260

Campbell, N. D., & Shaw, S. J. (2008). Incitements to discourse: Illicit drugs, harm reduction, and the production of ethnographic subjects. *Cultural Anthropology, 23*(4), 688–717.

Carrier, N., & Klantschnig, G. (2017). Quasilegality: Khat, cannabis and Africa's drug laws. *Third World Quarterly, 39*(2), 1–16. https://doi.org/10.1080/01436597.2017.1368383

Collins, R. (2004). *Interaction ritual chains / Randall Collins*. Princeton, NJ and Oxford: Princeton University Press.

Collins, R. (2011). Drug consumption: A social ritual? The examples of tobacco and cocaine. In G. Hunt, M. Milhet, & H. Bergeron (Eds.), *Drugs and Culture*. Aldershot: Ashgate.

Decorte, T. (2011). Blinding ourselves with science: The chronic infections of our thinking on psychoactive substances. In G. Hunt, M. Milhet, & H. Bergeron (Eds.), *Drugs and culture. knowledge, consumption and policy* (pp. 33–51). Farnham: Ashgate.

Dennis, F. (2016). Encountering "Triggers": Drug–Body–World entanglements of injecting drug use. *Contemporary Drug Problems, 43*(2), 126–141. https://doi.org/10.1177/0091450916636379

Dennis, F. (2017). Conceiving of addicted pleasures: A 'modern' paradox. *International Journal of Drug Policy, 49*, 150–159. https://doi.org/10.1016/j.drugpo.2017.07.007

Dennis, F., & Farrugia, A. (2017). Materialising drugged pleasures: Practice, politics, care. *International Journal of Drug Policy, 49*, 86–91. https://doi.org/10.1016/j.drugpo.2017.10.001

Dobkin de Rios, M. (2009). *The Psychedelic Journey of Marlene Dobkin de Rios: 45 Years with Shamans, Ayahuasqueros, and Ethnobotanists*. Simon and Schuster.

Dourish, P. (2016). Algorithms and their others: Algorithmic culture in context. *Big Data & Society, 3*(2), 205395171666512. https://doi.org/10.1177/2053951716665128

Drummond, D. C. (2000). What does cue-reactivity have to offer clinical research? *Addiction, 95*(8s2), 129–144. https://doi.org/10.1046/j.1360-0443.95.8s2.2.x

Duff, C. (2011). Networks, resources and agencies: On the character and production of enabling places. *Health & Place, 17*(1), 149–156. https://doi.org/10.1016/j.healthplace.2010.09.012

Duff, C. (2014). The place and time of drugs. *International Journal of Drug Policy, 25*(3), 633–639. https://doi.org/10.1016/j.drugpo.2013.10.014

Fleetwood, J. S. (2009). *Emotional work: Ethnographic fieldwork in prisons in Ecuador*. Glasgow: University of Glasgow.

Furst, R. T. (2000). The re-engineering of heroin: An emerging heroin "cutting" trend in New York City. *Addiction Research, 8*(4), 357–379.

Garmany, J. (2011). Drugs, violence, fear, and death: The necro- and narco-geographies of contemporary urban space. *Urban Geography, 32*(8), 1148–1166. https://doi.org/10.2747/0272-3638.32.8.1148

Glowacki, M. (2005). Food of the Gods or mere mortals? Hallucinogenic Spondylus and its interpretive implications for early Andean society. *Antiquity; Cambridge*. Retrieved from http://search.proquest.com/docview/217576617/abstract/F9F7335C9A194196PQ/1

Gomart, E. (2002). Methadone: Six effects in search of a substance. *Social Studies of Science, 32*(1), 93–135.

Gusfield, J. R. (1987). Passage to play: Rituals of drinking time in American society. In M. Douglas (Ed.), *Constructive drinking: Perspectives on drink from anthropology* (pp. 73–90). Cambridge: Cambridge University Press.

Haritavorn, N. (2014). Surviving in two worlds: Social and structural violence of Thai female injecting drug users. *International Journal of Drug Policy, 25*(1), 116–123. https://doi.org/10.1016/j.drugpo.2013.09.008

Hayward, K., & Hobbs, D. (2007). Beyond the binge in 'booze Britain': Market-led liminalization and the spectacle of binge drinking. *The British Journal of Sociology, 58*(3), 437–456. https://doi.org/10.1111/j.1468-4446.2007.00159.x

Hunt, G., & Frank, V. A. (2016). Reflecting on intoxication. In T. Kolind, B. Thom, & G. Hunt (Eds.), *The Sage handbook of drug and alcohol studies*. London: Sage.

Jensen, C., Forlini, C., Partridge, B., & Hall, W. (2016). Australian university students' coping strategies and use of pharmaceutical stimulants as cognitive enhancers. *Frontiers in Psychology, 7*. https://doi.org/10.3389/fpsyg.2016.00277

Lévi-Strauss, C. (1969). *The raw and the cooked: Introduction to a science of mythology* (Vol. 1). New York: Harper & Row.

Lucke, J. C., Bell, S., Partridge, B., & Hall, W. D. (2011). Deflating the neuroenhancement bubble. *AJOB Neuroscience, 2*(4), 38–43. https://doi.org/10.1080/21507740.2011.611122

MacAndrew, C., & Edgerton, R. B. (1969). *Drunken comportment: A social explanation*. Cambridge: Percheron Press.

Manderson, D. (1995). Metamorphoses: Clashing symbols in the social construction of drugs. *Journal of Drug Issues, 25*(4), 799–816. https://doi.org/10.1177/002204269502500410

Measham, F. (2004). The decline of ecstasy, the rise of 'binge' drinking and the persistence of pleasure. *Probation Journal, 51*(4), 309–326.

Measham, F., & Brain, K. (2016). 'Binge' drinking, British alcohol policy and the new culture of intoxication. *Crime, Media, Culture: An International Journal 1*(3): 262–283.

Mills, J. H. (2014). Globalizing ganja: The British Empire and international cannabis traffic c.1834 to c.1939. In *Consuming Habits*. https://doi.org/10.4324/9780203964118-16

Moyle, L., Childs, A., Coomber, R., & Barratt, M. J. (2019). #Drugsforsale: An exploration of the use of social media and encrypted messaging apps to supply and access drugs. *International Journal of Drug Policy, 63*, 101–110. https://doi.org/10.1016/j.drugpo.2018.08.005

Netherland, J., & Hansen, H. B. (2016). The war on drugs that wasn't: Wasted whiteness, "Dirty Doctors," and race in media coverage of prescription opioid misuse. *Culture, Medicine, and Psychiatry, 40*(4), 664–686.

Pardo, B. (2014). Cannabis policy reforms in the Americas: A comparative analysis of Colorado, Washington, and Uruguay. *International Journal of Drug Policy, 25*(4), 727–735. https://doi.org/10.1016/j.drugpo.2014.05.010

Parkin, S. G. (2013). *Habitus and drug using environments: Health, place and lived-experience*. Retrieved from https://www.dawsonera.com/abstract/9781409464938

Pennay, A. (2012). Carnal pleasures and grotesque bodies: Regulating the body during a 'big night out' of alcohol and party drug use. *Contemporary Drug Problems; London, 39*(3), 397–428, 346.

Robbins, T. (1969). Eastern mysticism and the resocialization of drug users: The Meher Baba cult. *Journal for the Scientific Study of Religion, 8*, 308–317.

Rodríguez, S., Fernández, M. C., Cepeda-Benito, A., & Vila, J. (2005). Subjective and physiological reactivity to chocolate images in high and low chocolate cravers. *Biological Psychology, 70*(1), 9–18. https://doi.org/10.1016/j.biopsycho.2004.10.001

Rosenberg, C. E. (2002). The Tyranny of diagnosis: Specific entities and individual experience. *The Milbank Quarterly, 80*(2), 237–260. https://doi.org/10.1111/1468-0009.t01-1-00003

Schüll, N. D. (2012). *Addiction by design: Machine gambling in Las Vegas*. Princeton University Press.

Scott, S. (2010). Revisiting the total institution: Performative regulation in the reinventive institution. *Sociology, 44*(2), 213–231.

Seddon, T. (2016). Inventing drugs: A genealogy of a regulatory concept. *Journal of Law and Society, 43*(3), 393–415. https://doi.org/10.1111/j.1467-6478.2016.00760.x

Smith, G. J. D., Bennett Moses, L., & Chan, J. (2017). The challenges of doing criminology in the big data era: Towards a digital and data-driven approach. *The British Journal of Criminology, 57*(2), 259–274. https://doi.org/10.1093/bjc/azw096

Stevens, A. (2007). Survival of the Ideas that Fit: An Evolutionary Analogy for the Use of Evidence in Policy. *Social Policy and Society* *6*(1): 25–35.
Strang, J., Griffiths, P., & Gossop, M. (1997). Heroin in the United Kingdom: Different forms, different origins, and the relationship to different routes of administration. *Drug and Alcohol Review, 16*(4), 329–337.
Taylor, A. (1993). *Women drug users: An ethnography of a female injecting community*. Oxford: Clarendon Press.
Windle, J. (2018). Why do South-east Asian states choose to suppress opium? A cross-case comparison. *Third World Quarterly, 39*(2), 366–384. https://doi.org/10.1080/01436597.2017.1376582
Zinberg, N. E. (1984). *Drug, set and setting: The basis for controlled intoxicant use*. New Haven, CT: Yale University Press.

5

Cultures of Intoxication: 'New' Psychoactive Substances

Fiona Hutton

Introduction

In recent years, drug-using repertoires have expanded to include intoxication via new psychoactive substances (NPS). The market for NPS such as BZP-based party pills (BZP-PPs[1]), mephedrone (Meow) and synthetic cannabis (Spice) has developed rapidly over the last decade or so in several westernised nations, alongside legislation to try and control the harms related to the use of these 'new' substances. Media discourse in relation to NPS such as mephedrone[2] has exaggerated both the extent of their use as well as their dangers with sensationalised reporting such as 'Legal drug teen ripped his scrotum off'[3] (Alexandrescu, 2014, p. 23). These dangers were noted by many as inflated with most NPS posing a low risk of harm to users (Chatwin, 2017). However, the landscape of NPS has changed somewhat since approximately 2016, with an increase

F. Hutton (✉)
School of Social and Cultural Studies, Institute of Criminology, Victoria University, Wellington, New Zealand
e-mail: fiona.hutton@vuw.ac.nz

F. Hutton (ed.), *Cultures of Intoxication*,
https://doi.org/10.1007/978-3-030-35284-4_5

in the potency and availability of NPS. Importantly, the demographics of users of NPS have also changed quite dramatically adding to the intensity of debates about 'Spice' (synthetic cannabis) in particular (Alexandrescu, 2019).

The issues surrounding NPS have become a global phenomenon, at least within westernised nations. In the US and Australia, as well as in New Zealand and the UK, NPS have become the focus of concerns about intoxication. In the US, these concerns have centred on use amongst high school seniors, with this group perceiving that synthetic cannabis (SC) and other synthetic drugs were less risky to use than illegal alternatives such as cannabis and ecstasy (Maxwell, 2014). Although there has been a recent reduction in SC use in the US context from 11.4% of high school leavers in 2011 to 5.2% in 2015, reported poisonings in the US have dramatically increased from 2668 in 2013 to 7779 in 2015 (Palamar & Barratt, 2016). This is despite the fact that NPS have been illegal in the US since 2012. Australian studies have found that although national prevalence is often low, there is increased use of NPS amongst high risk groups (Sutherland et al., 2016). Several Australian states banned the use of specific synthetic cannabinoids in 2011, in a flurry of legislation amid media hysteria, and in July 2011 eight cannabis agonists were made illegal, their possession being made a federal offence (Bright, Bishop, Kane, Marsh, & Barratt, 2013). The 2011 Global Drug Survey (GDS) conducted across several countries with 15,200 respondents found 16.8% of respondents had ever used SC, with 40.6% of these being used in the last 12 months (Winstock & Barratt, 2013). However, GDS respondents preferred natural cannabis over SC, with those expressing a preference for SC being in a minority. Despite this preference for natural cannabis, SC use continues for a number of reasons: avoiding detection in drug tests, for example, is often cited as a reason for using SC (Barratt, Cakic, & Lenton, 2013; Berry-Caban, Kleinschmidt, Rao, & Jenkins, 2012; Palamar & Barratt, 2016; Perrone, Helgesen, & Fischer, 2013; Winstock & Barratt, 2013), with availability and legal status also making SC and NPS attractive to users (Barratt et al., 2013). Although concerns about NPS have surfaced in several countries globally, the experiences in New Zealand are somewhat unique, both in terms of problems with, and legislative responses to, NPS. Therefore, the main focus of this chapter will be New Zealand, with other global experiences considered alongside this particular social and cultural setting, enabling a consideration of the impacts of NPS intoxication in the global context.

This chapter will focus on how shifts in the popularity of NPS, as well as who is using them, have meaning in terms of how intoxication is enacted, viewed and responded to. For example, what have the developments in the market for NPS meant in terms of intoxication? How are NPS related to intoxication in contemporary societies? Following the definition of intoxication in Chap. 1, for the purposes of this chapter, intoxication is defined as using a legal or illegal drug to alter one's state of consciousness, in order to change the way a person interacts with the world. Intoxication is also constructed here as having a purpose, for example, to have fun, to socialise or to ease trauma. In this chapter, it will be argued that the way intoxication via NPS is enacted in contemporary societies has become associated with specific social groups. Additionally, NPS intoxication is noted as a fluid changing phenomenon, although responses to NPS as intoxicants often remain fixed and rooted in prohibitionist policies and legislation. As a starting point for this discussion, it is important to consider what NPS are and how they have been defined.

'New' psychoactive substances were being developed as far back as the 1970s, so technically they are not 'new', as the United Nations Office on Drugs and Crime (UNDOC) notes in their definition of NPS;

> The term 'new' does not necessarily refer to new inventions—several NPS were first synthesised 40 years ago—but to substances that have recently emerged on the market and which have not been scheduled under the above Conventions [referring to current drug laws e.g. Misuse of Drugs Act 1975 in New Zealand]. (UNDOC, 2013, p. 2 cited in Measham & Newcombe, 2016, p. 578)

Implied in the above quote is that what is 'new' about NPS are the social and cultural contexts in which they are often used, particularly the popularity of mephedrone and synthetic cannabinoids, both of which have become synonymous with the term NPS in recent years. The complexities involved in defining NPS are also often hampered by the large number of substances that come under this type of classification. The

European Monitoring Centre for Drugs and Drug Addiction (EMCDDA) (2018, p. 4) defines NPS as follows;

> A broad range of drugs that are not controlled by the 1961 and 1971 United Nations drug control conventions but may pose similar threats to public health. Many of them are traded as 'legal' replacements to established controlled drugs such as cannabis, heroin, cocaine and MDMA.

For the purposes of this chapter, NPS will be defined as a broad range of substances that are not controlled under the 1961 and 1971 United Nations drug control conventions, often traded as 'legal' replacements to established controlled drugs such as cannabis, heroin, cocaine and 3,4-methylenedioxy-methamphetamine (MDMA). They are 'new' in the sense that they have recently come under scrutiny and have become associated with particular populations and contexts of use (e.g. mephedrone in clubbing cultures), rather than actually being new inventions.

New Psychoactive Substances: Background and Development

NPS have been in circulation for a number of years. In New Zealand, they have been widely available since about 2000 (Hutton, 2017), and in other countries, they have been 'on the scene' since approximately 2008 (Measham, Moore, Newcombe, & Welch, 2010). NPS have been referred to by a variety of names, including 'legal highs', 'herbal highs', 'Spice' (referring to synthetic cannabinoids) and 'Meow' (referring to mephedrone). NPS refer to substances that are synthetically developed often with the intention to mimic the effects of drugs that are currently illegal, such as ecstasy, amphetamines and cannabis. The World Drug Report (2018) notes that 803 NPS were reported from 2009 to 2017, with 426 NPS on the market in 2016. The complexity and diversity of this market is problematic, and the large number of NPS available means that tracking who uses what is increasingly difficult. However, while there are a diverse and wide-ranging number of NPS available, the market for these substances remains smaller than that of established illegal drugs such as cannabis, amphetamines and heroin (Chatwin, 2017; World Drug Report, 2018). The 2017 Global Drug Survey found that lifetime use of cannabis was 77.8%, while lifetime use of synthetic cannabis was 5.8%. Similarly lifetime use of MDMA was 33.5% with lifetime use of mephedrone only 1.9% (Winstock, Barratt, Ferris & Maier, 2017).

The attraction of NPS is that, originally at least, they were not illegal, but provided similar effects to illicit drugs. They were also attractive in contexts where illegal drugs were hard to access, or were of poor quality, and for those groups of people who wanted to become intoxicated without breaking the law or necessarily drinking alcohol. In the UK, mephedrone rose rapidly in popularity amongst drug-experienced clubbing polydrug users, driven in part by the decline in purity of illegal drugs such as ecstasy and cocaine. Availability and user satisfaction with the effects of mephedrone in comparison to other illegal drugs like ecstasy also contributed to its popularity (Measham et al., 2010). For other groups, the attractiveness of moving to use NPS included factors such as the inability for some synthetic cannabinoids to be detected in drug tests (Perrone et al., 2013; Ralphs, Williams, Askew, & Norton, 2017) and the intense dissociative high that is sought by some users (EMCDDA, 2018).

Polydrug use is also often a feature of intoxication, with people who use drugs (PWUD) combining particular substances for maximum effect, or for a required effect such as using cannabis or other sedatives like Valium to come down from the busy high of ecstasy, amphetamine or cocaine use in clubbing contexts (Hutton, 2006). Therefore, polydrug use is not necessarily wholly concerned with intoxication or becoming intoxicated, it is also related to soothing intoxicated bodies and managing the effects of intoxication. Research in the Australian context also notes that users of NPS use a range of other illicit drugs (Sutherland et al., 2016), with New Zealand, UK and US research noting similar findings (Hutton, 2010; Measham et al., 2010; Palamar & Acosta, 2015; Wilkins, Parker, Prasad, & Jawalkar, 2016).

Therefore, for some groups, NPS are another way of intensifying or adding to intoxication, and these substances are related to the search for intoxication by a variety of groups in diverse social and cultural contexts. However, different user groups are attracted to NPS for a variety of reasons. Mephedrone, for example, emerged as an addition to the drug-using repertoires for polydrug-using clubbers, in some instances replacing '*shit quality drugs*' for drug-experienced users, who were seeking the pleasures and benefits of intoxication within the night time economy (NTE) (regular mephedrone user cited in Measham et al., 2010, p. 17). The UK government's response to mephedrone was to ban it in 2010 and make it a Class B drug, a decision based on 'disproportionate reporting exaggerating the risk and harms of mephedrone, both to users and to broader society' that 'caused knee-jerk political responses and fear in the community' (Greenslade 2010 cited in Lancaster, Hughes, Spicer, Matthew-Simmons, & Dillon, 2011, p. 2). Tabloid newspapers in the UK such as the *Daily Mail* mounted a vocal campaign to ban mephedrone although this 'only pushed the drug underground and made things even more complicated for users' (Alexandrescu, 2014, p. 34), who enthusiastically incorporated it into their polydrug-using practices. Such media and political responses also meant that the drug doubled in price (Moore, Dargan, Wood, & Measham, 2013 cited in Alexandrescu, 2014, p. 34). McElrath and O'Neill (2011) in the Northern Irish context also noted the possibility of increased risks to users after the ban on mephedrone in 2010, and that the ban appeared not to have diminished demand for this popular 'legal high'. Participants in their research preferred mephedrone to poor quality ecstasy and cocaine and found their experiences of mephedrone use pleasurable, highlighting the demand for new and alternative ways to be intoxicated. Participants in a UK study by Measham, Wood, Dargan, and Moore (2011), focused on the gay club scene in London, also had high levels of mephedrone use, which continued past the banning of this 'legal high' in 2010, suggesting that legal status is only part of the story of intoxication: pleasure, availability and price are also significant.

Synthetic Cannabis

Synthetic cannabis (SC) is another NPS that has become popular in recent years. One of the first synthetic cannabinoids to be used as an intoxicating substance was developed by Professor John W. Huffman, the chemical structure being named after him—JWH-018 (Zawilska & Wojcieszak, 2013). Chemical compounds designed by Huffman for research purposes are now the main cannabimimetic compounds detected in many synthetic cannabis products such as Spice and K2. However, not all cannabinoids are responsible for the psychoactive effects associated with smoking cannabis. The cannabinoids 9-tetrahydrocannabinol (THC) and cannabidiol (CBD) are the key compounds in 'natural' cannabis. THC is the psychoactive compound that creates intoxicating effects when smoking cannabis, while CBD is a non-psychoactive cannabinoid which research has shown helps to reduce the negative effects of THC, and which also has potential medicinal benefits such as anti-inflammatory and antipsychotic properties, as well as the ability to protect neurons from damage or degeneracy (Medical Marijuana on the Mind, 2010; Niesink & Van Laar, 2013).

SC is often noted as having intense effects on users and part of the reason for this are the differences between 'natural' and SC. Cannabinoids attach to two types of receptors in the body: CB1 receptors, which are located mostly in the brain, as well as the nervous system and nerve endings, and CB2 receptors, which are located mostly within the immune system. The location of the CB1 receptors primarily in the brain means they are responsible for inducing the psychological effects associated with cannabis, while the CB2 receptors act largely as immune modulators (Gurney, Scott, Kacinko, Presley, & Logan, 2014). THC and synthetic cannabinoids act differently when binding to these CB receptors. THC is a partial agonist, while synthetic cannabinoids are full agonists; the difference being that a partial agonist does not induce a maximum response from the receptor when it binds to and activates it, whereas a full agonist can. Therefore, as full agonists, the potency of synthetic cannabinoids is much higher compared to 'natural' cannabis. Additionally, synthetic cannabinoids are originally in a solid form before being dissolved in organic solvents (acetone) and sprayed onto dry plant material (leaves, flowers, resin) to be smoked (Camp, 2011). Due to the way the cannabinoids are dissolved and sprayed, there is considerable inter- and intra-batch variability in terms of both the substances present and their quantity, producing varying levels of intoxication.

Synthetic cannabis (SC) is often associated with more marginalised and vulnerable populations (EMCDDA, 2018; World Drug Report, 2018), with SC cited as the most popular drug in UK prisons (Linnell,

Measham, & Newcombe, 2015). Perhaps of concern is that NPS are popular amongst certain groups who are attracted by their availability and low prices (Blackman & Bradley, 2017; EMCDDA, 2018; World Drug Report, 2018), often young inexperienced users, or those with multiple issues related to addiction and marginalisation. It is also often these kinds of users who experience adverse events from using synthetic cannabis (Amsterdam, Brunt, & Van Der Brink, 2015; Brown, 2017; Forrester et al., 2011). In the New Zealand context, synthetic cannabinoids[4] have similarly become associated with vulnerable groups such as those who are homeless, who are also suffering the most harms from the use of SC and for whom the intense high is often an escape from trauma. Sutherland et al. (2016) found in the Australian context that the group most likely to use synthetic cannabis were younger, more disadvantaged and were more likely to report trouble ceasing their drug use.

New Psychoactive Substances in New Zealand

In New Zealand, NPS became popular as illicit drugs such as ecstasy are often difficult to get hold of and are of poor quality. Therefore, for those immersed in the dance and festival scene and the night time economy (NTE), legal substances that claimed to have similar effects were immensely popular. The first wave of NPS to become popular in New Zealand were BZP-based party pills (BZP-PPs), which were popular from about 2000 onwards, among young dance club attendees. The NPS market developed particularly quickly in New Zealand, partly due to its geographical isolation and small population. Consequently, New Zealand has an underdeveloped illicit drugs market compared to European countries, making legal alternatives highly attractive (Cohen & Butler, 2011). BZP-PPs were often used when illicit drugs were unavailable or alongside other illicit substances as part of a polydrug-using repertoire (Butler & Sheridan, 2007; Hutton, 2010). However, BZP-PPs were not without controversy, with reports of adverse effects (Gee, Richardson, Woltersdorf, & Moore, 2005; Wilkins, Girling, Sweetsur, Huckle, & Huakau, 2006) and concerns over the fact that they were unregulated until 2005. BZP-PPs were eventually banned under the 2008 Misuse of Drugs

(Classification of BZP) Amendment Act, despite a lack of evidence that the harms were severe enough to warrant such action, and that the majority of submissions on the 2007 Bill supported regulation rather than prohibition (See Hutton, 2017 for a more detailed discussion). Almost immediately after the banning of BZP-PPs, new party pills without BZP in them became available, and 'Kronic'—a synthetic cannabis product—started causing similar concerns, receiving intense media attention, focusing on its availability and attractiveness to under 18s. 'Kronic' was banned in 2009, with another cannabis substitute, 'K2', taking its place. K2 was also then banned in 2011. This was despite a report by the Expert Advisory Committee on drugs, which could not identify any significant harm associated with synthetic cannabinoids to warrant their prohibition. Thus, the role of populism is particularly significant in debates about 'drugs', including NPS and SC (see Alexandrescu, 2014; Lancaster et al., 2011), with sensationalised media calls to 'get tough' leading to knee-jerk responses and blanket bans, as well as criticisms of politicians for their inaction in addressing perceived drug harms. For example, in an initial response to K2 and SC, Peter Dunne the then Associate Minister for Health in New Zealand (NZ) opted in 2011 to restrict the sale and supply of synthetic substances to those over 18. However, this did not last long, and Dunne made a U-turn following significant media attention, such as the media labelling him 'Dunne-Nothing' for not banning SC (Jones, 2011).

To try and address the 'cat and mouse' problem with NPS, namely that manufacturers simply tweak the chemical compounds of banned substances to produce NPS that are not controlled under drugs legislation, New Zealand introduced the Psychoactive Substances Act in 2013 (PSA, 2013). The PSA 2013 was hailed as a world leading piece of legislation, one that would reduce the harm from some drugs by regulating rather criminalising them. The onus would be on manufacturers to prove that their products were 'low risk' (See Wilkins et al., 2013). The PSA 2013 responded to the popularity of NPS in a NZ context, and the realisation that regulation of a chaotic NPS market was needed. However, any gains from taking this more nuanced approach to psychoactive substance use failed to materialise as the government executed a spectacular U-turn less than a year later and effectively banned all psychoactive substances previously made legal, through the Psychoactive Substances Amendment Act in 2014 (PSA, 2014). In response to the recent SC deaths, (see below) commentators have argued that the PSA 2013 and PSA 2014 meant that SC production and supply went underground with ongoing and tragic consequences for some users (Brown, 2017). It is also by no means certain that legislation to ban NPS is effective at managing harms from substance use. A number of scholars in this area suggest that, it may in fact increase the harms related to mephedrone (McElrath & O'Neill, 2011; Measham et al., 2010; Palamar & Barratt, 2016; Wood, Measham, & Dargan, 2012) and gamma-hydroxybutyrate (GHB) (EMCDDA, 2011), with more risky substitutes increasing in use, as well as decreases in purity of NPS alongside increases in prices.

Since approximately 2017, SC or 'synnies', as they are often referred to in New Zealand, have become a key issue in relation to debates about drug use and intoxication. New Zealand has suffered approximately 70 deaths to date from the use of synthetic cannabinoids since mid-2017, and ESR (Institute of Environmental Science and Research) testing data demonstrate that most of the synthetic compounds in 'synnies' are new substances, not leftovers from when psychoactive substances like 'Kronic' were legal in the New Zealand context. As noted by commentators when the PSA 2014 was introduced, the underground illegal market for NPS like synthetic cannabis flourished with tragic consequences. However, their use flourished amongst a different kind of population than had previously been associated with NPS, and as Brown (2017, p. 11) points out, SC use was '*concentrated among the marginalised and dispossessed. These are not recreational drug users*'. This concentration of use amongst already vulnerable populations highlights the social issues related to addiction and the use of drugs like SC: many people use these kinds of substances to mask their pain, and unless their pains are addressed, their addictions will remain the only way of coping with underlying trauma. Relatedly, the use of SC may also serve the soothing function noted earlier, for those whose use of NPS is related to trauma and structural disadvantage, whatever the results may look like to 'outsiders'.

Intoxication and Synthetic Cannabis

The users of 'synnies' that are suffering the most harms are very different from the more affluent, clubbing mephedrone users in the UK, and from the original users of NPS in the New Zealand context, a similar, polydrug-using population inhabiting the NTE. Due to the shift in intoxication related to NPS, and the headline grabbing 'spice zombies' noted by Alexandrescu (2019), intoxication via NPS has acquired a new level of stigma and is often viewed with disgust and as abject. Intoxication via some NPS has become problematised and associated with particular types of 'antisocial' users, as well as social issues such as addiction and homelessness. These populations are already seen as abject and their use of NPS and the way this is framed in media accounts emphasises their marginalisation and 'otherness'. After an initial flurry of headlines and commentaries, the issue has faded into the background, at least for most New Zealanders, with the issues related to intoxication via NPS such as SC remaining unaddressed. No early warning system to detect problematic substances is yet in place, leading commentators to argue that 'the suffering of marginalised people doesn't make headlines the way the pains of middle-class users do' (Brown, 2017, p. 13). Although, in response to a review of addiction services, the NZ government recently pledged 14 million over four years towards services to deal, in part, with addictions to drugs like SC (Wellbeing Budget, 2019). However, calls to 'get tough' have also been enshrined in the recently passed Misuse of Drugs Amendment Act 2019 that has made two synthetic cannabinoids AMB-FUBINACA and 5F-ADB class A drugs, in an effort to 'clamp down' on supply. This effectively sidelines much of the evidence related to the 'war on drugs' and its ineffectiveness in dealing with supply, as there will always be supply to meet demand. The 'escape hatch' offered by SC to some groups in society remains popular (Alexandrescu, 2019, p. 8), largely because the issues driving addictions to such substances are left unaddressed. Instead, harmful policies such as the drug testing of beneficiaries are introduced (in 2012 in New Zealand) that also encourage people to substitute arguably less harmful drugs for substances like SC that do not show up on drug tests (Perrone et al., 2013; Ralphs et al., 2017).

In the UK context, use of synthetic cannabinoids is concentrated amongst young people with the Crime Survey for England and Wales reporting that 1 in 40 (2.8%) of young adults aged 16–24 took an NPS in the previous year (Blackman & Bradley, 2017, p. 70). Similar to the New Zealand context, the use of synthetic cannabinoids and other NPS in the UK is often part of polydrug use and either used as a substitute for illegal drugs or alongside them (Blackman & Bradley, 2017; Hutton, 2017; Wilkins et al., 2016). A similar trajectory of NPS and synthetic cannabinoids has also been noted in the UK context, with initial use of NPS by more privileged populations engaging with the NTE. However, echoing the NZ experience, the use of synthetic cannabinoids in particular began gaining popularity amongst disadvantaged populations, those who were homeless, for example, after they fell out of favour with more privileged groups (Blackman & Bradley, 2017).

One explanation for this shift is that middle-class users tried NPS and SC, attracted by their legal status, but moved away from them as they were found to be poor substitutes for illegal drugs, or after having negative experiences. SC use also became stigmatised and associated with less advantaged and marginalised groups, lessening their attraction even further for wider drug-using populations. The UK market for NPS was also driven underground by the 2016 Psychoactive Substances Act, reducing their availability and any controls on dosing or harm reduction information that was given at point of sale in 'Headshops' (Blackman & Bradley, 2017). 'Spice' gained a foothold in disadvantaged populations who are often 'low in self-esteem [and] believe they have few life opportunities and positive outcomes' (Blackman & Bradley, 2017, p. 76), mirroring the situation in New Zealand, where synthetic cannabinoids or 'Spice' have become entrenched in similar groups. A documentary set in Manchester, UK, also noted that use of 'Spice' was primarily to 'reduce pain' (cited in Blackman & Bradley, 2017, p. 74), with users attracted by its cheapness and intense effects.

Of concern is that use of SC in New Zealand, as well as other countries, has become an attractive option for disadvantaged groups who want to experience intense intoxication and the escapism that this way of becoming intoxicated offers them. Further, for groups such as those in prison, the attraction also lies in the difficulties of detecting synthetic cannabinoids in drug testing regimes (Ralphs et al., 2017; Wilkins et al., 2016), emphasising the inadequacy of current responses to drug use, at least from a harm reduction perspective. As Ralphs et al. (2017, p. 66) note

> It is imperative that MDT (mandatory drug tests) policies are revised …an alternative solution, and one within our grasp is the removal of MDTs amongst those in custody at a minimum for cannabis detection….the removal of MDTs has the potential to significantly lessen the demand for synthetic cannabinoids as a replacement for other detectable substances and thus significantly diminish the market and associated harms.

Current drug policies such as drug testing are driving some populations, often those who are the most vulnerable, towards consumption of substances that are more dangerous than their legal counterparts (Glue et al., 2013; Noller, 2014). Additionally, the reasons why SC users may seek to escape and 'reduce pain' are left unacknowledged and unaddressed, with a tightening of the 'drug policy ratchet' (Stevens & Measham, 2014).

New Psychoactive Substances and Shifting Intoxications

Shifts in intoxication related to NPS demonstrate the ongoing search for the pleasures and benefits of intoxication. As Measham et al. (2010, p. 20) note, mephedrone's popularity was linked to the *desire for intoxication*, driven in part by concerns about purity and availability of illegal drugs. Users were unable to reach their desired states of intoxication via illegal drugs such as ecstasy and cocaine, creating ideal conditions for a cheap, effective, legal alternative. The New Zealand Illicit Drug Monitoring Survey (IDMS) in 2015 found that there was a decline in the availability of synthetic cannabis since the 2014 retail ban under the PSA 2014, most notably among users of party drugs such as MDMA (Wilkins, Prasad, Parker, Wong, & Rychert, 2017).

This suggests an ambivalence amongst recreational party drug users about SC linked to its unpredictable effects on levels of intoxication: SC simply did not fulfil the requirements for pleasurable intoxication for most users and is popularity waned when its legality was curtailed. More affluent groups that have experimented with NPS, like SC, appear to have simply returned to their use of illegal drugs when the effects of NPS were unpleasant or NPS were banned, removing the initial attraction of NPS, that they were legal (Bilgrei, 2016; Blackman & Bradley, 2017; Green, 2008). In the UK context, Hammersley (2010) argued that 'Spice' users, originally attracted to SC due it its legality, simply switched back to using cannabis once SC was made illegal, suggesting a similar temporary displacement for most users. For less affluent and more disadvantaged populations, the banning of synthetic cannabinoids in particular meant that their manufacture and distribution went underground, resulting in more potent products that were not only more harmful and risky for users but more attractive for those groups who wanted a temporary escape from their lives,

> These are people whose lives are so difficult they want to get *really* fucked up, and the Prime Minister needs to understand that some people's lives are so difficult that they just want to forget. (Ross Bell Director of the New Zealand Drug Foundation cited in https://thespinoff.co.nz/society/26-07-2017/we-havent-seen-deaths-like-this-in-ten-years-of-synthetics/)

A similar shift developed in the UK context, from niche experimental use of synthetic cannabis, to use by more disadvantaged populations as affluent users moved on to other substances (Blackman & Bradley, 2017). An analysis of drug forum discussions in Norway also noted a similar rejection of SC, after initial enthusiasm, with it being referred to as the 'heroin of cannabis', by one forum discussant (Bilgrei, 2016, p. 6).

Media coverage of 'Spice zombies' (Alexandrescu, 2018, 2019) in the UK has cemented the position of 'Spice' (synthetic cannabis) as a drug used by those with multiple problems and disadvantages. Therefore, intoxication in the context of NPS is exemplified in a variety of practices that are sought out by a diverse range of social groups. Intoxication may also be considered as pleasurable and beneficial for some groups and as a necessity for others. Thus, the meaning/s of intoxication are not fixed, which the exploration of NPS emphasises; using mephedrone in a recreational clubbing environment will produce different meanings, practices and experiences of intoxication, compared to using synthetic cannabinoids in the context of homelessness and deprivation.

Intoxication can therefore be used in a variety of ways, and the pleasures of using NPS such as mephedrone for *some* users are clear in the following example,

> Oh my god I took a whole capsule and I was off my face, I hadn't been like that for years. I've done pills for years and years and I've had nothing like that for a long time. ……and my friend said my eyes were rolling—she'd never seen me like that. <u>It was brilliant</u>. (Measham et al., 2010, p. 17, emphasis added)

The acceptability of *visible* intoxication is evident in this account, where rolling eyes and being 'really high' are desirable and sought after states, culturally acceptable between friends in this clubbing context. Being 'off your face' is an indicator of pleasure and of having a good time, although visible intoxication via NPS may not be as acceptable outside of this particular clubbing context. Alternatively, those intoxicated via SC represent visible and spectacular street-based intoxication, akin to Hebdige's (1979) spectacular subcultures, unavoidable to more privileged and less intoxicated spectators. Such '*spectacular intoxications*' are also positioned as unacceptable displays of abject bodies. The acceptability of altered states thus depends on the social and cultural position of the person who is intoxicated—the intoxications of more privileged populations are often accepted or avoid severe social sanctions, whilst the intoxicated bodies of 'spice zombies' are viewed with disgust (Alexandrescu, 2019).

'Spice zombies': New Psychoactive Substances and Stigma

Alexandrescu (2019) explores some of the issues related to synthetic cannabinoids and media images about users of SC or 'Spice zombies' as they have been referred to in media discourse. In common with the New Zealand context and the 2014 PSA, the 2016 Psychoactive Substances

Act (2016 PSA) in the UK imposed a blanket ban on all psychoactive substances, driving sales of substances like SC underground and increased use by those on the margins. The 2016 PSA also meant that NPS and SC were more dangerous with no controls on potency or ingredients, leading to unpredictable behaviour in some users after ingestion (Alexandrescu, 2019). As Stevens recently noted,

> The Psychoactive Substances Act has certainly not eliminated the supply or use of the substances it aimed to restrict. Nor has criminalising possession of synthetic cannabinoids by classifying them as a Class B substances under the Misuse of Drugs Act in December 2016 solved the problem. Quite the opposite: both the strength and price of these substances has increased since they were banned—a common effect of prohibition—leading to greater health harms and financial problems for users. (Stevens, 2018)

The 'Spice zombie' has become a potent symbol of problematic drug use and of the abject, lost SC 'addict'. In a media saturated age, images of SC users, often generated by the public (Alexandrescu, 2019), bring the issues related to addiction starkly into focus in the public domain, as well as into people's homes and living rooms (See for example, 'Killer chemicals: inside New Zealand's synthetic cannabis crisis', November, 2017). They reinforce the stigma associated with all forms of drug use, fuelling already embedded fears about drugs and their users and provide a visual symbol of marginalisation and despair. As Manderson (1995) notes, the symbols associated with drug use are powerful and long lasting, often intensifying stigma and exclusion.

The issue of stigma pervades many drug users' lives and is all too apparent in the debates around SC. Stigma related to the use of illicit drugs is damaging and far reaching for PWUD, with injecting drug users more stigmatised than other groups and often blamed for their problematic use of drugs (Lloyd, 2013). Stigma is also related to low self-esteem and poor health, with PWUD often internalising societal stigma, which becomes a barrier to treatment and harm reduction services (Ahern, Stuber, & Galea, 2007). The intense stigmatisation of SC users through the use of language such as 'spice zombies' further places them at the margins in a vicious cycle of addiction, trauma and structural disadvantage. Stigma in this instance reflects 'the political economy of stigma and its links to social exclusion' (Parker & Aggleton, 2003, cited in Tyler & Slater, 2018, p. 725), highlighting that the unequal power relations inherent in social stigma and *who* is stigmatised for doing *what* are crucial questions in these debates.

Conclusion

The meanings of intoxication related to NPS have changed over time and are dependent on the social, cultural and environmental contexts of the use of psychoactive substances to alter states of consciousness. The issues associated with the use of NPS such as BZP-PPS, mephedrone and 'Spice' demonstrate the variety of practices associated with intoxication. It also demonstrates the inadequacy of responses to 'intoxication', responses that fail to recognise the nuances involved in diverse intoxicating practices. The use of NPS moves along a continuum from recreational or experimental use to addicted, problematic intoxications. Mephedrone users are often experienced polydrug users, experimenting with mephedrone in the context of recreational drug use, defined as 'enjoying the desired effect of the drug and not presenting a risk to themselves or others' (Buchanan, 2008, p. 250). Recent SC users on the other hand are a population often struggling with multiple issues related to addiction and problematic drug use and for whom, intense intoxication is one way to cope with the pains in their lives.

The popularity and enthusiastic uptake (initially at least) of NPS demonstrates the embeddedness of intoxication within many westernised nations, the desire to become intoxicated evident in the uptake of a variety of NPS, alongside or in place of illicit substances. Although the attractiveness of NPS can be related to their legality, this is not the whole explanation for their popularity. A positive experience of intoxication is also important to users of substances, whether the substance is legal or illegal. As noted with mephedrone, the high level of intoxication was cited as especially pleasurable, and this was a key attraction for users, as well as its availability.

The shifts in intoxications related to NPS, and SC in particular, have meant that intoxication has become associated with marginalised groups, focusing the meanings of intoxication as an unacceptable and negative state. That the majority of intoxications, whether through legal or illegal drugs, are trouble free, unremarkable and often pleasurable is sidelined in these debates. What is clear in the development of a variety of NPS is that the most marginalised populations remain those who suffer the most drug harms (Stevens, 2011). The public health crisis brought on by SC has focused on the harms related to SC, often stigmatising and castigating SC users for their plight. Calls to 'get tough' are common and have been enshrined in the law in the New Zealand Misuse of Drugs Amendment Act 2019, despite the fact that this approach has proven ineffective in other contexts (Stevens, 2018), and that prohibition itself causes harms (Buchanan, 2008). Equally clear is that new and innovative approaches are urgently needed to address the addictions of those who remain marginalised due to structural disadvantage, poverty and stigma. Further, for those whose use of NPS remains within a recreational, experimental framework, an integrated early warning system to detect potentially risky substances, coupled with properly funded and widespread drug checking (see https://knowyourstuff.nz & https://wearetheloop.org), is an important harm reduction measure; further criminalisation and prohibition of NPS should be strenuously avoided.

Notes

1. BZP is short for benzylpiperazine, a substance that has stimulant properties similar to amphetamine but about one tenth the strength (Cohen & Butler, 2011). Party pills often, though not always, contained trifluoromethylphenylpiperazine (TFMPP) which supposedly mimicked the empathetic and energetic effects of ecstasy.
2. Mephedrone (4-methylmethcathinone) is a synthetic stimulant most similar chemically to amphetamines. It is a derivative of cathinone, a compound found in the plant called khat. https://www.thelancet.com/action/showPdf?pii=S0140-6736%2810%2960556-9.
3. This story was a fake and had originally been published on an Internet forum as a joke (Lancaster et al., 2011).

4. The word cannabinoid refers to every chemical substance, regardless of structure or origin, that joins the cannabinoid receptors of the body and brain, and that have similar effects to those produced by the Cannabis *sativa* plant (https://adf.org.au/drug-facts/cannabinoids/). Synthetic cannabis often refers to a specific product that contains synthetic cannabinoids such as B-FUBINACA, AMB-FUBINACA and JWH-122. Synthetic cannabinoids are substances most often applied to smokable plant material. The finished product is sometimes called synthetic cannabis or 'synnies' (https://www.drugfoundation.org.nz/info/drug-index/synthetic-cannabinoids/). Synthetic cannabinoids are also referred to as synthetic cannabis receptor agonists (SCRAs) (Alexandrescu, 2019).

References

Ahern, J., Stuber, J., & Galea, S. (2007). Stigma, discrimination and the health of illicit drug users. *Drug and Alcohol Dependence, 88*, 188–196.

Alexandrescu, L. (2014). Mephedrone, assassin of youth: The rhetoric of fear in contemporary drug scares. *Crime Media Culture, 10*, 23–37.

Alexandrescu, L. (2018). 'Ethnobotanicals' and 'Spice zombies': New psychoactive substances in the mainstream media. *Drugs: Education, Prevention and Policy, 25*, 356–364.

Alexandrescu, L. (2019). Streets of the 'spice zombies': Dependence and poverty stigma in times of austerity. *Crime, Media, Culture*. https://doi.org/10.1177/1741659019835274

Van Amsterdam, J., Brunt, T., & van den Brink, W. (2015). The adverse health effects of synthetic cannabinoids with emphasis on psychosis-like effects. *Journal of Psychopharmacology 29*, 254–63.

Barratt, M. J., Cakic, V., & Lenton, S. (2013). Patterns of synthetic cannabinoid use in Australia. *Drug and Alcohol Review, 32*(2), 141–146.

Berry-Caban, C., Kleinschmidt, P., Rao, D., & Jenikns, J. (2012, October–December). Synthetic cannabinoid and cathinone use among us soldiers. *The Army Medical Department Journal*, 19–23.

Bilgrei, O. (2016). From "herbal highs" to the "heroin of cannabis": Exploring the evolving discourse on synthetic cannabinoid use in a Norwegian Internet drug forum. *International Journal of Drug Policy, 29*, 1–8.

Blackman, S., & Bradley, R. (2017). From Niche to stigma-Headshops to prison: Exploring the rise and fall of synthetic cannabinoid use among young adults. *International Journal of Drug Policy, 40*, 70–77.

Bright, S., Bishop, B., Kane, R., Marsh, A., & Barratt, M. (2013). Kronic Hysteria: Exploring the intersection between Australian synthetic cannabis legislation, the media and drug related-harm. *International Journal of Drug Policy, 24*, 231–237.

Brown, R. (2017). We should have known. *Matters of Substance, 28*(3). New Zealand Drug Foundation. Wellington, 6–13.

Buchanan, J. (2008). Understanding and misunderstanding problem drug use. In R. Carnwell & J. Buchanan (Eds.), *Effective practice in health, social care & criminal justice: A partnership approach* (pp. 111–129). Maidenhead: Open University Press.

Butler, R., & Sheridan, J. (2007). Highs and lows: Patterns of use, positive and negative effects of benzylpiperazine-containing party pills (BZP-party pills) amongst young people in New Zealand. *Harm Reduction Journal, 4*, 1–10.

Camp, N. (2011). Synthetic cannabinoids. *Journal of Nursing, 37*, 292–293.

Chatwin, C. (2017). Assessing the 'added value' of European policy on new psychoactive substances. *International Journal of Drug Policy, 40*, 111–116.

Cohen, B., & Butler, R. (2011). BZP-party pills: A review of the research on benzylpiperazine as a recreational drug. *International Journal of Drug Policy, 22*, 95–101.

European Monitoring Centre for Drugs and Drug Addiction (EMCDDA). (2011). *Annual report 2011: The state of the drugs problem in Europe* (pp. 1–105). Luxembourg Publications Office of the European Union.

Evans-Brown, M., Gallegos, A., Christie, R., Sola, S., Almedia, A., Jorge, R., … Sedefov, R. (2018). *Fentanils and synthetic cannabinoids: Driving greater complexity into the drug situation* (pp. 1–25). European Monitoring Centre for Drugs and Drug Addiction (EMCDDA), Luxembourg Publications Office of the European Union.

Forrester, M. B., Kleinschmidt, K., Schwarz, E., & Young, A. (2011). Synthetic cannabinoid exposures reported to Texas poison centers. *Journal of Addictive Diseases, 30*, 351–358.

Gee, P., Richardson, S., Woltersdorf, W., & Moore, G. (2005). Toxic effects of BZP-based herbal party pills in humans: A prospective study in Christchurch New Zealand. *The New Zealand Medical Journal, 118*, 1–10.

Glue, P., Al-Shaqsi, S., Hancock, D., Gale, C., Strong, B., & Schep, L. (2013). Hospitalisation associated with use of the synthetic cannabinoid K2. *The New Zealand Medical Journal, 126*, 18–23.

Green, J. (2008). Partying on? Life after BZP-based party pills. *The New Zealand Medical Journal, 121*, 35–42.

Gurney, S., Scott, K., Kacinko, S., Presley, B., & Logan, B. (2014). Pharmacology, toxicology, and adverse effects of synthetic cannabinoid drugs. *Forensic Science Review, 26*, 26–53.

Hammersley, R. (2010). Dangers of banning spice and the synthetic cannabinoid agonists. *Addiction, 105*, 373.

Hebdige, D. (1979). *Subculture the meaning of style*. London: Routledge.

Hutton, F. (2006). *Risky pleasures? Club cultures and feminine identities*. Aldershot: Ashgate.

Hutton, F. (2010). Kiwis, clubs and drugs: Club cultures in Wellington New Zealand. *The Australian and New Zealand Journal of Criminology, 43*, 91–111.

Hutton, F. (2017). BZP-'Party pills', populism and prohibition: Exploring global debates in a New Zealand context. *Australian & New Zealand Journal of Criminology, 50*(2), 282–306.

Jones, N. (2011). *Designer drugs a cat and mouse game. New Zealand Herald*. Retrieved September 29, 2019, from https://www.nzherald.co.nz/nz/news/article.cfm?c_id=1&objectid=10738810

Lancaster, K., Hughes, C., Spicer, B., Matthew-Simmons, F., & Dillon, P. (2011). *Curiosity killed the M-Cat: An examination of illicit drugs and media*. Paper presented at the *ANZCCC:* The Australian and New Zealand Critical Criminology Conference 2010, Institute of Criminology, Sydney Law School, The University of Sydney, Australia.

Linnell, M., Measham, F., & Newcombe, R. (2015). *New psychoactive substances: The local picture, a research study and needs assessment for Blackburn with Darwen Council*. Manchester: Linnell Publications.

Lloyd, C. (2013). The stigmatization of problem drug users: A narrative literature review. *Drugs: Education, Prevention and Policy, 20*, 85–95.

Manderson, D. (1995). Metamorphoses: Clashing symbols in the social construction of drugs. *Journal of Drug Issues, 25*(4), 799–816.

Maxwell, J. (2014). Psychoactive Substances – Some new, some old: A scan of the situation in the U.S. *Drug and Alcohol Dependence, 134*, 71–77.

McElrath, K., & O'Neill, C. (2011). Experiences with mephedrone pre-and post-legislative controls: Perceptions of safety and sources of supply. *International Journal of Drug Policy, 22*, 120–127.

Measham, F., Moore, K., Newcombe, R., & Welch, Z. (2010). Tweaking, bombing, dabbing and stockpiling: The emergence of mephedrone and the perversity of prohibition. *Drugs and Alcohol Today, 10*, 14–21.

Measham, F., & Newcombe, R. (2016). 'What's so 'new' about new psychoactive substances? Definitions, prevalence, motivations, user groups and a proposed new taxonomy.'. In *The SAGE handbook of drug & alcohol studies – social science approaches* (pp. 576–596).

Measham, F., Wood, D., Dargan, P., & Moore, K. (2011). The rise in legal highs: Prevalence and patterns in the use of illegal drugs and first-and second-generation "legal highs" in South London gay dance clubs. *Journal of Substance Use, 16*, 263–272.

Medical Marijuana on the Mind. (2010). Harvard Mental Health Letter. Retrieved from http://www.health.harvard.edu/mind-and-mood/medical-marijuana-and-the-mind

Niesink, R., & Van Laar, M. (2013). Does cannabidiol protect against adverse psychological effects of THC? *Frontiers in Psychiatry, 4*, article 130, 1–8.

Noller, G. (2014). *Synthetic cannabinoid use in New Zealand: Assessing the harms* (Report #01). Auckland: The STAR Trust.

Palamar, J., & Acosta, P. (2015). Synthetic cannabinoid use in a nationally representative sample of US high school seniors. *Drug and Alcohol Dependence, 149*, 194–202.

Palamar, J., & Barratt, M. (2016). Synthetic cannabinoids: Undesirable alternatives to natural marijuana. *The American Journal of Drug and Alcohol Abuse, 42*, 371–373.

Perrone, D., Helgesen, R., & Fischer, R. (2013). United States drug prohibition and legal highs: How drug testing may lead cannabis users to spice. *Drugs, Education, Prevention and Policy, 20*, 216–224.

Psychoactive Substances Act. (2013). Retrieved from http://www.legislation.govt.nz/act/public/2013/0053/latest/DLM5042921.html?src=qs

Psychoactive Substances Amendment Act. (2014). Retrieved from http://www.legislation.govt.nz/act/public/2014/0024/latest/whole.html

Ralphs, R., Williams, L., Askew, R., & Norton, A. (2017). Adding Spice to the Porridge: The development of a synthetic cannabinoid market in an English prison. *International Journal of Drug Policy, 40*, 57–69.

Stevens, A. (2011). *Drugs, crime and public health: The political economy of drug policy*. London: Routledge.

Stevens, A. (2018). We predicted banning legal highs wouldn't work and a new review shows it's as bad as we feared. *The Conversation*. Retrieved August 28, 2019, from https://theconversation.com/we-predicted-banning-legal-highs-wouldnt-work-and-a-new-review-shows-its-as-bad-as-we-feared-104981

Stevens, A., & Measham, F. (2014). The 'drug policy ratchet': Why do sanctions for new psychoactive drugs typically only go up? *Addiction, 109*, 1226–1232.

Sutherland, R., Peacock, A., Whittaker, E., Roxburgh, A., Lenton, S., Matthews, A., … Bruno, R. (2016). New psychoactive substance use among regular psychostimulant users in Australia, 2010–2015. *Drug and Alcohol Dependence, 161*, 110–118.

Tyler, I., & Slater, T. (2018). Rethinking the sociology of stigma. *The Sociological Review Monographs, 66*, 721–743.

United Nations Office on Drugs and Crime (UNDOC). (2018). *World Drug Report.* United Nations Publication.

Wellbeing Budget. (2019). Taking mental health seriously. Retrieved from https://www.budget.govt.nz/budget/2019/wellbeing/mental-health/expanding-access.htm

Wilkins, C., Girling, M., Sweetsur, P., Huckle, T., & Huakau, J. (2006). *Legal party pill use in New Zealand: Prevalence of use, availability, health harms and 'gateway effects' of benzylpiperazine (BZP) and triflourophenylmethylpiperazine (TFMPP).* Auckland: Massey University.

Wilkins, C., Parker, K., Prasad, J., & Jawalkar, S. (2016). Do police arrestees substitute legal highs for other drugs? *International Journal of Drug Policy, 31*, 74–79.

Wilkins, C., Prasad, J., Parker, K., Wong, K., & Rychert, M. (2017). *Recent trends in illegal drug use in New Zealand 2006–2015: Findings from the 2006, 2007, 2008, 2009, 2010, 2011, 2012, 2013, 2014 and 2015 Illicit Drug Monitoring System (IDMS).* Auckland: SHORE & Whariki Research Centre, Massey University.

Wilkins, C., Sheridan, J., Adams, P., Russell, B., Ram, S., & Newcombe, D. (2013). The new psychoactive substances regime in New Zealand: A different approach to regulation. *Journal of Psychopharmacology, 27*, 584–589.

Winstock, A., & Barratt, M. (2013). Synthetic cannabis: A comparison of patterns of use and effect profile with natural cannabis in a large global sample. *Drug and Alcohol Dependence, 131*, 106–111.

Winstock, A., Barratt, M., Ferris, J., & Maier, L. (2017). Global Drug Survey 2017. Overview and highlights. Retrieved from https://www.globaldrugsurvey.com/wp-content/themes/globaldrugsurvey/results/GDS2017_key-findings-report_final.pdf

Wood, D. M., et al. (2012). 'Our favourite drug': Prevalence of use and preference for mephedrone in the London night-time economy 1 year after control. *Journal of Substance Use, 17*(2), 91–97.

Zawilska, B., & Wojcieszak, J. (2013). Spice/K2 drugs – More than innocent substitutes for marijuana. *International Journal of Neuropsychopharmacology, 17*, 1–17.

Websites

http://neptune-clinical-guidance.co.uk/wp-content/uploads/2016/07/Synthetic-Cannabinoid-Receptor-Agonists.pdf. Retrieved August 28, 2019.

https://interactives.stuff.co.nz/2017/09/killer-chemicals/index.html. Retrieved August 28, 2018.

6

Alcohol Mixed with Energy Drinks and Intoxication

Nicolas Droste, Amy Pennay, Amy Peacock, and Peter Miller

Introduction: A Holistic View of Alcohol Mixed with Energy Drinks Consumption and Intoxication

In the wider field of alcohol and other drug (AOD) research, substance use behaviours have been demonstrated as having many influences. It is widely acknowledged that substance use practices are shaped by many

---

N. Droste
School of Psychology, Deakin University, Geelong, VIC, Australia

A. Pennay
Centre for Alcohol Policy Research, La Trobe University, Melbourne, VIC, Australia

A. Peacock
National Drug and Alcohol Research Centre, University of New South Wales, Sydney, NSW, Australia

P. Miller (✉)
School of Psychology, Deakin University, Geelong Waterfront Campus, Geelong, VIC, Australia
e-mail: peter.miller@deakin.edu.au

F. Hutton (ed.), *Cultures of Intoxication*,
https://doi.org/10.1007/978-3-030-35284-4_6

factors that span genetic, cognitive, functional, pharmacological, social, cultural, historical, and environmental influences. Substance use might be driven by influences that are internal to the consumer, for example, for motives of mood management or relaxation, functional purposes such as endurance or reducing fatigue, or as a result of physiological dependence (e.g. Cooper, 1994; Martens, Rocha, Martin, & Serrao, 2008; Pennay, 2012). Alternatively, consumption choices may be influenced by factors external to the consumer, such as the perceived behaviour of peers, environmental contexts such as parties and licensed venues, and, more broadly, structural influences such as socio-economic status and other demographic factors (Hughes et al., 2012; Verkooijen, de Vries, & Nielsen, 2007). The pursuit of intoxication also plays an important influencing role in substance use (Hunt & Evans, 2008), a factor that is shaped by both internal (e.g. pleasure) and external (e.g. social and environmental) drivers.

Consuming alcohol mixed with energy drinks (AmED) has emerged as a popular substance use practice, as well as a public health concern, in the past decade, drawing widespread attention from research and policy sectors internationally (Australian and New Zealand Food Regulation Standing Committee, 2013; Pennay & Lubman, 2012b). Energy drinks have risen in popularity with consumers since their introduction to the US market in the mid-1990s (Reissig, Strain, & Griffiths, 2009), with research addressing AmED use appearing in peer-reviewed scientific journals around a decade later (e.g. Ferreira, de Mello, Pompeia, & Souza-Formigoni, 2004 ; Marczinski & Fillmore, 2006). In the years spanning from 2006 to 2018, more than 100 peer-reviewed commentaries, letters, research articles, and reviews on the topic of AmED consumption were published. This figure includes a number of systematic and narrative-based literature reviews (e.g. Benson, Verster, Alford, & Scholey, 2014; Ferré & O'Brien, 2011; Marczinski & Fillmore, 2014; McKetin, Coen, & Kaye, 2015; Peacock et al., 2014; Vida & Rácz, 2014).

Despite this flurry of activity to quantify the prevalence and correlated risks and harms of AmED consumption, researchers have, until recently, neglected to explore the role of pleasure and desired outcomes derived from AmED intoxication. Ultimately, this has led to a detailed portrait of the consumption patterns and harms associated with AmED use, but an incomplete overall picture of AmED intoxication in the literature, one which is decontextualised in terms of constellation of motives, functions, expectancies, and social environments that frame AmED consumption.

Intoxication is defined in the Merriam-Webster dictionary as (1) 'an abnormal state that is essentially a poisoning', (2) 'the condition of having physical or mental control markedly diminished by the effects of alcohol or other drugs', and (3) 'a strong excitement or elation'. In a discussion of public health discourse about harmful alcohol consumption, Keane (2009) argued that academic and policy efforts, choosing to focus exclusively upon intoxication in terms of the first two definitions, strongly linked to harm and risk outcomes, is futile. The everyday experiences of drinkers more commonly reflect intoxication as a positive, enhanced state, a form of bodily pleasure. Keane (2009, p. 138) argues:

> The model of intoxication as 'maladaptive behavioural or psychological changes' is based on a static and de-contextualised vision of human functioning. A phrase such as 'the individual cannot function within their normal range of physical/cognitive abilities' ignores the fact that from the perspective of the drinker at the social event, drinking reduces some capacities but enhances others which are probably more salient. He may not be able to operate machinery safely but he is able to talk and flirt with strangers, dance with abandon and forget his work worries. Intoxication is experienced as enhancement as well as diminishment.

In this chapter, we adopt the position of Keane (and others) that all aspects of intoxication are important to consider, including both diminished and enhanced capacities. In particular, the pursuit of pleasure through intoxication is central to understanding engagement in risky substance use practices (Goulding, Shankar, Elliott, & Canniford, 2009), of which AmED might be considered. Pleasure includes, but is not limited to, corporeal, cognitive, social, and emotional enhancement. Previous research on intoxication and pleasure has described the importance of social contexts and settings, as well as the importance of timing, sequencing, and drug combinations in maximising intoxication and pleasure (Duff, 2008; Hunt, Bailey, Evans, & Moloney, 2009; Olsen, 2009; Pennay, 2012). This literature highlights the complex and purposeful decision-making processes that often occur with respect to intoxication. In this chapter, we present an argument that the costs and benefits of AmED consumption are weighed by consumers as part of a decision-making process that is highly influenced by intoxication and pleasure, as well as a range of functional-, environmental-, social-, and individual-level considerations.

This chapter begins by providing a definition of energy drinks (EDs) and of AmED, followed by a summary of the current literature,[1] regarding consumption patterns and associated harms, and a summary of the observed physiological and behavioural effects of consumption. These observations are then contextualised within a framework of the consumers' social identity, environmental consumption contexts, and a functional approach to understanding what might be called the culture of AmED intoxication.

What Are Energy Drinks?

Developing an operationalised definition of energy drinks for the purpose of research is not as straightforward as it initially sounds. Energy drinks were originally brought to market in Austria in the 1980s, but first became popular following the introduction of Red Bull® to the US in 1997 (Reissig et al., 2009), with many more brands introduced over time, and sales in the US, Europe, and Australasia increasing greatly since then. Indeed, although reliable sales data are sparse and generally not released by industry, Australian data indicate that ED sales swelled from 2.8 million litres in 1997 to 13.9 million litres in 2006 (Levy & Tapsell, 2007).

Trying to separate energy drinks from other caffeinated drinks such as cola, tea, coffee, iced coffee, and sports drinks can be confusing, particularly if the definition is operationalised based on the most prominent ingredients. Caffeine is generally considered the primary active ingredient in an ED (Reissig et al., 2009), though, within their 'energy blends', most brands also contain the amino acid taurine, B vitamins, glucuronolactone, herbal extracts such as guarana and/or ginseng, and high levels of sugar in the form of glucose and/or sucrose. While these ingredients are readily available in other products, the unique contribution that EDs bring to the beverage market is a consequence of carefully advertised effects, branding, image management, and a common set of active ingredients that are largely consistent across brands (Zest Health Strategies, 2012). The most prominent distinguishing feature of energy drinks compared to other beverages is that they are defined in terms of the advertised effect of their primary active ingredients: caffeine and variations of the 'energy blend'. Energy drinks can only be properly defined and differentiated by incorporating both the active ingredients and the marketing of the product. As such, energy drinks are defined throughout this chapter as any caffeinated drink, which is advertised primarily as providing benefits to physical and mental performance, endurance, concentration, and/or stamina.

Alcohol Mixed with Energy Drinks: What Can Be Classified as Alcohol Mixed with Energy Drinks?

AmED is an alcoholic beverage category that has emerged in the past decade. The product has evolved rapidly and encompasses a wide variety of serving and consumption practices. At a basic level, AmED is available to consumers via the sale of pre-mixed packaged AmED products or by combining alcoholic drinks, typically spirits or liqueurs, with energy drinks as a mixer (Gunja & Brown, 2012; Jones, Barrie, & Berry, 2012; O'Brien, McCoy, Rhodes, Wagoner, & Wolfson, 2008; Pennay & Lubman, 2012a; Thombs et al., 2010). When AmED is prepared 'manually' by consumers or bartenders, the drink typically involves a shot of spirits (commonly vodka) mixed with ED in a glass as a mixer (Jones et al., 2012; Pennay & Lubman, 2012a). Other commonly reported AmED variants include 'bombs' (e.g. Jägerbombs and Skittle Bombs), which involve dropping a shot of the spirit Jägermeister or Cointreau, respectively, into a glass of ED, then rapidly consuming the combination in a single gesture (Jones et al., 2012; Pennay & Lubman, 2012a). Finally, consuming ED on their own during an alcohol session (e.g. a shot of spirits with an ED chaser or alternating between an alcoholic drink and ED) can also be considered AmED, as any pharmacological effects of the combination will still occur.

The scope of AmED available to consumers varies according to regulations and food standards in each country. At the time of writing, packaged pre-mixed AmED are still available for sale in Australia in the form of pre-mixed cans, and several other brands, but they are effectively prohibited in the US and many parts of Europe. Following the advice of scientists and health professionals, the US Food and Drugs Administration (FDA) declared that caffeine was an unsafe food additive to alcoholic beverages in November 2010, essentially banning the sale of pre-mixed AmED in the country (Arria & O'Brien, 2011; Siegel, 2011), although this does not preclude sale of these substances hand-mixed.

What Is Known About Alcohol Mixed with Energy Drinks Consumers and Consumption Patterns?

Compared to 'alcohol-only' consumers, AmED consumers are more likely to pursue and experience greater levels of alcohol-related intoxication and intoxication-related consequences. AmED consumers use alcohol more frequently, consume more alcohol per session, are more likely to binge drink alcohol or engage in heavy episodic drinking, and are more likely to use illicit drugs (Martz, Patrick, & Schulenberg, 2015; McKetin et al., 2015; Peacock et al., 2014). Further, AmED consumers exhibit greater propensity for risk-taking and, as such, are more likely to engage in drink driving, be involved in sexual or physical aggression or victimisation, experience alcohol-related injury, and engage in gambling (McKetin et al., 2015; Peacock et al., 2014; Pennay, Cheetham, et al., 2015). AmED users are more likely to be young and male, and some limited research suggests that AmED use is also associated with identifying as a sexual minority, living in a metropolitan area, or having limited or unknown income, each of which is a known risk factor associated with other harmful substance use behaviours (Bonar et al., 2015; Brache &

Stockwell, 2011; K. Brache, Thomas, & Stockwell, 2012; O'Brien et al., 2008; Pennay, Cheetham, et al., 2015).

So far, these are all the results of between-subject comparisons of alcohol consumers versus AmED consumers. However, among AmED consumers, within-subjects analyses comparing sessions of AmED versus sessions of alcohol only have been less consistent in both consumption and harm outcomes across the two types of session within the same individuals (Brache & Stockwell, 2011; de Haan, de Haan, van der Palen, Olivier, & Verster, 2012; Peacock, Bruno, & Martin, 2013; Peacock, Droste, Pennay, Lubman, et al., 2015; Price, Hilchey, Darredeau, Fulton, & Barrett, 2010; Woolsey, Waigandt, & Beck, 2010). The nuance of this design is important—while still being vulnerable to recall biases inherent in retrospective survey designs, within-group comparisons assist in controlling for individual consumer factors that are present in between-groups comparisons.

Longitudinal studies complicate matters further. In a series of papers, Patrick and colleagues (Patrick & Maggs, 2013; Patrick, Evans-Polce, & Maggs, 2014) overcame many of the limitations of cross-sectional research by using longitudinal data and within-subjects analyses (i.e. comparison of outcomes when the same individual consumed alcohol with and without ED) and cross-sectional designs to observe outcomes of AmED use (Patrick et al., 2014; Patrick & Maggs, 2013). Using a survey which tracked drinking behaviour amongst AmED consumers over 56 days, Patrick and Maggs (2013) reported that adding ED use to any given day of alcohol use was associated with an increase in negative drinking consequences that day, even after controlling for overall alcohol intoxication via an estimated blood-alcohol measure. Intoxication outcomes that were positively associated with AmED use included reporting a hangover, getting into trouble, and doing or saying something embarrassing.

In a follow-up study, the same authors surveyed a stratified sample of US college students over time (second year through to fourth year) to investigate the extent to which AmED use in the past month was associated with intoxication-related consequences, problems, and accidents over the following two years (Patrick et al., 2014). After controlling for demographic factors, both infrequent and frequent AmED use were associated with increased negative alcohol consequences (e.g. caused shame or embarrassment), and frequent use was further associated with serious alcohol problems and increased frequency of alcohol-related accidents (e.g. experienced serious injury/been hospitalised) compared to participants who had not consumed AmED (Patrick et al., 2014).

Using a similar data collection model in a US college student sample, Mallett, Scaglione, Reavy, and Turrisi (2015) collected baseline and 6-month follow-up data and subsequently described four classes of AmED consumers: non-users, initiators, discontinuers, and continuous users. Consistent with the literature, 'non-users' reported the lowest levels of risky drinking and alcohol-related consequences, whereas 'continuous' users recorded the highest levels. However, students who had initiated AmED use during the study period reported an abrupt increase in alcohol use and intoxication-related consequences between Time 1 and 6-month follow-up (measured using a standardised scale of physical, academic, social, and sexual consequences). Further, those who discontinued AmED use during the study period showed an increase from Time 1 to Time 2 in number of alcoholic drinks and frequency of drunkenness, but a reduction in alcohol-related consequences. The authors contend that the difference in trends between the initiator and discontinuer groups may imply a broader reduction in risk-taking overall amongst the discontinuer group (i.e. AmED and other alcohol-related risk-taking behaviour may be reduced simultaneously). Finally, in another survey of US college students using a 6-month follow-up model, AmED users identified at Time 1 reported at follow-up Time 2 an increased frequency of intoxication-related physical (e.g. 'have you felt very sick to your stomach or thrown up after drinking?'), sexual (e.g. 'have you gotten into sexual situations you later regretted?'), and academic ('Have you showed up late for work or school because of drinking, a hangover, or an illness caused by drinking?') consequences (Marzell, Turrisi, Mallett, Ray, & Scaglione, 2014).

Importantly, endorsement of particular AmED consumption motives has been associated with negative consumption and harm outcomes (Droste et al., 2014; Peacock, Droste, Pennay, Miller, et al., 2015). Hedonistic motives specific to sensation and pleasure-seeking have been associated with negative AmED-related consequences, including increased alcohol consumption, risk of alcohol dependence, and experience of aggressive incidents. Hedonistic motives for consumption—particularly those related to determined drunkenness—are not specific to AmED use and have been implicated in the use of various licit and illicit substances amongst young people (Keane, 2009; Measham, 2004a). These motives speak to a subgroup of AmED consumers for whom intoxication is a desired outcome, and this driver is reflected in measures of consumption outcomes.

In summary studies that monitored AmED consumption over time have linked AmED use to increased intoxication-related consequences at follow-up. Higher frequency of AmED use was also positively associated with increased reporting of intoxication-related consequences, and commencement of AmED consumption during the study period was associated with increased reporting of intoxication-related harms. While variability in risk-taking behaviour and negative consequences may also be influenced by shifts in environment, social contexts, other substance use behaviour, and individual personal factors, these findings lend support to the notion that AmED consumption may contribute to an increased propensity for risk-taking behaviour, harmful alcohol consumption, and experience of negative alcohol-related consequences. However, inconsistent results from within- and between-subject analyses suggest that the relationship between AmED consumption and alcohol outcomes is not immediately clear without exploring other factors, such as personality factors.

What Are the Acute Effects of Alcohol Mixed with Energy Drinks Intoxication?

Measurement of the subjective effects of AmED consumption suggests increased subjective ratings of stimulation and a reduced perception of the inebriating effects of alcohol compared to consuming alcohol alone (Ferreira, Tulio de Mello, Pompeia, & de Souza-Formigoni, 2006; Forward et al., 2017; Marczinski & Fillmore, 2006; Marczinski, Fillmore, Bardgett, & Howard, 2011; Marczinski, Fillmore, Henges, Ramsey, & Young, 2011). This phenomenon has been dubbed 'wide-awake drunkenness' by some researchers (e.g. Pennay, Miller, et al., 2015), a term that describes the perceived amelioration of the sedative effects of alcohol, whilst retaining other aspects of alcohol-related intoxication. This phenomenon has raised concerns regarding judgement of alcohol-related impairment and has implications for perceived ability while intoxicated to drive a vehicle or engage in other behaviours that may place the consumer at risk.

In addition, several experimental studies demonstrated a positive effect of AmED upon desire for more alcohol and rated liking of the alcoholic drink compared with when the participant consumed alcohol without ED (Marczinski, Fillmore, Henges, Ramsey, & Young, 2013; McKetin & Coen, 2014). Further, while very few studies have explored the experience of physiological side effects, dose-response analyses have indicated that during AmED sessions in the preceding 12 months, 59% of drinkers reported experiencing heart-racing symptoms, 39% experienced heart palpations, 43% experienced insomnia, and 20% experienced tremors, all of which occurred more frequently during AmED sessions compared to sessions of alcohol only, and all of which increased as the dose increased (Droste et al., 2017).

Findings concerning the potential for AmED to affect objectively measured cognitive performance outcomes are mixed. The balance of findings suggests that the use of ED may reduce alcohol-related impairment for some cognitive outcomes, particularly reaction time–based measures, and may increase likelihood of risk-taking behaviour (Marczinski & Fillmore, 2006; Marczinski, Fillmore, Bardgett, et al., 2011; Marczinski, Fillmore, Henges, et al., 2011; Peacock, Bruno, & Martin, 2013; Peacock, Bruno, Martin, & Carr, 2013). It is important to note that these effects are often dependent on the degree of intoxication, blood alcohol concentration (BAC) curve limb (i.e. ascending or descending), and volume of ED consumed (e.g. Peacock, Cash, & Bruno, 2015).

Intoxication and Pleasure: Social and Functional Motives for Alcohol Mixed with Energy Drinks Consumption

If AmED is associated with regular, unpleasant physiological side effects, and a trend towards increases in negative alcohol-related consequences, why do consumers choose to drink AmED?

Analysis of AmED consumption motives indicate that consumers are motivated to use AmED for a variety of social, functional, and hedonistic reasons (Brache et al., 2012; Ferreira et al., 2004; Jones et al., 2012; Marczinski, 2011; O'Brien et al., 2008; Peacock, Bruno, & Martin, 2013; Pennay & Lubman, 2012a). An early qualitative study reported that consumers used AmED for benefits such as wakefulness and energy; appealing taste; social bonding; to counteract the drowsy effects of alcohol; and to facilitate alcohol intoxication (Pennay & Lubman, 2012a). A systematic review of cross-sectional studies endorsed the findings of these last two benefits, with increased odds of self-reported stimulation-based outcomes and decreased odds of sedation-based physiological and psychological outcomes, relative to when alcohol was consumed alone. The authors concluded that mixing alcohol with energy drinks may exert a dual intoxication effect, increasing stimulation-based effects and reducing sedation-based outcomes (Peacock et al., 2014).

Based on survey data, motivations for AmED use have been factor analysed into four principle drivers: hedonistic, social, energy/endurance, and intoxication-reduction (Droste et al., 2014). In a further latent class analysis, four types of consumers were identified based on their motivations for AmED use: taste consumers, energy-seeking consumers, hedonistic consumers, and intoxication-management consumers (Peacock, Droste, Pennay, Miller, et al., 2015).

Putting taste aside, essentially, these studies suggest that AmED intoxication:

1. is pleasurable and fun in many ways—sensorially, physically, and socially;
2. is useful for 'managing intoxication'—the wide-awake drunkenness effect whereby the energy drink enhances the stimulation-based effects of alcohol and depresses the drowsy/sedative effects of alcohol, resulting in a more appealing alcohol intoxication; and
3. enhances sociability and social bonding through shared experiences and collaborative consumption practices (e.g. group rounds of Jägerbombs).

With respect to the first point—pleasure and hedonism—it appears that AmED intoxication, like many other forms of intoxication, is valued for its contribution to states of joy, happiness, excitement, and annihilation. Qualitative work with AmED users has suggested that AmED intoxication of this nature is most commonly linked to particular settings, particularly nightclubs, with other settings not so supportive of acute AmED intoxication practices such as group consumption of Jägerbombs. In this qualitative work, AmED consumption was seen to produce gregarious and extroverted behaviour among groups of consumers, but only in appropriate contexts (Droste et al., 2016). This supports findings of previous qualitative research where pleasure has been noted to operate within temporal, spatial, and social consumption limits, occurring within a framework where the costs and benefits are rationally weighed (Fry, 2011; Hunt et al., 2009; Measham, 2004a; Pennay, 2012).

With respect to the second point—intoxication management—it appears that AmED is used functionally to limit intoxication; in other words, to manage the drowsy or unappealing aspects of alcohol consumption. Alcohol consumers have long reported attempts to manage the perfect or ideal intoxication, for example, by maintaining the tipsy stage prior to uncontrolled states of inebriation (Measham & Brain, 2005; Zajdow & MacLean, 2014). Illicit drug consumers have also reported co-consuming illicit stimulants with alcohol to maximise pleasure and heighten or complement the intoxicating effects of alcohol and other drugs (Hunt et al., 2009; Pennay, 2012).

Finally, the importance of social contexts and social drinking motives suggests AmED enhances the pleasures of socialising. The link between substance use and enhanced social bonding has also commonly been reported by alcohol and illicit substance users (Pennay, 2010; Szmigin et al., 2008). In recent qualitative research, it was suggested that AmED consumers identified with a clear and consistent social identity that was distinct from other alcohol consumers, typified by outgoing behaviour, with AmED consumption observed to strengthen group cohesion (Droste, Pennay, et al., 2016). In the social psychology literature, group norms, group cohesion, and methods of conformity are often used to frame processes of consumer decision-making and can also be seen as mechanisms through which substance use performs a social function. Previous research has provided useful insights regarding the influence of social group processes upon substance use behaviour (e.g. Larimer, Turner, Mallett, & Geisner, 2004; Verkooijen et al., 2007).

Alcohol Mixed with Energy Drinks Consumers as a Distinct Social Group

The AmED literature suggests that AmED consumers have a greater propensity for risk-taking and harmful alcohol consumption overall—an important consumer-level factor in a model of AmED use. In qualitative interviews, AmED consumers have also positively self-identified as a distinctly high-risk subgroup of alcohol users, a novel finding that may help to explain higher levels of alcohol intoxication and risky behaviour among AmED consumers (Droste, Pennay, et al., 2016). AmED consumers identified with a clear and consistent social identity and described themselves as extroverted partygoers who binge drink, use illicit drugs, and are impulsive, fun, outgoing, and cool, amongst other traits. Further, these traits were positively distinguished from other 'out-group' alcohol consumers and patrons at licensed venues (Droste, Pennay, et al., 2016).

From this endorsement of a high-risk 'party-going' identity, it may be interpreted that the pattern of increased consumption and intoxication-related outcomes amongst AmED consumers is attributable to existing consumer factors rather than an effect of AmED. However, experimental studies have indicated that AmED may increase the desire for more alcohol and decrease the perception of intoxication, increase stimulation (Marczinski, Fillmore, Henges, et al., 2011; Marczinski et al., 2013; McKetin & Coen, 2014), and improve objectively measured cognitive and performance outcomes that may act as indicators of intoxication (Marczinski & Fillmore, 2006; C. A. Marczinski, Fillmore, Bardgett, et al., 2011; Peacock, Cash, & Bruno, 2015). These findings combined with AmED users' self-identification as high-risk alcohol consumers suggest that AmED may be functionally utilised by individuals who identify as extroverted partygoers to enable prolonged drinking sessions. Certainly, it is reported by consumers that combining alcohol with energy drinks enables them to drink for longer and maintain a desirable state of drunkenness for longer, maximising the ideal pleasure zone (Droste, Pennay, et al., 2016).

The functional endurance and energy-related motives endorsed by consumers imply a pharmacological effect that is generally also found in experimental literature (e.g. Marczinski, Fillmore, Henges, et al., 2011; Marczinski et al., 2013). Experimental designs have demonstrated that EDs may have ameliorating effects upon alcohol-related sedation and subjective intoxication. When AmED consumers positively self-identify as high-risk drinkers for whom outgoing, gregarious behaviour and intoxication are ideals, it follows that AmED may be valued as a tool for prolonged socialising, intoxication management, or increasing alcohol consumption. AmED consumers have also endorsed that AmED served a social function through the facilitation of celebratory drinking, competitive drinking games, group bonding, and social connectedness by 'bringing the group back together' (Droste, Pennay, et al., 2016). Qualitative research has suggested that AmED consumers report engaging in ritualised forms of consumption, particularly with respect to the consumption of Jägerbombs. This ritualised consumption served the purpose of re-emphasising group solidarity norms, maintaining group bonds, and allowing self-categorisation as the 'partygoer' identity by virtue of inclusion and shared experience of intoxication, social practices, and group processes (Droste, Pennay, et al., 2016).

The Role of Environment in Social Intoxication Cultures

AmED consumers have reported a relatively narrow range of social and environmental contexts where AmED use was deemed acceptable (Droste, Pennay, et al., 2016). From a social identity standpoint, many consumers indicated that their endorsement of the social 'in-group' prototype for AmED consumption was specific to being in the right social event or scenario, and that behaving in a manner that was consistent with this identity would be inappropriate in other scenarios (Droste, Pennay, et al., 2016). Only five papers have addressed the environmental and social contexts in which AmED are consumed (Jones et al., 2012; Peacock, Bruno, & Martin, 2013; Pennay & Lubman, 2012a; Price et al., 2010; Wells et al., 2013), and three of these addressed the context indirectly (Jones et al., 2012; Peacock, Bruno, & Martin, 2013; Price et al., 2010). Generally, discussion of AmED consumption contexts is cursory in the available literature, yet these five papers have shown that the majority of AmED consumption takes place either prior to or during attendance at licensed nightlife venues.

AmED consumption most commonly occurs in venues where intoxication is highest, and which project a permissive 'anything goes' atmosphere (Droste, Miller, Pennay, Zinkiewicz, & Lubman, 2016), similarly described in previous research as encompassing swearing, overt sexual contact, rowdiness, underage patrons, and generally poor decorum expectancies (Hughes et al., 2011; Quigg et al., 2014). Consumers endorse the appropriateness of time and place as an explanation of the environments where AmED use occurs, and that AmED use must align with the desired outcome of the social event. For many, AmED use is associated with 'big nights' and the pursuit of intoxication in party contexts, with consumers matching their AmED use to suitable environmental contexts (Droste, Pennay, et al., 2016).

Research has highlighted the importance of context and setting in maximising intoxication and pleasure, a concept previously referred to as the risk environment—a space—whether social or physical—in which a variety of factors interact to increase the chances of drug-related harm (Rhodes, 2002). For example, participants attending San Francisco dance parties reported using different drugs in particular combinations in keeping with parameters and timing that they had predetermined. Participants suggested that certain drug combinations were inherently time sensitive and that synchronising the timing of different drugs was an important factor in both maximising pleasure and reducing risk (Hunt et al., 2009). Australian research with party drug users has reflected on the importance of contextual pleasures such as the corporeal experience of space and 'feeling' of the music (Duff, 2008), as well as the importance of social setting in determining the appropriate substance in the appropriate amount in the appropriate space (Pennay, 2012). Similarly, AmED consumers' endorsement and adoption of a 'party' social identity in nightclub settings can be considered as the adoption of a context-specific identity that allows individuals to engage in hedonistic, raucous behaviour, and loss of control, in situations where doing so is socially acceptable. Previously, researchers have identified nightclubs and other private parties as spaces and scenarios where partygoers may engage in socially endorsed recklessness—where alcohol and other substances may be consumed for the purposes of achieving intoxication and a controlled loss of control (Lindsay, 2009; Measham, 2004b; Pennay, 2012). In a study exploring AmED consumption contexts using observational research inside licensed venues, AmED was strongly linked to environments where heavy intoxication and risky drinking practices took place, but it was not predictive of these factors in a multivariate model (Droste, Pennay, et al., 2016). Taking into account that AmED consumption does not predict intoxication in multivariable models accounting for a range of environmental and demographic factors (see also Pennay, Miller, et al., 2015), it may be concluded that AmED consumption is more frequent in high intoxication scenarios and environments that align with consumer motives and expectancies for AmED use.

It is perhaps unsurprising that AmED consumers report hedonistic- or intoxication-driven motives for consumption, or energy and endurance motives to prolong partying; motives which have commonly been described in previous research (Peacock, Bruno, & Martin, 2013). These motives naturally align with venues such as nightclubs, where patrons engage in 'calculated hedonism', a phenomenon that describes de-stressing, escapism, deliberate recklessness, sexual and social fulfilment, or enjoying the effect of substances in particular bars, pubs, and clubs (Szmigin et al., 2008). These findings lend further support to the notion that AmED use may be purposefully targeted by consumers if their motives and expectancies align with the appropriate environmental context, for example, venues that are more permissive and compatible with intoxicated practices.

Previous sociological explorations of recreational drug use, determined drunkenness, and nightclub environments portray these behaviours and contexts as a necessary construction through which partygoers express the 'controlled loss of control' or an escape from the surveillance and regulation of modern consumer society (Measham, 2004b). Within these spaces and by pursuing intoxication, substance use is the method through which consumers and groups practice a time-out from cultural expectancies of self-regulation (Measham, 2004b). This terminology allows for the phenomenon of young people engaging in excessive alcohol consumption (i.e. determined drunkenness), while also having this behaviour contained to a specific environment, time, and social scenario (Measham, 2004a). This behaviour is not necessarily 'out of control' or irrational, but rather a controlled loss of control within appropriate spaces (clubs, private parties) where high-level intoxication and a deregulated body are deemed an appropriate transgression of cultural norms, despite increased risk of adverse consequences (Pennay, 2012). Drinking to deliberately get drunk, or 'determined drunkenness', is idealised as fun, spontaneous, and free, and it is actively pursued by many young drinkers (Keane, 2009). Outside of these environmental and social contexts, or without consideration of structural influences, the deliberate attainment of intoxication may appear irrational to outsiders.

Conclusions

AmED are typically consumed by high-risk alcohol consumers in contexts where elevated alcohol use is commonplace and where intoxication is regularly a desired outcome. AmED consumers positively self-identify as high-risk drinkers and identify as outgoing, fun, and highly sociable in party and nightclub environments. Despite a high frequency of self-reported negative physiological side effects, AmED consumers continue to engage in AmED use due to the importance they place upon the desired effects of the drink, be they social, functional, or purely pharmacological.

A core question in the AmED literature has been whether EDs interact with alcohol to affect consumption outcomes and behaviour and levels of intoxication. We suggest that researchers seeking to generalise the findings of laboratory studies to the consumption of AmED in naturalistic scenarios must consider the social, functional, and environmental drivers of AmED use, and their interplay. Regardless of the pharmacological effects or behavioural outcomes that may be demonstrated in laboratory settings, the current body of research suggests AmED use commonly occurs within specific environmental contexts (e.g. nightclubs or private parties) where intoxication is most often a key motivation for use.

Note

1. For readers seeking a more comprehensive summary of the available research, we refer to a growing number of systematic and narrative-based literature reviews (e.g. Benson et al., 2014; Ferré & O'Brien, 2011; Marczinski & Fillmore, 2014; McKetin et al., 2015; Peacock et al., 2014; Vida & Rácz, 2014).

References

Arria, A. M., & O'Brien, M. C. (2011). The "high" risk of energy drinks. *Journal of the American Medical Association, 305*(6), 600–601. https://doi.org/10.1001/jama.2011.109

Australian and New Zealand Food Regulation Standing Committee. (2013). *Food regulation policy options paper: The regulation of caffeine in foods*. FRSC Caffeine Working Group.

Benson, S., Verster, J. C., Alford, C., & Scholey, A. (2014). Effects of mixing alcohol with caffeinated beverages on subjective intoxication: A systematic review and meta-analysis. *Neuroscience and Biobehavioral Reviews, 47*, 16–21. https://doi.org/10.1016/j.neubiorev.2014.07.008

Bonar, E. E., Cunningham, R. M., Polshkova, S., Chermack, S. T., Blow, F. C., & Walton, M. A. (2015). Alcohol and energy drink use among adolescents seeking emergency department care. *Addictive Behaviors, 43*, 11–17. https://doi.org/10.1016/j.addbeh.2014.11.023

Brache, K., & Stockwell, T. (2011). Drinking patterns and risk behaviors associated with combined alcohol and energy drink consumption in college drinkers. *Addictive Behaviors, 36*(12), 1133–1140. https://doi.org/10.1016/j.addbeh.2011.07.003

Brache, K., Thomas, G., & Stockwell, T. (2012). *Caffeinated alcoholic beverages in Canada: Prevalence of use, risks and recommended policy responses*. Ottawa: Canadian Centre on Substance Abuse.

Cooper, M. L. (1994). Motivations for alcohol use among adolescents: Development and validation of a four-factor model. *Psychological Assessment, 6*(2), 117–128. https://doi.org/10.1037/1040-3590.6.2.117

de Haan, L., de Haan, H., van der Palen, J., Olivier, B., & Verster, J. (2012). Effects of consuming alcohol mixed with energy drinks versus consuming alcohol only on overall alcohol consumption and negative alcohol-related consequences. *International Journal of General Medicine, 5*(1), 953–960. https://doi.org/10.2147/IJGMS38020

Droste, N., Miller, P., Pennay, A., Zinkiewicz, L., & Lubman, D. I. (2016). Environmental contexts of combined alcohol and energy drink use: Associations with intoxication in licensed venues. *International Journal of Drug Policy, 36*, 58–66. https://doi.org/10.1016/j.drugpo.2016.06.016

Droste, N., Peacock, A., Bruno, R., Pennay, A., Zinkiewicz, L., Lubman, D. I., & Miller, P. (2017). Combined use of alcohol and energy drinks: Dose relationship with self-reported physiological stimulation and sedation side effects. *Addictive Behaviors, 71*, 68–74. https://doi.org/10.1016/j.addbeh.2017.02.031

Droste, N., Pennay, A. E., Lubman, D. I., Zinkiewicz, L., Peacock, A., & Miller, P. (2016). The right place at the right time: The social contexts of combined alcohol and energy drink use. *Drugs: Education, Prevention and Policy*, 1–12. https://doi.org/10.3109/09687637.2016.1156650

Droste, N., Tonner, L., Zinkiewicz, L., Pennay, A., Lubman, D. I., & Miller, P. (2014). Combined alcohol and energy drink use: Motivations as predictors of consumption patterns, risk of alcohol dependence, and experience of injury and aggression. *Alcoholism: Clinical and Experimental Research, 38*(7), 2087–2095. https://doi.org/10.1111/acer.12438

Duff, C. (2008). The pleasure in context. *International Journal of Drug Policy, 19*(5), 384–392. https://doi.org/10.1016/j.drugpo.2007.07.003

Ferré, S., & O'Brien, M. C. (2011). Alcohol and caffeine: The perfect storm. *Journal of Caffeine Research, 1*(3), 153–162. https://doi.org/10.1089/jcr.2011.0017

Ferreira, S. E., de Mello, M. T., Pompeia, S., & Souza-Formigoni, M. L. O. (2004). Can energy drinks affect the effects of alcoholic beverages? A study with users. *Revista da Associacao Medica Brasileira, 50*(1), 48–51. https://doi.org/10.1590/S0104-42302004000100034

Ferreira, S. E., Tulio de Mello, M., Pompeia, S., & de Souza-Formigoni, M. L. (2006). Effects of energy drink ingestion on alcohol intoxication. *Alcoholism: Clinical and Experimental Research, 30*(4), 598–605. https://doi.org/10.1111/j.1530-0277.2006.00070.x

Forward, J., Akhurst, J., Bruno, R., Leong, X., VanderNiet, A., Bromfield, H., … Peacock, A. (2017). Nature versus intensity of intoxication: Co-ingestion of alcohol and energy drinks and the effect on objective and subjective intoxication. *Drug and Alcohol Dependence, 180*, 292–303. https://doi.org/10.1016/j.drugalcdep.2017.08.013

Fry, M.-L. (2011). Seeking the pleasure zone: Understanding young adult's intoxication culture. *Australasian Marketing Journal (AMJ), 19*(1), 65–70. https://doi.org/10.1016/j.ausmj.2010.11.009

Goulding, C., Shankar, A., Elliott, R., & Canniford, R. (2009). The Marketplace Management of Illicit Pleasure. *Journal of Consumer Research, 35*(5), 759–771. https://doi.org/10.1086/592946

Gunja, N., & Brown, J. A. (2012). Energy drinks: Health risks and toxicity. *Medical Journal of Australia, 196*(1), 46–49. https://doi.org/10.5694/mja11.10838

Hughes, K., Quigg, Z., Bellis, M. A., Calafat, A., van Hasselt, N., Kosir, M., … Juan, M. (2012). Drunk and disorganised: Relationships between bar characteristics and customer intoxication in European drinking environments. *International Journal of Environmental Research and Public Health, 9*(11), 4068–4082. https://doi.org/10.3390/ijerph9114068

Hughes, K., Quigg, Z., Eckley, L., Bellis, M., Jones, L., Calafat, A., … van Hasselt, N. (2011). Environmental factors in drinking venues and alcohol-related harm: The evidence base for European intervention. *Addiction, 106(Suppl 1)*, 37–46. https://doi.org/10.1111/j.1360-0443.2010.03316.x

Hunt, G., & Evans, K. (2008). "The great unmentionable": Exploring the pleasures and benefits of ecstasy from the perspectives of drug users. *Drugs (Abingdon, England), 15*(4), 329–349. https://doi.org/10.1080/09687630701726841

Hunt, G. P., Bailey, N., Evans, K., & Moloney, M. (2009). Combining different substances in the dance scene: Enhancing pleasure, managing risk and timing effects. *Journal of Drug Issues, 39*(3), 495–522. https://doi.org/10.1177/002204260903900303

Jones, S., Barrie, L., & Berry, N. (2012). Why (not) alcohol energy drinks? A qualitative study with Australian university students. *Drug and Alcohol Review, 31*(3), 281–287. https://doi.org/10.1111/j.1465-3362.2011.00319.x

Keane, H. (2009). Intoxication, harm, and pleasure: An analysis of the Australian National Alcohol Strategy. *Critical Public Health, 19*, 135–142. https://doi.org/10.1080/09581590802350957

Larimer, M. E., Turner, A. P., Mallett, K. A., & Geisner, I. M. (2004). Predicting drinking behavior and alcohol-related problems among fraternity and sorority members: Examining the role of descriptive and injunctive norms. *Psychology of Addictive Behaviors, 18*(3), 203–212. https://doi.org/10.1037/0893-164X.18.3.203

Levy, G., & Tapsell, L. (2007). Shifts in purchasing patterns of non-alcoholic, water-based beverages in Australia, 1997–2006. *Nutrition & Dietetics, 64*(4), 268–279. https://doi.org/10.1111/j.1747-0080.2007.00223.x

Lindsay, J. (2009). Young Australians and the staging of intoxication and self-control. *Journal of Youth Studies, 12*(4), 371–384. https://doi.org/10.1080/13676260902866520

Mallett, K. A., Scaglione, N., Reavy, R., & Turrisi, R. (2015). Longitudinal patterns of alcohol mixed with energy drink use among college students and their associations with risky drinking and problems. *Journal of Studies on Alcohol and Drugs, 76*(3), 389–396. https://doi.org/10.15288/jsad.2015.76.389

Marczinski, C. A. (2011). Alcohol mixed with energy drinks: Consumption patterns and motivations for use in U.S. college students. *International Journal of Environmental Research and Public Health, 8*(*8*), 3232–3245. https://doi.org/10.3390/ijerph8083232

Marczinski, C. A., & Fillmore, M. T. (2006). Clubgoers and their trendy cocktails: Implications of mixing caffeine into alcohol on information processing and subjective reports of intoxication. *Experimental and Clinical Psychopharmacology, 14*(4), 450–458. https://doi.org/10.1037/1064-1297.14.4.450

Marczinski, C. A., & Fillmore, M. T. (2014). Energy drinks mixed with alcohol: What are the risks? *Nutrition Reviews, 72*(*Suppl 1*), 98–107. https://doi.org/10.1111/nure.12127

Marczinski, C. A., Fillmore, M. T., Bardgett, M. E., & Howard, M. A. (2011). Effect of energy drinks mixed with alcohol on behavioral control: Risks for college students consuming trendy cocktails. *Alcoholism: Clinical and Experimental Research, 35*(7), 1282–1292. https://doi.org/10.1111/j.1530-0277.2011.01464.x

Marczinski, C. A., Fillmore, M. T., Henges, A. L., Ramsey, M. A., & Young, C. R. (2011). Effects of energy drinks mixed with alcohol on information processing, motor coordination and subjective reports of intoxication. *Experimental and Clinical Psychopharmacology, 20*(2), 129–138. https://doi.org/10.1037/a0026136

Marczinski, C. A., Fillmore, M. T., Henges, A. L., Ramsey, M. A., & Young, C. R. (2013). Mixing an energy drink with an alcoholic beverage increases motivation for more alcohol in college students. *Alcoholism: Clinical and Experimental Research, 37*(2), 276–283. https://doi.org/10.1111/j.1530-0277.2012.01868.x

Martens, M. P., Rocha, T. L., Martin, J. L., & Serrao, H. F. (2008). Drinking motives and college students: Further examination of a four-factor model. *Journal of Counseling Psychology, 55*(2), 289–295. https://doi.org/10.1037/0022-0167.55.2.289

Martz, M. E., Patrick, M. E., & Schulenberg, J. E. (2015). Alcohol mixed with energy drink use among U.S. 12th-grade students: Prevalence, correlates, and associations with unsafe driving. *Journal of Adolescent Health, 56*(5), 557–563. https://doi.org/10.1016/j.jadohealth.2015.01.019

Marzell, M., Turrisi, R., Mallett, K., Ray, A. E., & Scaglione, N. M. (2014). Combining alcohol and energy drinks: An examination of psychosocial constructs and alcohol outcomes among college students using a longitudinal design. *Addiction Research and Theory, 22*(2), 91–97. https://doi.org/10.3109/16066359.2013.804510

McKetin, R., & Coen, A. (2014). The effect of energy drinks on the urge to drink alcohol in young adults. *Alcoholism: Clinical and Experimental Research, 38*(8), 2279–2285. https://doi.org/10.1111/acer.12498

McKetin, R., Coen, A., & Kaye, S. (2015). A comprehensive review of the effects of mixing caffeinated energy drinks with alcohol. *Drug and Alcohol Dependence, 151*, 15–30. https://doi.org/10.1016/j.drugalcdep.2015.01.047

Measham, F. (2004a). The decline of ecstasy, the rise of 'binge' drinking and the persistence of pleasure. *Probation Journal, 51*(4), 309–326. https://doi.org/10.1177/0264550504048220

Measham, F. (2004b). Play space: Historical and socio-cultural reflections on drugs, licensed leisure locations, commercialisation and control. *International Journal of Drug Policy, 15*(5–6), 337–345. https://doi.org/10.1016/j.drugpo.2004.08.002

Measham, F., & Brain, K. (2005). 'Binge' drinking, British alcohol policy and the new culture of intoxication. *Crime, Media, Culture: An International Journal, 1*(3), 262–283.

O'Brien, M. C., McCoy, T. P., Rhodes, S. D., Wagoner, A., & Wolfson, M. (2008). Caffeinated cocktails: Energy drink consumption, high-risk drinking, and alcohol-related consequences among college students. *Academic Emergency Medicine, 15*(5), 453–460. https://doi.org/10.1111/j.1553-2712.2008.00085.x

Olsen, A. (2009). Consuming e: Ecstasy use and contemporary social life. *Contemporary Drug Problems, 36*(1–2), 175–191. https://doi.org/10.1177/009145090903600109

Patrick, M. E., Evans-Polce, R. J., & Maggs, J. L. (2014). Use of alcohol mixed with energy drinks as a predictor of alcohol-related consequences two years later. *Journal of Studies on Alcohol and Drugs, 75*(5), 753–757. https://doi.org/10.15288/jsad.2014.75.753

Patrick, M. E., & Maggs, J. L. (2013). Energy drinks and alcohol: Links to alcohol behaviors and consequences across 56 days. *Journal of Adolescent Health, 54*(4), 454–459. https://doi.org/10.1016/j.jadohealth.2013.09.013

Peacock, A., Bruno, R., & Martin, F. H. (2013). Patterns of use and motivations for consuming alcohol mixed with energy drinks. *Psychology of Addictive Behaviors, 27*(1), 202–206. https://doi.org/10.1037/a0029985

Peacock, A., Bruno, R., Martin, F. H., & Carr, A. (2013). The impact of alcohol and energy drink consumption on intoxication and risk-taking behavior. *Alcoholism: Clinical and Experimental Research, 37*(7), 1234–1242. https://doi.org/10.1111/acer.12086

Peacock, A., Cash, C., & Bruno, R. (2015). Cognitive impairment following consumption of alcohol with and without energy drinks. *Alcoholism: Clinical and Experimental Research, 39*(4), 733–742. https://doi.org/10.1111/acer.12680

Peacock, A., Droste, N., Pennay, A., Lubman, D. I., Miller, P., Newcombe, D., & Bruno, R. (2015). Self-reported risk-taking behavior during matched-frequency sessions of alcohol versus combined alcohol and energy drinks consumption: Does co-ingestion increase risk-taking? *Alcoholism: Clinical and Experimental Research, 39*(5), 911–918. https://doi.org/10.1111/acer.12700

Peacock, A., Droste, N., Pennay, A., Miller, P., Lubman, D. I., & Bruno, R. (2015). Typology of alcohol mixed with energy drink consumers: Motivations for use. *Alcoholism: Clinical and Experimental Research, 39*(6), 1083–1092. https://doi.org/10.1111/acer.12729

Peacock, A., Pennay, A., Droste, N., Bruno, R., & Lubman, D. (2014). 'High' risk? A systematic review of the acute outcomes of mixing alcohol with energy drinks. *Addiction, 109*(10), 1612–1633. https://doi.org/10.1111/add.12622

Pennay, A. (2010). *"What goes up must go down": Exploring the harms experienced by a group of heavy ecstasy users in Melbourne and discussing the implications for harm reduction*. Paper presented at the 3rd International MDMA Conference, Melbourne, Australia.

Pennay, A. (2012). Carnal pleasures and grotesque bodies: Regulating the body during a 'big night out' of alcohol and party drug use. *Contemporary Drug Problems, 39*(Fall), 397–428. https://doi.org/10.1177/009145091203900304

Pennay, A., Cheetham, A., Droste, N., Miller, P., Lloyd, B., Pennay, D., … Lubman, D. I. (2015). An examination of the prevalence, consumer profiles, and patterns of energy drink use, with and without alcohol, in Australia. *Alcoholism: Clinical and Experimental Research, 39*(8), 1485–1492. https://doi.org/10.1111/acer.12764

Pennay, A., & Lubman, D. (2012a). Alcohol and energy drinks: A pilot study exploring patterns of consumption, social contexts, benefits and harms. *BMC Research Notes, 5*(369). https://doi.org/10.1186/1756-0500-5-369

Pennay, A., & Lubman, D. I. (2012b). More Australian research needed into alcohol and energy drinks. *Drug and Alcohol Review, 31*(7), 928–929. https://doi.org/10.1111/j.1465-3362.2012.00483.x

Pennay, A., Miller, P., Busija, L., Jenkinson, R., Droste, N., Quinn, B., … Lubman, D. I. (2015). 'Wide Awake Drunkenness'? Investigating the association between alcohol intoxication and stimulant use in the night-time economy. *Addiction, 110*(2), 356–365. https://doi.org/10.1111/add.12742

Price, S. R., Hilchey, C. A., Darredeau, C., Fulton, H. G., & Barrett, S. P. (2010). Energy drink co-administration is associated with increased reported alcohol ingestion. *Drug and Alcohol Review, 29*(3), 331–333. https://doi.org/10.1111/j.1465-3362.2009.00163.x

Quigg, Z., Hughes, K., Bellis, M. A., van Hasselt, N., Calafat, A., Košir, M., … Goossens, F. X. (2014). Incidents of harm in European drinking environments and relationships with venue and customer characteristics. *International Journal of Alcohol and Drug Research, 3*(4), 7. https://doi.org/10.7895/ijadr.v3i4.180

Reissig, C. J., Strain, E. C., & Griffiths, R. R. (2009). Caffeinated energy drinks – A growing problem. *Drug and Alcohol Dependence, 99*, 1–10. https://doi.org/10.1016/j.drugalcdep.2008.08.001

Rhodes, T. (2002). The 'risk environment': A framework for understanding and reducing drug-related harm. *International Journal of Drug Policy, 13*(2), 85–94.

Siegel, S. (2011). The Four-Loko effect. *Perspectives on Psychological Science, 6*(4), 357–362. https://doi.org/10.1177/1745691611409243

Szmigin, I., Griffin, C., Mistral, W., Bengry-Howell, A., Weale, L., & Hackley, C. (2008). Re-framing 'binge drinking' as calculated hedonism: Empirical evidence from the UK. *International Journal of Drug Policy, 19*(5), 359–366. https://doi.org/10.1016/j.drugpo.2007.08.009

Thombs, D. L., O'Mara, R. J., Tsukamoto, M., Rossheim, M. E., Weiler, R. M., Merves, M. L., & Goldberger, B. A. (2010). Event-level analyses of energy drink consumption and alcohol intoxication in bar patrons. *Addictive Behaviors, 35*(4), 325–330. https://doi.org/10.1016/j.addbeh.2009.11.004

Verkooijen, K. T., de Vries, N. K., & Nielsen, G. A. (2007). Youth crowds and substance use: The impact of perceived group norm and multiple group identification. *Psychology of Addictive Behaviors, 21*(1), 55–61. https://doi.org/10.1037/0893-164X.21.1.55

Vida, K., & Rácz, J. (2014). Prevalence and consequences of the consumption of alcohol mixed with energy drinks: A literature review. *Journal of Caffeine Research, 5*(1), 11–30. https://doi.org/10.1089/jcr.2014.0022

Wells, B. E., Kelly, B. C., Pawson, M., LeClair, A., Parsons, J. T., & Golub, S. A. (2013). Correlates of concurrent energy drink and alcohol use among socially active adults. *The American Journal of Drug and Alcohol Abuse, 39*(1), 8–15. https://doi.org/10.3109/00952990.2012.720320

Woolsey, C., Waigandt, A., & Beck, N. C. (2010). Athletes and energy drinks: Reported risk-taking and consequences from the combined use of alcohol and energy drinks. *Journal of Applied Sport Psychology, 22*, 65–71. https://doi.org/10.1080/10413200903403324

Zajdow, G., & MacLean, S. (2014). "I just drink for that tipsy stage": Young adults and embodied management of alcohol use. *Contemporary Drug Problems, 41*(4), 522–535. https://doi.org/10.1177/0091450914567123

Zest Health Strategies. (2012). *Review of evidence on the effects and international regulation of caffeinated energy drinks*. Canberra: Department of Health and Ageing.

Part II

Diverse Intoxications

7

Sexualities and Intoxication: "To Be Intoxicated Is to Still Be Me, Just a Little Blurry"—Drugs, Enhancement and Transformation in Lesbian, Gay, Bisexual, Transgender and Queer Cultures

Kiran Pienaar, Dean Murphy, Kane Race, and Toby Lea

K. Pienaar (✉)
Department of Sociology, Faculty of Arts, School of Social Sciences, Monash University, Clayton, VIC, Australia
e-mail: kiran.pienaar@monash.edu

D. Murphy • K. Race
Department of Gender and Cultural Studies, University of Sydney, Sydney, NSW, Australia

T. Lea
German Institute for Addiction and Prevention Research (DISuP), Catholic University of Applied Sciences, North Rhine-Westphalia, Germany

Centre for Social Research in Health, The University of New South Wales, Sydney, NSW, Australia

F. Hutton (ed.), *Cultures of Intoxication*,
https://doi.org/10.1007/978-3-030-35284-4_7

Introduction

The everyday lives of Western consumers are filled with chemicals and pharmaceutical agents that are understood to perform a number of different functions. In particular, they are used to prevent and treat disease, modify bodies, enhance pleasure and, importantly for the purposes of this chapter, 'change the experience of the self in the world' (Bancroft, 2009, p. 5). Nowhere is this trend more evident than in the modification of gender and sexuality. Pharmaceuticals have become key technologies for the modification of sexed and gendered experience. For example, the clinical use of hormones is a common component of gender transition procedures (Stryker & Whittle, 2006). Similarly, in other domains of everyday life, pharmaceutical companies have developed medications that promise to transform sex and enhance lifestyle ('sexuopharmaceuticals' such as Viagra and other erectile dysfunction medications), making the use of substances for therapeutic purposes difficult to disentangle from their use for recreational and personal enhancement purposes (Race, 2009).

In line with these developments, since the 'decade of dance' in the 1990s, illicit drugs have become an increasingly familiar component of everyday culture. Illicit drug use is known to be more prevalent among lesbian, gay, bisexual, transgender and queer (LGBTQ) populations, with drug researchers describing them as 'early adopters' at the 'forefront of emergent drug trends' (Measham, Wood, Dargan, & Moore, 2011; Roxburgh, Lea, de Wit, & Degenhardt, 2016). The use of stimulants such as crystal methamphetamine has also given rise to new sexual cultures among gay men, and is associated with a range of risks (including human immunodeficiency virus [HIV] infection and drug dependence), and the emergence of new harm-reduction efforts in response (Bourne, Reid, Hickson, Torres-Rueda, & Weatherburn, 2015; Race, 2015). Here, stimulants may be used in combination with therapeutic agents (such as sexuopharmaceuticals and HIV pre-exposure prophylaxis [PrEP]) to enhance sexual experience in a manner that again mixes recreational and therapeutic functions (Holt, 2009). High rates of substance use have also been documented among lesbian and bisexual women and among transgender individuals (Leonard, Lyons, & Bariola, 2015; Roxburgh et al., 2016), but the contexts, meanings and effects of these practices remain underexplored. More specifically, little is known about the role of drug use and the pursuit of particular drug effects (such as intoxication) in transforming sexual and gendered experience.

This chapter aims to respond to these openings in the literature by exploring the dynamics of drug consumption among a diverse sample of LGBTQ Australians, with a particular focus on its role in the making of sexual and gendered identities. Drawing on 32 in-depth interviews with LGBTQ consumers, it explores how sexual and gender-diverse Australians:

1. experience drug consumption and intoxication;
2. give meaning to drug effects, including intoxication;
3. pursue particular drug effects to transform their experience of gender and/or sexuality; and
4. reproduce, complicate and disrupt norms of gender and sexuality through their consumption practices.

Given their collective history of using different drugs for a wide range of purposes, LGBTQ communities are a particularly significant site for exploring the place of drugs and intoxication in social life. More specifically, investigating drug consumption in the context of sexuality and gender variance affords unique insights into the multiplicity and range of consumption practices, and their significance for gender and sexual identities.

Intoxication, Gender and Sexuality

Within the social science literature on intoxicants, the role of drinking and intoxication in enhancing masculinity is well recognised (Hinote & Webber, 2012; Peralta, 2007). However, early social scientific accounts focussed almost exclusively on men's drinking practices and largely neglected consideration of women's experiences and the gendered meanings of intoxication more generally. In the last 30 years, a growing body of feminist social science research has explored women's drinking practices and the gendered meanings and norms surrounding intoxication (Griffin, Szmigin, Bengry-Howell, Hackley, & Mistral, 2013; Measham, 2002). This critical feminist literature offers valuable insights into the gendered dimensions of intoxication, although much remains unknown about experiences of intoxication among LGBTQ people, whose gender and sexual expression may complicate dominant norms.

Indeed, research that addresses the gendered and sexual dynamics of substance use among LGBTQ people is limited, with a few notable exceptions (e.g. Emslie, Lennox, & Ireland, 2017; Hunt, Antin, Sanders, & Sisneros, 2018; Race, 2011, 2015). Within this body of literature are studies of gay men's drug use in the 1990s and early 2000s, which explore its implications for HIV risk, health education and harm-reduction interventions (Reback, 1997; Southgate & Hopwood, 2001; Weatherburn et al., 1993). Some scholars writing at that time were critical of the normative framing of gay men's drug use as 'risky' and argued for a more nuanced understanding of sexualised drug use and the risk calculus it entails (Rhodes & Cusick, 2002; Westhaver, 2005). However, more recent research has tended to frame LGBTQ substance use as a pathology or problem with mainstream alcohol and other drug (AOD) studies characterising substance use among LGBTQ people as significantly higher and presenting greater risk than use among cisgender, heterosexual people (Hughes, 2011; Newcomb, Ryan, Greene, Garofalo, & Mustanski, 2014). The emphasis in these studies on prevalence rates, earlier age of initiation, risk and 'misuse' often frames LGBTQ drug consumption as risky, deviant and problematic. By explaining drug use amongst sexual and gender minorities as a response to stigma, marginalisation and increased prevalence of mental health issues, these accounts tend to reduce it to an individual pathology, associated with other problems. Not only does this understanding overlook the other social and structural issues contributing to increased AOD consumption amongst LGBTQ people, it also neglects the pleasures and benefits substance use can afford. Importantly for our purposes, such research does not address the generative role of drugs in shaping sexuality and gender and in contributing to alternative socio-sexual cultures. Hunt et al. make this point in relation to LGBTQ alcohol use, but we suggest that it applies to queer drug use more generally:

> When a focus on queer alcohol use is reduced to problems and pathologies, important structural and sociological issues are neglected and under-theorized, including the meanings and pleasures of alcohol consumption, the experiences of intoxication, and the relationships between alcohol use, social groups, sexuality, sociability, notions of space, and identity constructions. (2018, p. 3)

Apart from the often pathologising framing of drug use in mainstream AOD research, much research on intoxication tends to focus on *youth drinking* and the related phenomena of 'drinking cultures' (Järvinen & Room, 2007) and 'cultures of intoxication' (Griffin et al., 2013). While contributing valuable perspectives on the gendering of youth drinking cultures (Hutton, Wright, & Saunders, 2013; Leyshon, 2008), and the pleasures of intoxication for young people (Murphy, Wilson, & Moore, 2017; Niland, Lyons, Goodwin, & Hutton, 2013), this literature leaves open questions about the experiences and meanings of intoxication in relation to other substances and for people of diverse ages.

With the exception of the feminist literature cited above, mainstream AOD research has also tended to ignore important developments in gender and queer theory and 'continues to be dominated by a heteronormative and binary gender discourse that considers masculinity and femininity exclusively as opposites and associates them with essentially male and female sexed bodies' (Hunt et al., 2018, p. 2). Building on these critiques and taking up the call by Hunt and Antin (2017, p. 7) to 'step outside the confines of binary normative notions of gender', this chapter aims to generate much-needed new insights into the lived experiences of LGBTQ people who consume drugs to transform their gender and/or sexual experience.

Performativity and Drug 'Effects'

Our analysis applies concepts from the fields of gender studies, and science and technology studies (STS), to theorise the relations between drugs, intoxication, gender and sexuality. A key concept underpinning our work is 'performativity'. First elaborated by Judith Butler (1999) in her influential book *Gender Trouble*, the notion of performativity challenges the sex-gender distinction and its assumption of a 'natural' body that pre-exists its inscription by culture. This familiar view, Butler argues, relies on a problematic conception of the body as an inert blank slate on which culture inscribes its mark in the form of gender. Challenging this understanding, Butler's performativity refigures gender as an iterative effect of discourse, produced through the repetition of discursive practices. In other words, Butler credits language (or discourse) with having constitutive power. As Salih (2007, p. 56) puts it, 'gender identities are constructed and constituted by language, which means that there is no gender identity that precedes language'. The notion of performativity has since been elaborated by feminist science studies scholar Barad (2003), whose work offers an expanded account of performativity that engages the role of both material and discursive practices in the process of materialisation. Applied to this study, 'performativity' refers to the constitutive role of material and discursive phenomena in making realities. In the context of LGBTQ drug use, these phenomena may include the body, gender, sex, desire, play, risk, care and pleasure.

Our conception of drugs and their 'effects' aligns with the notion of performativity but is also informed by work in the field of STS. Challenging the commonplace view of drugs as stable entities with unique chemical properties that act to produce certain effects, we proceed on the understanding that the action of drugs and their purported effects are produced in relation to various other actors, contexts and practices (Race, 2014). On this rethinking, the effects of a particular drug are not inherent properties of that substance, but they are shaped by networks of other phenomena usually thought to be separate from, if not irrelevant to, the drug itself (Fraser, Moore, & Keane, 2014). Within this approach, the materiality of drugs is understood to be emergent, rather than fixed. That is, drugs and their effects are brought into being and changed in their encounters with other phenomena including individual bodies, gender norms, sexual practices, pleasure and intimacy. In line with this view, we define 'intoxication' as the ways in which individuals use psychoactive substances to '*manage, maintain or change the experience of the self in the world*' (Bancroft, 2009, p. 5, emphasis added). Importantly, like other drug effects, intoxication is socioculturally constituted: it materialises in relation to an array of sociocultural factors including the social setting in which a drug is consumed, its legal status and cultural norms governing its use.

This relational approach to drugs has informed recent AOD research on topics such as drinking practices and 'alcohol effects' (Hart, 2015; Poulson, 2015), contexts of illicit drug use (Dilkes-Frayne, 2016; Farrugia, 2015) and addiction (Fraser et al., 2014; Pienaar et al., 2015). Building on this literature and its commitment to challenging pharmacological determinism, the analysis presented here tracks the variety of forces and actors that produce the phenomena of intoxication, sexuality and gender in highly specific and contextually contingent ways.

Methods

This chapter is based on data from interviews with 32 self-identified LGBTQ participants from a larger qualitative study that explores the use of substances among LGBTQ Australians to transform aspects of sexual and gender experience. Participants were recruited through the newsletters and networks of Australian LGBTQ organisations, social media posts (e.g. Facebook and Twitter), leafleting in LGBTQ health clinics and social venues as well as chain referrals. Prospective participants were screened for eligibility and to ensure diversity across age, gender, sexuality, ethnic background and drug types.

The 32 eligible participants comprised people of diverse genders and sexualities, aged between 18 and 66 years, living in New South Wales or Victoria, Australia. All described ongoing use of a range of licit and illicit drugs including alcohol, HIV antiretrovirals, hormones, cannabis, methamphetamine, methylenedioxy-methamphetamine (MDMA) and gamma-hydroxybutyrate/gamma-butyrolactone (GHB/GBL). The study was approved by the University of Sydney Human Research Ethics Committee (Approval number: 2017/735). All participants provided informed written consent. Interviews were conducted in person in urban New South Wales or Victoria, Australia, and involved a dual-method approach aimed at expanding the depth of the interview data. The interview method included a mapping exercise in which participants were asked to plot the substances they consume, and indicate the frequency of consumption (see Fig. 7.1).

The maps functioned as an elicitation and rapport-building technique for the in-depth interviews: participants were asked to identify which substances on their map were most closely related to transforming their sexual and/or gender experience, and they were then asked a series of open-ended questions about their drug use, its relevance to their gender and/or sexual experience, what they perceive particular drugs 'do' for them, their experiences of 'intoxication' (and the meanings they associate with this term) and how they manage drug use to maximise benefits and minimise potential harms.

Interviews were audio-recorded and professionally transcribed verbatim before being checked for accuracy. To protect participant identities, each was given a pseudonym and all identifying details were removed from the transcripts. The interviews were analysed using an iterative inductive approach in which the research team drew up a preliminary list

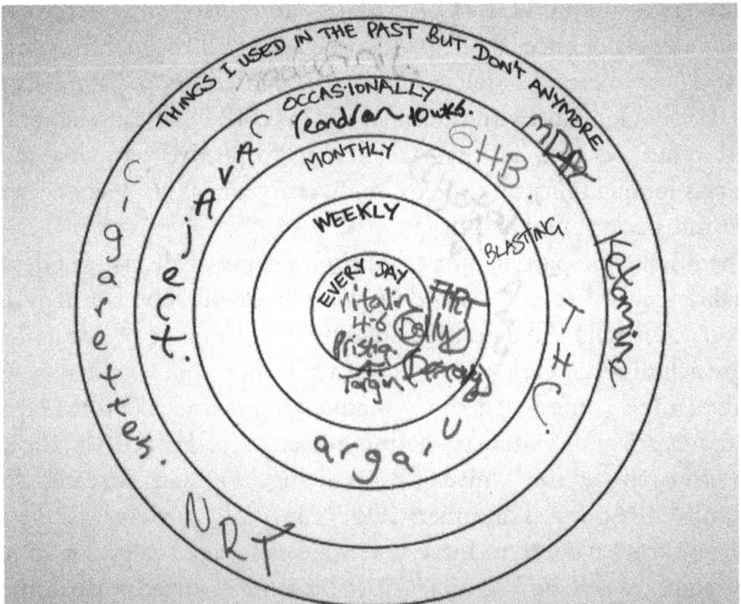

Fig. 7.1 Example of participant map. Dalston (44, gay, cis man)

of codes based on the aims of the study, as well as knowledge of key debates and past research. These codes were then tested on a subset of data, and supplementary codes were added across the data set to capture a wider range of themes derived from the interviews themselves. The data were coded using the software programme NVivo.

We use the following conventions when presenting qualitative data in the chapter: **Bold text** indicates interviewer speech; square brackets indicate words that have been edited for the purposes of clarity or de-identification in the original verbatim transcript (e.g. [this city]); ellipses [...] indicate that some words from the transcript have been omitted. Accompanying each quotation is basic information about the participant quoted, including their **age, and their self-identified sexuality and gender**, for example, *Mira* ***(25, queer, trans woman)***.[1]

In the analysis that follows, we begin by exploring the ways in which LGBTQ drug consumers articulate intoxication in terms of the meanings they ascribe to it. We then consider accounts of intoxication in sexual contexts, emphasising the ways in which drug use enhances pleasure, increases stamina and transforms the experience of the sexual-gendered body. In doing so, we highlight the performativity of drug practices in terms of how they are said to alter experiences of the body, the self and its relation to others. Finally, we discuss the dynamics of intoxication and gender, highlighting the role of drug use in materialising gender beyond the male/female binary. We argue that in the context of LGBTQ cultures, drug practices generate sensual pleasures, altered subjectivities and novel forms of sociality that are otherwise inaccessible or unintelligible. We conclude by reflecting on the implications of our findings for LGBTQ health policy and service provision.

Analysis

Ontologies of Intoxication

To explore the meanings that LGBTQ consumers ascribe to 'intoxication', participants were asked to describe their associations with the term and how it relates to their own experiences of particular drug effects. Unsurprisingly, given the cultural links between intoxication and alcohol use, many participants connected it exclusively to the effects of excessive drinking:

> If you say, 'you are intoxicated', I say you're pissed on alcohol. I wouldn't associate that with any form of drug-taking at all […] If you're intoxicated, it means that […] you've had too much alcohol.
>
> Devon (53, gay, cis man)

> **I: When I say the word 'intoxication' what comes to mind?** […]
>
> R: I would say alcohol. That is, I mean, that's the only kind of setting that I would hear the word used, especially like 'intoxication' is specifically like, 'you are too drunk, you must leave the premises'.
>
> Benjamin (37, gay, cis man)

Invoking the etymology of 'intoxication' from the Latin *intoxicātus* meaning 'steeped in poison' (Rivas, 2015), the concept was seen as carrying connotations of toxicity. Several questioned these connotations on the basis that they obscure the 'fun' and pleasures that drug use can afford:

> 'Intoxicated' for me kind of goes back to toxicity. And we talk about toxicity as this kind of very negative thing, that's an awful thing. So being intoxicated ultimately is […] toxic, it's horrible. That's a very awkward descriptor, I find, for that because I don't like to think of my experiences, you know, the ones I'm enjoying as negative or as toxic […] From a clinical stance, sure, you're putting weird substances in your body that have some kind of toxicity and toxic effect, but as […] a user of those substances, they're fun, they're fun things.
>
> Dudley (38, gay, cis man)

> I guess the word 'intoxicated' to me […] just doesn't describe the experience. And […] the person who uses the word, 'intoxicated' is […] either pretending or have no experience of actually being under the influence of some sort of drug […] Just trying to sort of box it off […] *I think it's just state change and there are so many different ways of changing one's state, whether it's through the influence of some sort of chemical or you know like*

meditation or breath work or dreaming or whatever. Like they're all just, it's all just, state change. It's all just part of that spectrum of consciousness.

Nico (40, queer, non-binary person, emphasis added)

Nico's comment resonates with the broad definition of intoxication proposed by Bancroft (2009) as involving a range of practices aimed at changing one's consciousness, including prayers, psychotherapy, ritual scarring and, of course, the use of drugs. Like Nico, many participants commented on the transformative effects of drugs on their subjectivity and consciousness. Drug use was described not only as a means of altering consciousness but as softening the hard edges of reality. This is perhaps best captured by Byron (27, gay, cis man) who states that 'to be intoxicated [...] is to still be me, just a little blurry'. This blurring invokes the notion of the boundary between the self and the world becoming less clear, which for marginalised groups might be considered a particularly welcome effect.

Consistent with some of the sociological literature on the benefits and transformative effects of drug use (Duff, 2008; Peralta, 2008), several participants emphasised the ways in which consuming their preferred drug transports them beyond the domain of everyday life, enabling the suspension of social norms and the possibility of greater emotional openness:

> With MDMA and LSD, I will pre-emptively warn [my friends]. I'll be like, 'Hey so I'm going to be intoxicated tonight, do not be surprised if I send you a long-winded rambling message about how much I love you', which has happened and will happen again in the future.
>
> (Mira, 25, queer, trans woman)

This sense of connection was a common theme in participants' accounts of drug practices, whether in relation to connecting with friends, sexual partners or indeed with oneself. A number of participants spoke of the ways in which the experience of intoxication prompted self-reflection and greater self-awareness. This was particularly salient for several of the study's gender-diverse participants in relation to lysergic acid diethylamide (LSD), as the following quotes illustrate:

> LSD tends to make me internalise sort of lessons about myself and really work through them; [It helps with] personal realisations, that kind of thing.
>
> Roux (22, homoromantic,[2] trans woman)

> LSD has been really good [...] for me unpacking a lot of things in terms of my gender and sexuality. Like stuff that I may not even be aware that I'm holding on to. I've kind of like described LSD in terms of like how it interacts with trauma [...] Trauma is like this red-hot pan: if you touch it sober, it will burn you because that's what trauma does. But LSD is kind of this soft cushion that allows you to interact with it safely [...] and often times lets you talk through it a lot, especially within yourself.
>
> Mira (25, queer, trans woman)

When asked which term(s) they use to capture the effects of the drugs they consume, many participants eschewed the word 'intoxication' to articulate their experiences because of its negatively freighted meanings, lack of specificity and its association with clinical and public health discourses which construct intoxication as harmful and risky (Keane, 2009). Instead, they opted for more positive, colloquial terms to describe the desired effects of their preferred drugs, such as 'mellow', 'enhanced' (Arya, 57, polyamorous, genderqueer person), 'high' (Enzo, 18, gay, trans man), 'rolling' (Benjamin, 37, gay, cis man), 'wired' (Bertie, 32, gay, cis man) and 'sparkly' (Emery, 43, queer, non-binary person). Participants commonly pointed out the specificity of the terms they use, highlighting that they vary according to the drug, mode of administration and the setting in which it is consumed:

> I would say 'high' for weed [...] For the others, it really depends. Like, for LSD it's 'tripping', for MDMA 'rolling' [...] It's sort of different terminology for everything [...] 'shrooms would also be 'tripping'. Like 'tripping' is like psychedelics [...] There is pretty much always a word that I can use that's going to sum it up.
>
> Maddox (19, queer, non-binary person)

The range of terms participants used to articulate particular drug effects highlight the contingency and specificity of drug experiences, which are not captured by the generic, negatively freighted concept of 'intoxication'. As Bancroft (2009, p. 194) puts it, 'Intoxicants are social substances, and intoxication is a social practice...These technologies of the self produce very different meanings, actions and experience depending on the substance, its form and the conditions of its consumption'.

Drug-Mediated/Enhanced Pleasures: Intoxication, Play and Sex

Many of our participants took drugs in sexual contexts and described the dynamics between particular chemical practices and the experience of sex. Sexualised drug use was valued for its capacity to generate new ways of relating to sexual partners, to experiment with what the body can do and to express gender. A key theme in participants' accounts of sexualised drug use was the role of intoxicants in enhancing the experience of sex by amplifying the intensity and pleasure of play sessions:

> I just still love having sex on MDMA [...] Like you'd come home from the club, you're feeling a lot kind of sweaty and clammy and a little bit tired, and then I might like smoke a joint or have a bong. And that kind of like brings back but also takes off the edge and then you just have this kind of crazy sex.
>
> Julian (33, queer, cis man)

> [Crystal meth] has an immediate impact on me, it just totally, totally overwhelms me with sexual feelings [...] and desire and every possible warm, wonderful feeling.
>
> Van (66, gay, cis man)

Elaborating on the sexual effects of their preferred drugs, some participants commented that these drugs increase their sexual confidence, prowess and comfort:

> I feel like sexually [GHB] makes me feel really empowered and confident, which has been fun. It kind of makes sex more comfortable for me if I'm

> bottoming[3] as well […] I've probably found that I can have like much longer sex in terms of comfort when I've been on GHB.
>
> Avery (31, gay, fluid cis man)

Others described how crystal methamphetamine increases sexual endurance and creates a 'sensuously dilated temporality' (Race, forthcoming) in which sexual encounters are extended beyond the point of orgasm:

> [Crystal] lengthens [play sessions] time-wise, definitely, yeah. And even if you do come, you still want to keep going and going […] So you can quite easily go for 12 or 24 or 36 hours. And […] if you do come, that doesn't make you stop and think, 'Okay, now I'm going to make you a cup of tea and have a cigarette', if you know what I mean. You still want to keep going.
>
> Corey (59, gay, cis man)

These accounts of drug-enhanced sexual pleasures resonate with popular media depictions of 'chemsex', although without the negative, sensationalised undertones all too often present in popular representations (e.g. the 2015 documentary *Chemsex*; Flynn, 2015). Indeed, as other scholars have observed, in popular representations of chemsex, the combination of sex, drugs and digital media (notably 'hookup applications') is depicted as giving rise to 'horrible monsters "the walking dead" (Fairman & Gogarty, 2015)—in a frenzy of cultural production that seizes upon the most disturbing casualties of this mix of practices' (Race, 2017, p. 129; see also Race, Lea, Murphy, & Pienaar, 2016). Not only are such depictions overdetermined and one-dimensional, they disavow the possibility that sexualised drug use, though not without risks, can actually contribute to sexual pleasure, intimacy and connection. In contrast to these normative popular discourses, our participants' accounts emphasise the generative effects of drugs and, in so doing, challenge the negative associations with both sexualised drug use and intoxication.

Particularly valued for some LGBTQ consumers was the capacity of particular intoxicants to enhance and transform the experience of the body. This was especially striking for some gender-diverse participants who described how drugs allow them to connect with their bodies in ways that 'remove a lot of gender dysphoria', enable self-acceptance and enhance the experience of sex. One participant commented on this in some depth:

> I've had sex on both MDMA and LSD wildly [...] I like both for different reasons actually because MDMA is amazing at removing a lot of gender dysphoria [...] I have a very complicated relationship with my genitals especially with their functionality because a lot of time [my gender] doesn't match with that [...] But with MDMA it just feels great [...] because you know, you don't have that same anxiety. You don't have that same internal narrative. It allows you to connect to your physical form and your sexuality a lot easier [...] It's just like MD is good for [...] accepting the equipment that I have now [...] And universally it has been a deeply emotional experience. There's a lot of crying usually, because just like overwhelming happiness. It' just like, 'Oh my god, something like this feels so good and so right' [...] So often, you can feel like that you're mismatched wires [...] and just for a little while to feel like everything just works, that is an amazingly fun experience and good emotionally.
>
> Mira (25, queer, trans woman)

Nico, a 40-year-old non-binary participant, makes a similar point in relation to alcohol, describing it as 'hugely beneficial' in helping overcome internalised homophobia and enjoy physical intimacy:

> So one of my girlfriends, when we first started being intimate [...] alcohol was hugely beneficial for me because there was so much shame, like internalised queer-phobia around [...] my feelings of desire for her. I just felt deeply ashamed and [...] when we were intimate, I would completely get out of my body and into my head [...] and that was such a disconnected experience it wasn't enjoyable for either of us. But when I was under the influence of drugs, I felt that shame melt away, I could just be in my body and experience it as the sensual, pleasurable experience that it was. Like without having any of those stories in my head about who we supposedly were and what we were doing, and it just felt good.
>
> Nico (40, queer, non-binary person)

Importantly, participants routinely emphasised that the consumption of their preferred drugs enabled particular sexual practices and pleasures that were otherwise inaccessible or even unthinkable while sober. In other words, our participants' accounts illuminate the performativity of drugs, their capacity to transform the body and the self in significant and often very affirming ways. They point to the role of intoxication in generating novel modes of sociality, sexual connections and sensual pleasures that transcend oppressive sexual and gender norms. For many of our participants, certain drug settings and practices effectively produced them as new or different kinds of subjects, transforming them from a member of a stigmatised group to an agentive, desiring sexual subject.

Intoxication in the Making of Gender

Our focus on the role of psychoactive drugs in shaping gender emerged from the responses of our gender-diverse participants, many of whom commented on the significance of particular drugs for transforming their gender identity. In reflecting on the relationship between chemical practices and gender transformation, Mira, a 25-year-old trans woman, described the therapeutic effects of illicit drug use, characterising it as a 'deeply personally affirming and transcendent experience':

> I think that trans people have a very unique position to hold on a lot of topics, but especially with recreational drug use because it's not just about having a great time, and not just like getting munted at the club and being a sloppy mess [...] It can be a [...] deeply personally affirming and transcendent experience [...] It's very easy to categorize recreational narcotics as being like a bunch of young kids going out, getting fucked and having fun. It's just like, 'No, it means a lot more to people'. It can mean coming to terms with your trauma. It can mean working through other emotional or mental health issues. It can mean having a moment of respite from the world feeling like it's trying to kill you. It can mean having a moment where you actually feel good about yourself for the first time in your life [...] But it means a lot to me and I don't think that I would be the person that I am today and as well-rounded and as developed as a human being as I would be if I hadn't had these experiences.
>
> Mira (25, queer, trans woman)

Another participant, Maddox, offers a similar account of the therapeutic value of intoxication, specifically in relation to the use of MDMA and how it facilitates a sense of bodily ease that they otherwise do not experience:

> [MDMA] lifts all of me up and I am able to be like, 'Okay, this is my body and I feel good in it' […] like I […] forget my main issues with my body and I think about the good things. And sometimes I will get really vain. Like I will take a bunch of selfies or something. I go, 'Oh, I look so good' […] like the way that I feel in [my body] like the smoothness, like the freedom […] If I am high in some way it […] really affects like how I look at [my body] and how I experience it, and it will make me feel better.
>
> Maddox (19, queer, non-binary person)

Here, intoxication provides a release (or as Mira puts it, a 'respite') from the self, an experience that has been characterised as 'self-forgetting' (Zajdow, 2010, p. 223). The accounts offered by Mira and Maddox challenge the common narrative of drug use as driven by self-centred hedonism. Not only does this dominant narrative demonise the use of intoxicants, it also reinforces a series of binary distinctions between medications/drugs, therapeutic/recreational use, pain/pleasure and legitimate/illegitimate. As Malins (2017, p. 129) notes, 'western medicine likes to forcibly construct and maintain [a binary] separation, framing pharmaceutical treatment for pain as empirically distinct from the illegitimate pleasures of illicit drugs'. As these accounts make clear, in reality, these distinctions do not hold: illicit drugs can be used therapeutically, just as pharmaceutical drugs can be used for recreational and pleasure-seeking purposes. Indeed, both licit and illicit drugs may be used for pain relief and pleasure at the same time. If these purposes are not treated as mutually exclusive, we can avoid reproducing the stigmatising associations of illicit drug use with hedonistic pleasure, dependence and loss of control (valentine & Fraser, 2008).

For a number of gender-diverse participants, the experience of intoxication was profoundly transformative insofar as it aligned their sense of self with their gendered body, allowing them to suspend doubts and worries about their gender expression. Others, such as Julian, credited drug use with helping him to accept his non-normative gender expression or what he calls his 'more feminine side':

> I haven't always been as comfortable with the more feminine side of me. But now I guess I understand that my more feminine qualities are actually just part of my masculinity […] Like being the sissy boy or being the effeminate boy growing up […] and not liking things that boys liked or were supposed to like, like sports and that kind of stuff […] *Maybe in some ways, my drug use was about coming to terms [and finding ….] self-acceptance […] of how my gender is expressed* [….in terms of things like being] emotional, soft […] having like a gay voice, liking to bottom, the enjoyment of the arts.
>
> Julian (33, queer, cis man, emphasis added)

Our participants' accounts of the role of drugs in transforming their sense of self, facilitating a sense of bodily ease and enabling free expression of gender identity are consistent with the recognition that intoxication allows a temporary release from social norms (Bancroft, 2009). However, while critical AOD research has amply demonstrated the role of intoxicants in offering an escape from the normative social order, relatively few studies have explored the significance of intoxication for transforming gender and sexual identity (for some examples, see Preciado, 2013; Race, 2015; Race et al., 2016). Our analysis contributes to this literature by charting the role of LGBTQ drug use in shaping sociosexual encounters and gender expression.

Remaking Intoxication: Beyond Harm, Risk and Pathology

In this chapter, we have tracked some of the ways in which drug use and experiences of intoxication shape LGBTQ identities and modes of sociability, without reifying drugs and their effects as fixed. Instead, the discussion has sought to explore the role of drug practices in forming, and transforming, the gender and sexual identities of LGBTQ people, with a particular focus on the corporeal and sensory pleasures that psychoactive drugs afford in the context of sex, sociability and intimacy. Writing about gay disco culture, Race highlights the significance of intoxication in the materialisation of socio-sexual encounters: 'No longer simply a mechanism to assuage guilt or enable sexual coupling, intoxication emerges as one aspect of a culture of playful participation and socio-sexual interaction that has a particularity of its own' (2011, p. 37). Building on this understanding, we see drug use as one practice among many that helps to materialise LGBTQ cultures and identities, rather than threatening only to erode them. By extension, we suggest that the proximity of pleasure, risk, care and intimate experimentation as prominent concerns within LGBTQ cultures offer new ways of thinking about the place of drugs and intoxication in social life.

As the accounts presented here show, the pursuit of pleasure and a desire to alter the experience of the self in the world are key reasons why many LGBTQ people are attracted to drug use. The eagerness of participants to dissociate their positive experiences of psychoactive drug use from intoxication, with its negative connotations, is understandable. But a question remains about the risks and benefits of endorsing such a move. Contrary to the AOD literature, intoxication could be understood to apply to processes set in motion by any substance with pharmacokinetic effects, including medications, rather than limited to psychoactive drug consumption. Maintaining that intoxication is implicated in the full range of drug effects, including beneficial effects such as pleasure or the restoration of health, may have specific advantages, insofar as it enacts the identity of drugs and medications as ambivalent, their particular effects an outcome of the specific relations and practices that a given occasion of consumption entails. This understanding could have the benefit of engendering an approach to drug consumption that attends more carefully to the full range of possibilities that drug consumption, of any sort, necessarily entails.

Such a rethinking has significant implications for drug policy and service provision. Unless harm-reduction efforts take the desires for pleasure and self-(trans)formation seriously, they will fail to engage with the concerns of LGBTQ consumers. Notably, LGBTQ health organisations in the jurisdictions covered by this study already have a number of innovative projects built on consumers' embodied experiences, which address the pleasures, benefits and transformative value of drug use, alongside its potential risks and harms (Burgess, Parkhill, Wiggins, Ruth, & Stoové, 2018; Gonçalves, Kolstee, Ryan, & Race, 2016; Stardust, Kolstee, Joksic, Gray, & Hannan, 2018). Critical drugs scholars have long argued for the need to recognise the pleasures of drug use and have critiqued the normative public health emphasis on drug-related risks and harms, arguing that it fails to resonate with embodied experiences of drug use (Moore, 2008; Race, 2009). As Malins puts it in a recent article on the place of desire and pleasure in drug practices:

> [W]hen everyday embodied experiences of drugs (as positive, pleasurable, life-affirming) fail to resonate in official discourses about them (as harmful, dangerous, unhealthy), stigma and shame are likely to increase while trust in practical, health-affirming drug messages and services is sure to diminish. Acknowledgement of pleasure, then, is crucial to understanding and adequately responding to issues related to drug use. (2017, p. 127)

Echoing this call, we highlight the pressing need for drug policy and practice to recognise not only the pleasures of drugs but also their generative role in producing socio-sexual intimacies and self-transformation in LGBTQ cultures. To do so is to begin to reckon with the complexity of drug use, its performative dimensions and the dynamic relations of gender, sexuality, pleasure and risk that shape lived experiences of drug use.

Acknowledgements The research reported in this chapter was funded by an Australian Research Council Discovery Grant (DP170101373), awarded to Kane Race, Toby Lea and Kiran Pienaar. It also benefited from the support of the Gender and Cultural Studies Program, Faculty of Arts, University of Sydney; the Faculty of Arts, Monash University and the University of New South Wales. The interviews were conducted by Dean Murphy, Kiran Pienaar and David Vakalis. The study benefited from the expertise of an advisory panel and the assistance of Australian LGBTIQ organisations. The authors thank the editor for comments on earlier drafts of this chapter. They also thank the participants for generously sharing their stories and insights—without them this research would not be possible.

Notes

1. Cisgender refers to a person whose gender conforms to the sex they were assigned at birth. For example, a cis man is a man who identifies as male and was assigned a male sex at birth. Transgender describes a person who identifies with a gender that does *not* align with the sex they were assigned at birth, for example, a trans woman is a woman who was assigned a male sex at birth but identifies as female. Genderqueer is sometimes used as an umbrella term for gender non-conforming or non-binary identities (e.g. agender, bigender and genderfluid). It describes a person who does not identify with the male/female binary and whose gender expression does not fit into a static identity category.
2. 'Homoromantic' refers to being attracted to someone of the same sex in a romantic but not necessarily sexual way.
3. 'Bottoming' refers to being the receptive partner during anal sex.

References

Bancroft, A. (2009). *Drugs, intoxication and society*. Cambridge: Polity Press.

Barad, K. (2003). Posthumanist performativity: Toward an understanding of how matter comes to matter. *Signs: Journal of Women in Culture and Society, 28*(3), 801–831.

Bourne, A., Reid, D., Hickson, F., Torres-Rueda, S., & Weatherburn, P. (2015). Illicit drug use in sexual settings ('chemsex') and HIV/STI transmission risk behaviour among gay men in South London: Findings from a qualitative study. *Sexually Transmitted Infections, 91*(8), 564–568. https://doi.org/10.1136/sextrans-2015-052052

Burgess, K., Parkhill, G., Wiggins, J., Ruth, S., & Stoové, M. (2018). Re-wired: Treatment and peer support for men who have sex with men who use methamphetamine. *Sexual Health, 15*(2), 157–159. https://doi.org/10.1071/SH17148

Butler, J. (1999). *Gender trouble: Feminism and the subversion of identity*. London: Routledge.

Dilkes-Frayne, E. (2016). Drugs at the campsite: Socio-spatial relations and drug use at music festivals. *International Journal of Drug Policy, 33*, 27–35. https://doi.org/10.1016/j.drugpo.2015.10.004

Duff, C. (2008). The pleasure in context. *International Journal of Drug Policy, 19*(5), 384–392. https://doi.org/10.1016/j.drugpo.2007.07.003

Emslie, C., Lennox, J., & Ireland, L. (2017). The role of alcohol in identity construction among LGBT people: A qualitative study. *Sociology of Health and Illness*, 1–15. https://doi.org/10.1111/1467-9566.12605
Fairman, W. & Gogarty, M. (Directors). (2015). Chemsex, UK: Vice Production.
Farrugia, A. (2015). "You can't just give your best mate a massive hug every day": Young men, play and MDMA. *Contemporary Drug Problems, 42*(3), 240–256.
Flynn, P. (2015, November 22). Addicted to chemsex: 'It's a horror story'. *The Guardian*. Retrieved from https://www.theguardian.com/world/2015/nov/22/addicted-to-chemsex-gay-drugs-film
Fraser, S., Moore, D., & Keane, H. (2014). *Habits: Remaking addiction*. Basingstoke: Palgrave Macmillan.
Gonçalves, D. M., Kolstee, J., Ryan, D., & Race, K. (2016). Harm reduction in process: The ACON Rovers, GHB, and the art of paying attention. *Contemporary Drug Problems, 43*(4), 314–330. https://doi.org/10.1177/0091450916661821
Griffin, C., Szmigin, I., Bengry-Howell, A., Hackley, C., & Mistral, W. (2013). Inhabiting the contradictions: Hypersexual femininity and the culture of intoxication among young women in the UK. *Feminism & Psychology, 23*(2), 184–206.
Hart, A. (2015). Assembling interrelations between low socioeconomic status and acute alcohol-related harms among young adult drinkers. *Contemporary Drug Problems, 42*(2), 148–156.
Hinote, B. P., & Webber, G. R. (2012). Drinking toward manhood: Masculinity and alcohol in the Former USSR. *Men and Masculinities, 15*(3), 292–310. https://doi.org/10.1177/1097184x12448466
Holt, M. (2009). 'Just take Viagra': Erectile insurance, prophylactic certainty and deficit correction in gay men's accounts of sexuopharmaceutical use. *Sexualities, 12*, 746–764. https://doi.org/10.1177/1363460709346112
Hughes, T. (2011). Alcohol use and alcohol-related problems among sexual minority women. *Alcoholism Treatment Quarterly, 29*(4), 403–435.
Hunt, G., & Antin, T. (2017). Gender and intoxication: From masculinity to intersectionality. *Drugs: Education, Prevention and Policy*, 1–9. https://doi.org/10.1080/09687637.2017.1349733
Hunt, G., Antin, T., Sanders, E., & Sisneros, M. (2018). Queer youth, intoxication and queer drinking spaces. *Journal of Youth Studies*, 1–21. https://doi.org/10.1080/13676261.2018.1508826

Hutton, F., Wright, S., & Saunders, E. (2013). Cultures of intoxication: Young women, alcohol, and harm reduction. *Contemporary Drug Problems, 40*(4), 451–480.

Järvinen, M., & Room, R. (Eds.). (2007). *Youth drinking cultures: European experiences* (Vol. 13). Aldershot: Ashgate Publishing.

Keane, H. (2009). Intoxication, harm and pleasure: An analysis of the Australian National Alcohol Strategy. *Critical Public Health, 19*(2), 135–142. https://doi.org/10.1080/09581590802350957

Leonard, W., Lyons, A., & Bariola, E. (2015). *A closer look at private lives 2: Addressing the mental health and wellbeing of lesbian, gay, bisexual, and transgender (LGBT) Australians*. Melbourne: Australian Research Centre in Sex, Health and Society (ARCSHS), La Trobe University.

Leyshon, M. (2008). 'We're stuck in the corner': Young women, embodiment and drinking in the countryside. *Drugs: Education, Prevention and Policy, 15*(3), 267–289. https://doi.org/10.1080/09687630801920286

Malins, P. (2017). Desiring assemblages: A case for desire over pleasure in critical drug studies. *International Journal of Drug Policy*. https://doi.org/10.1016/j.drugpo.2017.07.018

Measham, F. (2002). "Doing Gender" – "Doing Drugs": Conceptualizing the gendering of drugs cultures. *Contemporary Drug Problems, 29*(2), 335–373. https://doi.org/10.1177/009145090202900206

Measham, F., Wood, D. M., Dargan, P. I., & Moore, K. (2011). The rise in legal highs: Prevalence and patterns in the use of illegal drugs and first- and second-generation "legal highs" in South London gay dance clubs. *Journal of Substance Use, 16*(4), 263–272. https://doi.org/10.3109/14659891.2011.594704

Moore, D. (2008). Erasing pleasure from public discourse on illicit drugs: On the creation and reproduction of an absence. *International Journal of Drug Policy, 19*(5), 353–358.

Murphy, D. A., Wilson, J. C., & Moore, D. (2017). Playing hard: Young men's experiences of drinking in inner-city Melbourne. *Journal of Sociology, 53*(2), 398–412.

Newcomb, M. E., Ryan, D. T., Greene, G. J., Garofalo, R., & Mustanski, B. (2014). Prevalence and patterns of smoking, alcohol use, and illicit drug use in young men who have sex with men. *Drug and Alcohol Dependence, 141*(Supplement C), 65–71. https://doi.org/10.1016/j.drugalcdep.2014.05.005

Niland, P., Lyons, A. C., Goodwin, I., & Hutton, F. (2013). “Everyone can loosen up and get a bit of a buzz on”: Young adults, alcohol and friendship practices. *International Journal of Drug Policy, 24*(6), 530–537. https://doi.org/10.1016/j.drugpo.2013.05.013

Peralta, R. L. (2007). College alcohol use and the embodiment of hegemonic masculinity among European American Men. *Sex Roles, 56*(11), 741–756. https://doi.org/10.1007/s11199-007-9233-1

Peralta, R. L. (2008). “Alcohol allows you to not be yourself”: Toward a structured understanding of alcohol use and gender difference among gay, lesbian, and heterosexual youth. *Journal of Drug Issues, 38*(2), 373–399. https://doi.org/10.1177/002204260803800201

Pienaar, K., Fraser, S., Kokanovic, R., Moore, D., Treloar, C., & Dunlop, A. (2015). New narratives, new selves: Complicating addiction in online alcohol and other drug resources. *Addiction Research and Theory, 23*(6), 499–509.

Poulson, M. (2015). Embodied subjectivities: Bodily subjectivity and changing boundaries in post-human alcohol practices. *Contemporary Drug Problems, 42*(1), 3–19.

Preciado, B. (2013). *Testo Junkie: Sex, drugs, and biopolitics in the pharmacopornographic era*. New York: The Feminist Press at City University New York.

Race, K. (2009). *Pleasure consuming medicine: The queer politics of drugs*. Durham, NC: Duke University Press.

Race, K. (2011). Party animals: The significance of drug practices in the materialisation of urban gay identity. In S. Fraser & D. Moore (Eds.), *The drug effect: Health, crime and society* (pp. 35–56). Cambridge: Cambridge University Press.

Race, K. (2014). Complex events: Drug effects and emergent causality. *Contemporary Drug Problems, 41*(3), 301–334.

Race, K. (2015). ‘Party and Play’: Online hook-up devices and the emergence of PNP practices among gay men. *Sexualities, 18*(3), 253–275.

Race, K. (2017). *The gay science: Intimate experiments with the problem of HIV*. London/New York: Routledge.

Race, K. (forthcoming). A lifetime on drugs. In S. Herring & L. Wallace (Eds.), *Long term*. Durham: Duke University Press.

Race, K., Lea, T., Murphy, D., & Pienaar, K. (2016). The future of drugs: Recreational drug use and sexual health among gay and other men who have sex with men. *Sexual Health*. https://doi.org/10.1071/SH16080

Reback, C. (1997). *The social construction of a gay drug: Methamphetamine use among gay & bisexual males in Los Angeles. Report for the City of Los Angeles.* Los Angeles: AIDS Coordinator.

Rhodes, T., & Cusick, L. (2002). Accounting for unprotected sex: Stories of agency and acceptability. *Social Science & Medicine, 55*(2), 211–226. https://doi.org/10.1016/S0277-9536(01)00162-9

Rivas, J. (2015). Intoxication and toxicity in a 'Pharmacopornographic Era': Beatriz Preciado's Testo Junkie. In E. Brennan & R. Williams (Eds.), *Literature and intoxication: Writing, politics and the experience of excess* (pp. 147–159). London: Palgrave Macmillan.

Roxburgh, A., Lea, T., de Wit, J., & Degenhardt, L. (2016). Sexual identity and prevalence of alcohol and other drug use among Australians in the general population. *International Journal of Drug Policy, 28*, 76–82.

Salih, S. (2007). On Judith Butler and performativity. In K. Lovas & M. Jenkins (Eds.), *Sexualities and communication in everyday life: A reader* (pp. 55–68). Thousand Oaks, CA and London: Sage Publications.

Southgate, E., & Hopwood, M. (2001). The role of folk pharmacology and lay experts in harm reduction: Sydney gay drug using networks. *International Journal of Drug Policy, 12*(4), 321–335. https://doi.org/10.1016/S0955-3959(01)00096-2

Stardust, Z., Kolstee, J., Joksic, S., Gray, J., & Hannan, S. (2018). A community-led, harm-reduction approach to chemsex: Case study from Australia's largest gay city. *Sexual Health, 15*(2), 179–181. https://doi.org/10.1071/SH17145

Stryker, S., & Whittle, S. (2006). *The transgender studies reader*. New York: Routledge.

valentine, k., & Fraser, S. (2008). Trauma, damage and pleasure: Rethinking problematic drug use. *International Journal of Drug Policy, 19*(5), 410–416. https://doi.org/10.1016/j.drugpo.2007.08.001

Weatherburn, P., Davies, P. M., Hickson, F. C., Hunt, A. J., McManus, T. J., & Coxon, A. P. (1993). No connection between alcohol use and unsafe sex among gay and bisexual men. *Aids, 7*(1), 115–119.

Westhaver, R. (2005). 'Coming out of your skin': Circuit parties, pleasure and the subject. *Sexualities, 8*(3), 347–374. https://doi.org/10.1177/1363460705053338

Zajdow, G. (2010). 'It blasted me into space': Intoxication and an ethics of pleasure. *Health Sociology Review, 19*(2), 218–229. https://doi.org/10.5172/hesr.2010.19.2.218

8

Ethnicities and Intoxication

Sarah Herbert and Tim McCreanor

Introduction

Alcohol use and often intoxication are features of everyday life for many as learnt behaviours determined by the values, attitudes and norms within cultures, and shaped by social environments (Babor et al., 2010; Bancroft, 2009). Understandings of intoxication, in this instance, from alcohol, are thus located within particular historical, social, cultural and political contexts (Kelly, Advocat, Harrison, & Hickey, 2011) and mean different things to different people. When and where we consume alcohol, the quantities and types of alcohol we consume, who we engage with and our expected outcomes of alcohol use are all determined by such contexts;

S. Herbert (✉)
Te Kupenga Hauora Māori, The University of Auckland,
Auckland, New Zealand
e-mail: sarah.herbert@auckland.ac.nz

T. McCreanor
SHORE & Whariki Research Centre, College of Health, Massey University,
Auckland, New Zealand

F. Hutton (ed.), *Cultures of Intoxication*,
https://doi.org/10.1007/978-3-030-35284-4_8

which are dynamic, fluid and complex (Borlagdan et al., 2010; Social Issues Research Centre [SIRC], 1998). For the purpose of this chapter, alcohol intoxication is understood to change a person's sense of self in the world and may act as a behaviour modifier, a mediator of social relations or to enhance collective and peer experiences (Bancroft, 2009).

Conversely, and just as importantly, while drinking to intoxication is a persistent feature of alcohol cultures in Aotearoa (New Zealand Law Commission [NZLC], 2010), it is widely recognised as causing psychological and psychomotor performance impairment (New Zealand Medical Association [NZMA], 2015) and is strongly and clearly linked to harmful outcomes (NZLC, 2010; NZMA, 2015). In many countries, alcohol use is also the "leading preventable cause of premature mortality, disability and social harm" (Randerson, Casswell, & Huckle, 2018, p. 14). The impacts of alcohol intoxication are diverse, ranging from having valued social functions to negative and harmful health outcomes. This chapter recognises the multiplicity of functions and impacts that alcohol intoxication serves.

Alcohol Use and Intoxication in Aotearoa

There is a long history of intoxication in Aotearoa originating from colonisation, particularly the heavy, frequent and public alcohol use among European male colonialists (Hutt, 1999; McEwan, Campbell, & Swain, 2010). During the temperance movement in the 1870s, concepts of manhood among colonialist men were challenged because their widespread behaviour of public intoxication and heavy alcohol use, which was often accompanied by violence, swearing, gambling and prostitution (Phillips, 1996), caused much concern in general society. Thus, the prohibition campaign focused on 'civilising' the Pākehā *(New Zealander of European descent)* male and ensuring his behaviour became more respectable, suggesting that visible and heavy intoxication practices and associated behaviours were at odds with accepted societal values at that time. In contrast, among women, there was an expectation to maintain sobriety, purity and nurturing behaviours and values, thus alcohol use and intoxication was not encouraged (Hutton & Wright, 2015).

By the 1900s, prohibition was still sought by many, and alcohol intoxication was regarded a serious social problem (Phillips, 1996). This led to a number of legislative restrictions on alcohol use, including the 6 o'clock closing of pubs (public house licensed to sell alcohol) which began during World War One in 1917 (Cagney, 2006; McEwan et al., 2010; Phillips, 1996). While the aim was to restrict alcohol use, what resulted was the '6 o'clock swill' phenomena, where men attempted to drink as much beer as possible before the pub closed (Cagney, 2006; McEwan et al., 2010), thus aiding in the continuation of intoxication and binge drinking alcohol use among men. In 1967, when 6 o'clock closing of pubs ceased, changes to gendered expectations of alcohol use occurred. Women began to visit the pub, which subsequently changed to become more inviting for women to consume alcohol there (Phillips, 1996). Wine also became increasingly popular for men and women, which not only challenged masculine stereotypes of 'beer drinking men' but also led to more frequent alcohol use among women (McEwan et al., 2010).

In contemporary Aotearoa, alcohol is commonly used to facilitate social interactions, is viewed as a symbol of hospitality and, an important marker in celebratory events (Cagney, 2006). Similarly, intoxication is widely accepted, viewed as part of everyday life and generally tolerated (Cagney, 2006; Lyons & Willott, 2008). In 2014, among a sample of 4000 New Zealand adults, more than half (53%) agreed with the idea that binge drinking is part of the 'kiwi' culture (Gray, Gordon, & Newcombe, 2015). Much of this may be explained by Aotearoa having liberal alcohol laws, which is believed to have fostered an alcohol-based, leisure economy in many urban centres that is characterised by heavy alcohol use (McEwan, Swain, & Campbell, 2011) and minimal social shame among intoxicated individuals (Lyons, Emslie, & Hunt, 2014). This has generated an 'alcogenic' environment (NZMA, 2015) in which alcohol use and intoxication are widely viewed as acceptable, enjoyable, and even socially sanctioned (Lyons & Willott, 2008; NZMA, 2015; Randerson et al., 2018).

Specifically, research shows that among some groups such as young people, there is a phenomenon whereby people 'drink to get drunk' (Hutton & Wright, 2015; Lyons et al., 2014), or with the intention of becoming intoxicated (Hutton & Wright, 2015; McEwan et al., 2011), otherwise coined "determined drunkenness" (Measham & Brain, 2005, p. 268). Further, research suggests that, in general, people are not concerned about the health effects of alcohol use (Cagney, 2006; Lyons & Willott, 2008), are generally reluctant to limit their alcohol use (Lyons & Willott, 2008) and believe it is acceptable to get drunk (McEwan et al., 2011).

In Aotearoa, alcohol is one of the leading causes of premature mortality, disability and social harm (NZMA, 2015; Randerson et al., 2018). The cost of which was estimated in 2005 at $5.3 billion dollars per year (Randerson et al., 2018). Researchers highlight the increasing unease about the harmful effects of alcohol on the lives of particular groups, including young people (Lyons et al., 2014; McCreanor et al., 2015), the elderly (Herbert, 2012; Towers, Sheridan, Newcombe, & Szabo, 2018) and Māori (Bramley et al., 2003; Clark et al., 2013; Herbert, 2012; Herbert & Stephens, 2015; Ministry of Health [MoH], 2016).

Alcohol legislation and policy seek to control and reduce alcohol-related harm as a result of this 'culture of intoxication' (Measham, 2006; NZLC, 2010). However, as McCreanor, Moewaka-Barnes, Kaiwai, Borell, and Gregory (2008) point out, understanding intoxication requires consideration of "a complex interplay of personal, cultural, historical, political and other contextual factors" (p. 938). The NZLC (2010) asserts that in order to combat the current culture of intoxication, serious examination and redevelopment of alcohol policy is necessary, including reviewing the legal age for purchasing alcohol, opening hours of liquor outlets, and, taxation and price of alcohol. Further, as D'Abbs (2015) emphasises, policy to change alcohol behaviours is generally met with resistance, particularly "when imposed by the more powerful on the less powerful" (p. 121). Some argue that such efforts may indeed have little relevance to, or effectiveness within, indigenous populations (Brady, 2000; Gray & Saggers, 2005; Herbert, Stephens, & Forster, 2017). Harmful alcohol use among Māori, for example, remains unchanged over the last two decades (MoH, 2009, 2016), reflecting consistent patterns of indigenous alcohol use over time (Saggers & Gray, 1998).

The most recent findings from the New Zealand Health Survey on alcohol use (MoH, 2019) suggest disparate patterns of alcohol use between Māori and non-Māori continue into the present. Approximately 80% of the population drank alcohol in the past year, with no disparity between Māori and non-Māori. However, the survey also shows that nearly 20% consume alcohol in a hazardous manner that "carries a risk of harming the drinker's physical or mental health or having harmful social effects on the drinker or others" (MoH, 2019). The data also show that 32% of Māori adults drink in this way, and that adjusting for age and gender, they are 1.6 times more likely to do so than non-Māori adults (MoH, 2019). Given the internationally robust findings about the role of alcohol in preventable mortality and morbidity, it seems inevitable that these markers of use and intoxication are deeply implicated in the long-standing health disparities that have defined the ethnic population health landscape since reliable data were first collected in 1950 (Ajwani, Blakely, Robson, Tobias, & Bonne, 2003; StatsNZ, 2014).

Alcohol Use and Intoxication Among Indigenous Peoples

Many indigenous populations had little or no exposure to alcoholic beverages prior to contact with Europeans. Māori in Aotearoa (Brady, 2000; Saggers & Gray, 1998), Aboriginal peoples in Canada (Saggers & Gray, 1998) and Australia (Brady, 2000; Saggers & Gray, 1998), and First Nations tribes in the United States (Brady, 2000) were all effectively alcohol free. When colonial settlers introduced alcohol to these indigenous groups, it was often met with resistance (Awatere, Casswell, Cullen, Gilmore, & Kupenga, 1984; Saggers & Gray, 1998). Historically, alcohol was often used as a means of exchange by colonial settlers, which appears to have spread the integration of alcohol into indigenous societies (Cagney, 2006; Saggers & Gray, 1998; Sargent, 1983).

In contemporary colonial societies such as those named earlier, problematic use is routinely drawn on to explain the negative impact alcohol has on the health and well-being of indigenous peoples (Awatere et al., 1984; Durie, 2004; Saggers & Gray, 1998). The influence of European settlers is widely theorised as causal in problematic alcohol use among these groups (Marie, Fergusson, & Boden, 2012; Saggers & Gray, 1998), casting it as coping or escape mechanisms in the face of the brutality of colonisation (MacLachlan, 2015; Marie et al., 2012; Saggers & Gray,

1998). Settler patterns of heavy drinking likely modelled unsafe practices among those who had yet to establish their own cultural norms and practices (Brady, 2000; Saggers & Gray, 1998).

Culture is argued to influence the development of individual and collective alcohol use and behaviours related to intoxication (Maclachlan, 2015). Although the exact nature of this relationship is varied, it has been theorised that alcohol use is influenced by culture-related factors including acculturative stress, problems associated with oppression and racism (Winter, Riordan, Surace, & Scarf, 2019), alienation from one's culture, identity conflict, intergenerational conflict and a sense of powerlessness among indigenous and minority ethnic groups (Cagney, 2006). Conversely, culture and having a strong sense of cultural identity are understood to mitigate problem alcohol use (Whitbeck, Chen, Hoyt, & Adams, 2004). However, in general, there is a scarcity of literature exploring the influence of culturally specific factors on alcohol use and intoxication, and further research is needed to understand this relationship more clearly.

Discriminatory legislation used by colonial governments (e.g. Aotearoa, Canada and Australia), which sought to prohibit and control alcohol use, has also contributed to problematic alcohol use among indigenous people both historically (Brady, 2000; D'Abbs, 2015; Hutt, 1999; Saggers & Gray, 1998) and in contemporary society (e.g. Northern Territory, Australia) (D'Abbs, 2017). Often, under the guise of 'protecting' their health and well-being, such legislation was viewed among indigenous people as unfair because it lacked acknowledgement of their citizenship and implied a sense of inferiority through the provision of separate standards for indigenous people's alcohol use (Brady, 2000; Cagney, 2006; Eggleston, 1974). Indigenous alcohol use was thus viewed as stigmatising compared to non-indigenous people's use, which was socially sanctioned by the government (Eggleston, 1974). Such framing results in biased representations of indigenous alcohol use practices that contribute to the dominant framing of indigenous people's alcohol use as problematic (Sargent, 1983; Spicer, Novins, Mitchell, & Beals, 2003).

Biases in the reporting of indigenous people's alcohol use have also been identified (Cagney, 2006; Sargent, 1983; Spicer et al., 2003), which have led to misconceptions that indigenous people misuse alcohol simply because they do not conform to western ideas of acceptable alcohol use (Spicer et al., 2003; Whitbeck, Chen, Hoyt, & Adams, 2004). These representations contribute to negative stereotypes of indigenous alcohol use as inevitably bad, hazardous or as having detrimental health and social effects (Saggers & Gray, 1998). Sustained media representations of intoxication of Aboriginal peoples in Australia are understood to have contributed to the stereotype that assumes all Aborigines are hopeless drunks. Similarly, the 'drunken Indian' trope draws on constructions of American and Canadian First Nations as regularly tied into bingeing, intoxication, spendthrift and alcohol-fuelled socialising (Spicer et al., 2003; Whitbeck et al., 2004). Despite a lack of empirical evidence (Spicer et al., 2003) and research that highlights the diversity of alcohol use among indigenous populations (e.g. Herbert et al., 2017; Herbert, Stephens & Forster, 2018a; Spicer et al., 2003), such representations persist in the problematising of indigenous people's alcohol use.

This overview provides some insight into current understandings of indigenous people's alcohol use, the prevailing focus on problematic alcohol use, the biases in the reporting of indigenous people's alcohol use and the stereotypes that have meant that indigenous people's alcohol use is understood as problematic. While alcohol use and its destructive impact on indigenous societies must be acknowledged, understanding wider social and cultural aspects is also vital. There has been minimal exploration of indigenous perspectives of alcohol use, including their own understandings of their use, intoxication, drinking patterns and the functions of alcohol within indigenous communities.

Alcohol Use and Intoxication Among Māori

Māori did not escape the worldwide pattern of alcohol usage that has plagued indigenous people in the wake of Western colonisation (Durie, 2004, p. 125).

Alcohol use among Māori is fundamentally linked to colonial history from its introduction by Pākehā settlers (Awatere et al., 1984; Hutt, 1999; Saggers & Gray, 1998), to the undeniable and negative effects it has had on Māori health and well-being (Durie, 2004; Marie et al., 2012; Moewaka-Barnes, McPherson, & Bhatta, 2003). Initially, Māori had a strong aversion to alcohol, referring to it as 'waipiro' or stinking water (Awatere et al., 1984; Saggers & Gray, 1998). By 1840 however, many Māori chiefs had expressed concerns about the extent and effects of alcohol use observed among both Māori and Pākehā (Awatere et al., 1984; Hutt, 1999; Saggers & Gray, 1998).

Meanwhile, alcohol was steadily incorporated into Māori social life in the 1840s, suggesting a gradual change in the social norms of alcohol use among Māori. However, heavy alcohol use and intoxication were still predominantly Pākehā practices, as were the majority of alcohol-related offenses (Awatere et al., 1984; Hutt, 1999). In 1847, and in response to Māori concerns about alcohol, Governor Grey introduced the Sale of Spirits to Natives Ordinance Act, which prohibited Māori from buying and selling alcohol (Awatere et al., 1984; Durie, 2004; Hutt, 1999). This legislation couched alcohol as a Māori problem and was also viewed by many Māori as discriminatory because only Māori alcohol use was being controlled. Further, the Act granted Pākehā sole control over the distribution and use of alcohol, thereby minimising the collective ability of Māori to develop successful ways of dealing with the impact of alcohol in their communities (Awatere et al., 1984; Hutt, 1999).

From the 1860s, the number of Māori-led initiatives seeking to restrict alcohol increased as the negative consequences, presumably relating to heavy use and/or intoxicated individuals, became more widely recognised. For example, in te rohe Pōtae *(the King Country),* Pōtatau Te Wherowhero *[the first Māori king]* initiated what eventually became the Māori wardens' scheme (Fleras, 1981). He appointed wātene Māori *(Māori wardens)* to be responsible for preventing alcohol from entering marae *(traditional meeting place/s of Māori)* and controlling the supply of alcohol in Māori communities and licensed hotels (Fleras, 1981).

Many Māori also joined temperance movements that supported the prohibition of alcohol from the 1860s through to the early twentieth century. These Māori-led responses to alcohol, in combination with the developing temperance movement in Aotearoa, led to an increase in sobriety observed within many Māori communities during the 1870s–1880s (Awatere et al., 1984). More broadly, these responses suggest that alcohol misuse, intoxication and the deleterious effects of alcohol were not acceptable within Māori communities. Further, they illustrate a strong awareness among Māori of the negative impacts alcohol was having in their communities. Indeed, at this point in history, it was widely acknowledged that alcohol was linked to cultural, social and spiritual degradation within Māori communities (Awatere et al., 1984; Hutt, 1999).

By the 1900s, alcohol was understood to be contributing to widespread social problems in society, and attention turned to local-level responses seeking to address the issues (Walker, 1984). Prominent Māori leaders including Maui Pōmare and Apirana Ngata began speaking more publicly about Māori and alcohol and associated matters (Hutt, 1999; Walker, 1984). Ngata, who was chairman of Horouta/East Coast council at the time, initiated the first by-law in 1901, which included banning alcohol on marae (Hutt, 1999). In 1911, he persuaded the Horouta Māori Council to run a poll for prohibition which, with the support of many in his iwi, Ngāti Porou, led to complete prohibition across the East Coast district until 1922 (Hutt, 1999).

However, while many from Ngāti Porou supported Ngata's prohibition campaigns, some became increasingly frustrated at his efforts. In 1920, Ngata's uncle, Tamati Kaiwai, wrote an anti-prohibition haka *(posture dance)* 'Poropeihana' *(prohibition)*, directly challenging his nephew (Awatere et al., 1984). In general, this haka is interpreted as articulating frustration among Ngāti Porou who did not support prohibition, but, at times, Ngata himself led Poropeihana to "dampen the personal sting" (Hutt, 1999, p. 67), suggesting he shared some empathy towards his people and their frustrations, despite being a clear and strong supporter of prohibition. Ngata is still recognised as being a strong advocate and leader who was effective in his efforts to minimise alcohol use among Māori in the early 1900s.

The 1920s–1950s saw much diversification of alcohol use among Māori. For example, while alcohol was increasingly present during important events at some marae, it was prohibited at others including Turangawawae marae in Ngaruawahia, when Te Puea forbade any alcohol from entering the marae in 1929 (Hutt, 1999). In the 1930s, while heavy alcohol use was observed among many military personnel, including Māori, drinking in the general population decreased as a result of the Depression (Hutt, 1999). In 1948, the Licensing Amendment Bill repealed all previous and discriminatory alcohol legislation, thereby providing Māori and Pākehā equal access to alcohol (Awatere et al., 1984; Ebbett & Clarke, 2010; Fleras, 1981; Hutt, 1999). At the same time, many Māori began migrating to urban areas in search of work (Hutt, 1999). Together, these factors improved Māori access and opportunities to engage in alcohol use, which led to an observed increase in Māori alcohol use and intoxication (Hutt, 1999). Indeed, Fleras (1981) notes that 'drunkenness and disorderly conduct' had been singled out as requiring attention in the 1945 Māori Social and Economic Advancement Act, suggesting problem alcohol use was already prevalent in Māori communities. This Act provisioned the establishment of the office of Māori Wardens; one task of which was to police alcohol use among Māori using a 'by Māori, for Māori' approach, thus highlighting a Māori-led management system of alcohol use.

In 1962, Māori warden roles were formalised, albeit in a voluntary capacity, in the Māori Community Development Act (1962). This Act led to the establishment of an association of Māori wardens, providing them legislative authority to regulate alcohol use within tribal districts (Durie, 2004; Hutt, 1999). However, as agents of social control, Māori wardens were expected to prevent trouble associated with intoxicated Māori, but not to interfere with alcohol sales and profit at licensed hotels. Unsurprisingly, Māori wardens were often met with ambivalence by both Māori and hotel proprietors (Awatere et al., 1984; Durie, 2004; Fleras, 1981). From the mid-1950s onwards, Māori alcohol use began to reflect the alcohol use practices of Pākehā, leading to more widespread acceptance among Māori of the role of alcohol in everyday life (Hutt, 1999).

In contemporary Aotearoa, alcohol use is generally considered a 'normal' part of everyday social life among Māori (Cagney, 2006; Durie, 2004). Alarmingly, however, there is much alcohol-related harm occurring within the Māori population. In 2000, the first and only Māori National Alcohol Survey— *Te Ao Waipiro*—was conducted. This survey assessed drinking patterns and alcohol-related problems among 1992 Māori, aged 13–65 years (Moewaka-Barnes et al., 2003). Of concern, findings highlight that most alcohol consumption within this sample (76%) occurred during heavier drinking occasions and that Māori people, especially Māori women, suffer significantly more harm than non-Māori as a result of alcohol use (Moewaka-Barnes et al., 2003). The disproportionate burden of alcohol-related harm among Māori compared to other groups in the population is well documented (Bramley et al., 2003; Clark et al., 2013: MoH, 2019).

Disparities in alcohol-related harm between Māori and non-Māori remain unchanged over time. One explanation for this may be the primary framing of alcohol use among indigenous peoples, including Māori, as problematic and harmful (Inter-Agency Committee on Drugs, 2015; SIRC, 1998) by health authorities. Accordingly, alcohol policy often focuses on prevention or harm minimisation strategies at the individual level (Inter-Agency Committee on Drugs, 2015), including restricting alcohol use, binge drinking and intoxication among individuals (Inter-Agency Committee on Drugs, 2015). On the other hand, these weak measures are traded off by politicians against far more effective approaches based on regulation, taxation and controls that reduce population-level consumption and harm (Babor et al., 2010). While the individual focus may elicit some success in reducing problematic alcohol use and harm, alcohol use statistics show that alcohol policy and interventions among Māori are failing, with minimal change in harmful alcohol use observed over the last 20 years (MoH, 2009, 2016), suggesting the need for more to be done.

Māori understandings of alcohol use and intoxication are of critical importance in understanding the nuances of Māori drinking cultures and provide one avenue for more effectively reducing harms arising from alcohol use among Māori. To date, research indicates that alcohol use among Māori is diverse (Clarke & Ebbett, 2010; Herbert, Forster, McCreanor, & Stephens, 2017; Herbert & Stephens, 2015; Herbert, Stephens, & Forster, 2018a, 2018b; Muriwai, Huckle, & Romeo, 2018) and often prompted by social motivations (Awatere et al., 1984; Clarke & Ebbett, 2010; Herbert, Forster, et al., 2017; Herbert et al., 2017, 2018a, 2018b; Hutton & Wright, 2015; Muriwai, Huckle, & Romeo, 2018).

In particular, Herbert (2017), explored broad, socially shared meanings of alcohol use from the perspectives of older Māori. Comprising three separate but related studies, the overarching findings suggest diverse Māori drinking cultures, which are embedded in four key social contexts:

a sporting culture, a working culture, the context of family and Māori culture (Herbert, Forster, et al., 2017). Further, Māori understandings of their alcohol use were contextualised within three key themes including "Not all Māori are problem drinkers", "There is good Māori alcohol use" and "Alcohol is not the problem" (Herbert et al., 2018a), supporting the need to shift away from problematic framing of Māori alcohol use.

Important social factors were also found to influence Māori alcohol use across the lifetime including kaumātua *(respected elder/s)* status, tikanga *(Māori protocols and practices)*, whānau *(family)*, religion and finances along with special occasions such as weddings and birthdays, and other events such as tangi, first alcohol use experiences, a change in social milieu, parental roles and responsibilities, changing social roles and responsibilities and the impact of ageing (Herbert et al., 2017). Interestingly, whānau alcohol use was constructed as 'good' or socially acceptable, among kaupapa whānau *(groups with a common purpose)*, suggesting Māori understandings of the positive functions of alcohol use that may drive intoxication. Additionally, whanaungatanga, described as socialising, connectedness and communicating, was also important in determining Māori alcohol use and Māori engagement in social environments where alcohol is present (Herbert et al., 2018b). These findings build on previous research, recognising the socialising or whanaungatanga-related functions of alcohol use among Māori (Awatere et al., 1984; Clarke & Ebbett, 2010).

Interestingly, tikanga was identified as dictating acceptable alcohol use practices among Māori. Tikanga provides guidelines for behaviour, conduct and expectations (Mead, 2003), and this may be understood as promoting health and safety in the context of alcohol use by ensuring the safer use of alcohol. Specifically, participants in Herbert, Forster, et al. (2017) study often described their role as kaumātua in enforcing this tikanga, thus emphasising the importance of Māori cultural roles, such as kaumātua, in relation to alcohol use. Participants indicated wanting to be good role models for younger generations, and this related to the idea of reducing their alcohol consumption. This finding suggests that being abstemious or engaging in minimal alcohol use is synonymous with being seen as a good role model. The importance of kaumātua roles in the context of alcohol use is useful to consider because there may be potential for kaumātua to assist in reinforcing tikanga, which supports safer alcohol use as well as providing important role modelling for younger generations. However, future research should explore this potential in further detail.

Further, the physical locations of alcohol use may be important. Herbert et al. (2018b) identified the home and the Returned Services Association establishments as locations which support whanaungatanga and thus contribute to older Māori engagement in social environments where alcohol is present. Similarly, research highlights pubs and hotels as being popular locations for drinking among Māori (Awatere et al., 1984; Herbert et al., 2017). Interestingly, while the marae was once a popular location for alcohol use among Māori in the past, research suggests this is not the case in contemporary society, and that alcohol use is more likely to occur in the home (Herbert et al., 2017, 2018a; Muriwai et al., 2018).

Cultural identity is understood to influence alcohol use among Māori (Clarke & Ebbett, 2010; Herbert & Stephens, 2015; Waldon, 2004; Winter et al., 2019). For example, Winter et al.'s (2019) research highlights a relationship between hazardous drinking among Māori and experiences of racial discrimination. Clarke and Ebbett (2010) found that Māori cultural identity influenced frequency of drinking among Māori and suggested that Māori who have a strong cultural identity may attend more social occasions involving alcohol use. Similarly, findings from a study by Herbert and Stephens (2015) suggest a stronger Māori cultural identity may support particular drinking behaviours among older Māori although caution the need for further research to explore this relationship.

In a study exploring alcohol use practices among young Māori and Pacific women, Hutton and Wright (2015) found that participants drank alcohol to achieve "a desired state of intoxication" (p. 108). Further practices such as preloading; drinking alcohol before going out to licensed premises, and sideloading; drinking alcohol that was purchased elsewhere whilst at a bar or club, were normalised within these participants and their peer groups. Such findings reinforce broader contemporary alcohol use cultures within Aotearoa that revolve around intoxication and 'determined drunkenness' (Hutton & Wright, 2015; Measham & Brain, 2005). Moreover, McCreanor et al. (2015) highlight behaviours such as preloading, as a "growing concern in Aotearoa" (p. 1). Despite this,

Hutton and Wright (2015) caution that analysis of Māori alcohol use must be contextualised within "contemporary cultures of intoxication" (p. 104), whilst also attending to the cultural context where Māori often occupy vulnerable positions as a result of colonisation. They also highlight the tensions young Māori women face as they navigate both their own culture and that of the dominant 'kiwi' culture, in relation to alcohol use.

Drawn together, research exploring the social and cultural context of Māori alcohol use and intoxication to date suggest a complex range of factors at play. The key social contexts and diverse influences on Māori alcohol use, including the roles of tikanga, kaumātua status, physical locations of Māori alcohol use, cultural identity and motivations for drinking alcohol, all work to influence Māori alcohol use and intoxication in various ways. Future research could usefully consider how the social locations of Māori alcohol use contribute to understandings of intoxication and alcohol use practices. Understanding the changes in socialising practices among Māori that involve alcohol use as people age and within different social contexts would also provide more comprehensive accounts of the social location of Māori alcohol use.

Further, detailed exploration of how those social factors listed above work to influence particular types of alcohol use, including hazardous alcohol use, binge drinking and intoxication would be useful. Similarly, future research could explore the ways in which the physical location, Māori cultural identity and kaumātua status may influence different types of alcohol use and intoxication behaviours among Māori at various ages and stages across the lifetime.

Conclusion

As this chapter highlights, at a population level, alcohol use practices involving intoxication are well established and long-standing in the context of Aotearoa, with origins in early European male colonists' drinking behaviours. In the contemporary setting of Aotearoa, it is understood that we are immersed in a widely accepted alcogenic environment in which about 80% of the population drink, and roughly 20% use alcohol in diverse and harmful ways. This culture of intoxication contributes to an interwoven and complex array of health and social issues that causes preventable morbidity and mortality, social disruption, damage to the economy/work and a multi-billion-dollar annual health bill, with particular groups such as the young, the elderly and Māori being most impacted by alcohol and its associated harms. While alcohol legislation and policy have sought to control and reduce alcohol-related harm over time, this has had limited impact, highlighting an urgent need to consider broader contextual factors influencing alcohol use as well as serious scrutinising of existing alcohol policy. For Māori, in particular, there has been limited effectiveness from these efforts, with results from the New Zealand Health Survey (MoH, 2019) highlighting ongoing disparities in alcohol-related harm between Māori and non-Māori.

The historical context of indigenous people's alcohol use is discussed to highlight the ways in which alcohol was introduced and incorporated into indigenous societies. The focus on harmful alcohol use and the negative impacts of such has dominated much research, theorising and understanding of indigenous people's alcohol use. However, biases in the representation of indigenous people's alcohol use have been identified, which have led to misconceptions and stereotyping of indigenous people's alcohol use, resulting in narrow understandings of indigenous alcohol practices. Attending to the wider contextual factors of indigenous alcohol use is necessary, alongside indigenous understandings of alcohol use and its functions within indigenous communities. Such approaches can provide more nuanced understandings of indigenous people's alcohol use, allowing for improved ways in which to reduce consumption and harmful use.

The history of Māori alcohol use shows that the early efforts at self-determination by Māori communities have been subverted across time, and rejuvenation of these approaches in response to colonisation may have a place in efforts to prevent and reduce future alcohol-related harms in Māori communities. In contemporary Aotearoa society, Māori alcohol use has been influenced by the broader alcohol use cultures at play so that alcohol use is generally considered a natural part of everyday social life in Māori communities. Despite this, the disproportionate and significant alcohol-related harm among Māori is well documented with a multitude of broader contextual factors understood to be influencing Māori alcohol use, including cultural identity, physical and social locations of alcohol use and motivations for alcohol use.

To conclude, given the differences in alcohol use profiles and alcohol-related harm between Māori and others in Aotearoa, the topic of Māori alcohol use is an area of critical concern. Such disparities highlight the failings of existing alcohol policy and alcohol interventions among Māori and point to a need for Māori self-determination in policy development in this area of social life. Attending to the broader contextual factors, which influence Māori alcohol use as well as exploring Māori and indigenous meanings of alcohol use and intoxication, may lead to the development of more grounded, comprehensive, culturally effective and appropriate alcohol policy and interventions. More broadly, efforts must go towards substantially changing current legislation if it is to have any significant impact on alcohol use and related harms as well as shifting majority views about alcohol use, which has led to a 'culture of intoxication' in Aotearoa.

References

Ajwani, S., Blakely, T., Robson, B., Tobias, M., & Bonne, M. (2003). *Decades of disparity: Ethnic mortality trends in New Zealand 1980–1999*. Wellington, New Zealand: Ministry of Health, Public Health Intelligence Group and University of Otago.

Awatere, D., Casswell, S., Cullen, H., Gilmore, L., & Kupenga, D. (1984). *Alcohol and the Māori people*. Auckland, New Zealand: Alcohol Research Unit, School of Medicine, University of Auckland.

Babor, T., Caetano, R., Casswell, S., Edwards, G., Giesbrecht, N., Graham, K., … Rossow, I. (2010). *Alcohol: No ordinary commodity, Research and public policy* (2nd ed.). Oxford: Oxford University Press.

Bancroft, A. (2009). *Drugs, intoxication and society*. Cambridge, UK: Polity Press.

Borlagdan, J., Freeman, T., Duvnjak, A., Lunnay, B., Bywood, P. T., & Roche, A. M. (2010). *From ideal to reality: Cultural contradictions and young people's drinking*. National Centre for Education and Training on Addiction, Flinders University, Adelaide, Australia: DrinkWise Australia Ltd.

Brady, M. (2000). Alcohol policy issues for indigenous people in the United States, Canada, Australia and New Zealand. *Contemporary Drug Problems, 27*(3), 435–509.

Bramley, D., Broad, J., Harris, R., Reid, P., Jackson, R., Ameratunga, S., … Wells, S. (2003). Differences in patterns of alcohol consumption between Māori and non-Māori in Aotearoa (New Zealand). *New Zealand Medical Journal, 116*(1184), 1–17.

Cagney, P. (2006). *A healthy drinking culture: A search and review of international and New Zealand literature.* Retrieved from http://www.hpa.org.nz/sites/default/files/imported/field_research_publication_file/Report_on_NZ_drinking_culture.pdf

Clark, T. C., Robinson, E., Crengle, S., Sheridan, J., Jackson, N., & Ameratunga, S. (2013). Binge drinking among Māori secondary school students in New Zealand: Associations with source, exposure, and perceptions of alcohol use. *The New Zealand Medical Journal, 126*, 70–84.

Clarke, D., & Ebbett, E. (2010). Māori identification, drinking motivation and mental health. *International Journal of Mental Health and Addiction, 8*(2), 145–159. https://doi.org/10.1007/s11469-009-9215-3

D'Abbs, P. (2015). Reform and resistance: Exploring the interplay of alcohol policies with drinking cultures and drinking practices. *Contemporary Drug Problems, 42*(2), 118–129. https://doi.org/10.1177/0091450915587535

D'Abbs, P. (2017, June). *Alcohol policy in the Northern Territory: Towards a critique and refocusing – A submission to the Northern Territory alcohol policies and legislation review.* Retrieved from https://alcoholreform.nt.gov.au/__data/assets/pdf_file/0011/436916/dAbbs,-Peter-Submission.pdf

Durie, M. (2004). *Mauri Ora: The dynamics of Māori health.* New York, NY: Oxford University Press.

Ebbett, E., & Clarke, D. (2010). Māori identification, alcohol behaviour and mental health: A review. *International Journal of Mental Health Addiction, 8*, 214–231. https://doi.org/10.1007/s11469-009-9200-x

Eggleston, E. (1974). Legal controls on alcohol. In B. S. Hetzel, M. Dobbin, L. Lippmann, & E. Eggleston (Eds.), *Better health for Aborigines? Report of a National Seminar at Monash University* (pp. 53–65). St. Lucia, Queensland: University of Queensland Press.

Fleras, A. (1981). Māori wardens and the control of liquor among the Māori of New Zealand. *The Journal of the Polynesian Society, 90*(4), 495–513.

Gray, D., & Saggers, S. (2005). The evidence base for responding to substance misuse in Indigenous minority populations. In T. Stockwell, P. J. Gruenewald,

J. W. Toumbourou, & W. Loxley (Eds.), *Preventing harmful substance use* (pp. 381–393). Chichester: John Wiley & Sons Ltd.

Gray, R., Gordon, C., & Newcombe, R. (2015). *Perceptions of drinking culture in New Zealand. [In Fact]*. Wellington, New Zealand: Health Promotion Agency Research and Evaluation Unit.

Herbert, S. (2012). *Alcohol use and older Māori people: Reason for further investigation?* Refereed proceedings of the Manawatū Doctoral Research Symposium, 2, 51–58. Retrieved from http://hdl.handle.net/10179/4959

Herbert, S. (2017). *He tirohanga taurahere tangata: The social context of older Māori alcohol use in Aotearoa*. Doctoral thesis, Massey University, Palmerston North, New Zealand. Retrieved from https://mro.massey.ac.nz/handle/10179/12882

Herbert, S., Forster, M., McCreanor, T., & Stephens, C. (2017). The social context of alcohol use among Māori in Aotearoa/New Zealand: Reflections of life experiences of alcohol use by older Māori. *International Journal of Indigenous Health, 12*(1), 57–74. https://doi.org/10.18357/ijih121201716904

Herbert, S., & Stephens, C. (2015). Alcohol use and older Māori in Aotearoa. *Journal of Ethnicity in Substance Abuse, 14*(3), 1–19. https://doi.org/10.1080/15332640.2014.993786

Herbert, S., Stephens, C. V., & Forster, M. (2017). Socially based trajectories of alcohol use among indigenous Māori in Aotearoa/New Zealand. *Critical Public Health*, 1–10. https://doi.org/10.1080/09581596.2017.1378424

Herbert, S., Stephens, C. V., & Forster, M. (2018a). Older Māori understandings of alcohol use in Aotearoa/New Zealand. *International Journal of Drug Policy, 54*, 123–129. https://doi.org/10.1016/j.drugpo.2018.01.017

Herbert, S., Stephens, C. V., & Forster, M. (2018b). It's all about whanaungatanga: Alcohol use and older Māori in Aotearoa. *AlterNative*, 1–9. https://doi.org/10.1177/1177180118785381

Hutt, M. (1999). *Te iwi Māori me te inu waipiro: He tuhituhingā hītori (Māori & alcohol: A history)*. Wellington, New Zealand: Health Services Research Centre/Alcohol Advisory Council.

Hutton, F., & Wright, S. (2015). 'You don't ditch your girls': Young Māori and Pacific women and the culture of intoxication. *Critical Public Health, 25*(1), 101–119. https://doi.org/10.1080/09581596.2014.946886

Inter-Agency Committee on Drugs. (2015). *National drug policy 2015 to 2020*. Wellington, New Zealand: Ministry of Health.

Kelly, P., Advocat, J., Harrison, L., & Hickey, C. (2011). *Smashed! The many meanings of intoxication and drunkenness*. Australia: Monash University Publishing.
Lyons, A., & Willott, S. (2008). Alcohol consumption, gender identities and women's changing social positions. *Sex Roles, 59*(9–10), 694–712. https://doi.org/10.1007/s11199-008-9475-6
Lyons, A. C., Emslie, C., & Hunt, K. (2014). Staying 'in the zone' but not passing the 'point of no return': Embodiment, gender and drinking in mid-life. *Sociology of Health and Illness, 36*(2), 264–277. https://doi.org/10.1111/1467-9566.12103
MacLachlan, M. (2015). Culture, empowerment and health. In M. Murray (Ed.), *Critical health psychology* (pp. 125–143). China: Palgrave Macmillan.
Marie, D., Fergusson, D. M., & Boden, J. M. (2012). The links between ethnicity, cultural identity and alcohol use, abuse and dependence in a New Zealand birth cohort. *Alcohol and Alcoholism, 47*(5), 591–596. https://doi.org/10.1093/alcalc/ags070
McCreanor, T., Lyons, A., Moewaka-Barnes, H., Hutton, F., Goodwin, I., & Griffin, C. (2015). 'Drink a 12 box before you go': Pre-loading among young people in Aotearoa New Zealand. *Kotuitui: New Zealand Journal of Social Sciences*. https://doi.org/10.1080/1177083X.2015.1037314
McCreanor, T., Moewaka-Barnes, H., Kaiwai, H., Borell, S., & Gregory, A. (2008). Creating intoxigenic environments: Marketing alcohol to young people in Aotearoa New Zealand. *Social Science & Medicine, 67*, 938–946. https://doi.org/10.1016/j.socscimed.2008.05.027
McEwan, B., Campbell, M., & Swain, D. (2010). New Zealand culture of intoxication: Local and global influences. *New Zealand Sociology, 25*(2), 15–37.
McEwan, B., Swain, D., & Campbell, M. (2011). Controlled intoxication: The self-monitoring of excessive alcohol use within a New Zealand tertiary student sample. *The New Zealand Medical Journal, 124*(1336), 68–74.
Mead, H. M. (2003). *Tikanga Māori: Living by Māori values*. Wellington, New Zealand: Huia Publishers.
Measham, F. (2006). The new policy mix: Alcohol, harm minimisation, and determined drunkenness in contemporary society. *International Journal of Drug Policy, 17*(4), 258–268. https://doi.org/10.1016/j.drugpo.2006.02.013
Measham, F., & Brain, K. (2005). 'Binge drinking, British alcohol policy and the new culture of intoxication. *Crime Media Culture, 1*(62), 262–283. https://doi.org/10.1177/1741659005057641
Ministry of Health. (2009). *Alcohol use in New Zealand: Key results of the 2007/08 New Zealand alcohol and drug use survey*. Wellington, New Zealand: Author.

Retrieved from http://www.health.govt.nz/publication/alcohol-use-new-zealand-key-results-2007-08-new-zealand-alcohol-and-drug-use-survey

Ministry of Health. (2016). *Annual update of key results 2015/16: New Zealand health survey.* Wellington, New Zealand: Author. Retrieved from http://www.health.govt.nz/publication/annual-update-key-results-2015-16-new-zealand-health-survey

Ministry of Health. (2019). *Annual data explorer 2017/18: New Zealand health survey.* Retrieved from https://minhealthnz.shinyapps.io/nz-health-survey-2017-18-annual-data-explorer/_w_0811ceee/_w_a8ced35d/_w_ee07803c/#!/explore-indicators

Moewaka-Barnes, H., McPherson, M., & Bhatta, K. (2003). *Te Ao Waipiro 2000: Māori National Alcohol Survey*. Auckland, New Zealand: The Whariki Research Group, Massey University & The Alcohol and Public Health Research Unit, University of Auckland.

Muriwai, E., Huckle, T., & Romeo, J. (2018). *Māori attitudes and behaviours towards alcohol.* Wellington: Health Promotion Agency.

New Zealand Law Commission. (2010). *Alcohol in our lives: Curbing the harm. Law Commission Report, No. 114.* Wellington, New Zealand: New Zealand Law Commission. Retrieved from https://www.lawcom.govt.nz/sites/default/files/projectAvailableFormats/NZLC%20R114.pdf

New Zealand Medical Association. (2015). *Reducing alcohol-related harm. [Policy briefing].* Retrieved from https://www.tttpho.co.nz/wp-content/uploads/2016/10/Alcohol-Briefing18.may_.FINAL_.pdf

Phillips, J. (1996). *A man's country? The image of the pākehā male, a history.* Auckland, New Zealand: Penguin Books.

Randerson, S., Casswell, S., & Huckle, T. (2018). Changes in New Zealand's alcohol environment following implementation of the Sale and Supply of Alcohol Act (2012). *New Zealand Medical Journal, 131*(1476), 14–23.

Saggers, S., & Gray, D. (1998). *Dealing with alcohol: Indigenous usage in Australia, New Zealand and Canada.* Cambridge, UK: Cambridge University Press.

Sargent, M. (1983). The production of drug problems: Creating and controlling consumers. In R. A. Bush (Ed.), *Exploring the alcohol and drug crime link: Society's response* (pp. 35–44). Canberra City, Australia: Australian Institute of Criminology.

Social Issues Research Centre. (1998). *Social and cultural aspects of drinking.* Oxford, UK: Author.

Spicer, P., Novins, D. K., Mitchell, C. M., & Beals, J. (2003). Aboriginal social organization, contemporary experience and American Indian adolescent alcohol use. *Journal of Studies on Alcohol, 64*, 450–457.

Statistics New Zealand. (2014). *Complete New Zealand period life tables – Time-series summaries. Life expectancy by age and sex 1950–2014*. Retrieved from http://archive.stats.govt.nz/browse_for_stats/health/life_expectancy/nz-period-life-tables-info-releases.aspx

Towers, A., Sheridan, J., Newcombe, D., & Szabo, A. (2018). *The longitudinal patterns of alcohol use in older New Zealanders*. Wellington, New Zealand: Health Promotion Agency.

Waldon, J. (2004). Oranga Kaumātua: Perceptions of health in older Māori people. *Social Policy Journal of New Zealand, 23*, 167–180.

Walker, R. (1984). The genesis of Māori activism. *The Journal of the Polynesian Society, 93*(3), 267–281.

Whitbeck, L. B., Chen, X. J., Hoyt, D. R., & Adams, G. W. (2004). Discrimination, historical loss and enculturation: Culturally specific risk and resiliency factors for alcohol abuse among American Indians. *Journal of Studies on Alcohol, 65*(4), 409–418.

Winter, T., Riordan, B., Surace, A., & Scarf, D. (2019). Association between experience of racial discrimination and hazardous alcohol use among Māori in Aotearoa New Zealand. *Addiction*. https://doi.org/10.1111/add.14772

9

Femininities and Intoxication

Fiona Hutton

Introduction

Historically, intoxication has been a key part of many societies, with both pre-modern and contemporary societies enthusiastically engaging in intoxication practices. Intoxication was often related to festivals celebrating a variety of gods pre-Christianity or, in more contemporary times, embedded in leisure, socialising and identity construction (Walton, 2001). However, particular groups that are engaged in intoxicating practices are often viewed with alarm, and one of these groups are women (e.g. see Kohn, 1992). Intoxication or the use of alcohol and other drugs (AOD) by women is often viewed ambiguously. Historically, women were a relatively invisible group in terms of 'drug use', although when they did start becoming visible, their intoxication was often viewed with concern. It should be acknowledged though that much of the research about AOD is situated in westernised nations such as those in Europe,

F. Hutton (✉)
School of Social and Cultural Studies, Institute of Criminology,
Victoria University, Wellington, New Zealand
e-mail: fiona.hutton@vuw.ac.nz

F. Hutton (ed.), *Cultures of Intoxication*,
https://doi.org/10.1007/978-3-030-35284-4_9

the UK, Australia, New Zealand and the US. As noted in Chap. 1, this means that a particular historical, social and cultural context is often discussed, as well as a focus on the experiences of particular groups. Indigenous women's drinking is often absent from debates about the historical context of intoxication, although in the New Zealand context Māori[1] women's drinking was positioned as problematic, and they were not permitted to drink alcohol at all except on doctor's orders (Park, 1995). However, research that does focus on ethnicity often notes strict gendered traditions. For example, Pasifika[2] men usually drank alcohol away from villages and women and children after it was introduced to Pasifika cultures by European settlers (Hutton & Wright, 2015), and in Gray and Nosa's (2009) research, it was considered disrespectful for Niuean women to drink alcohol in front of parents and older males. Young Pasifika and Māori women in New Zealand also have to negotiate a 'dual cultural context' (Bayley & Hurcombe, 2010, p. 13), alongside their management of femininities. For these groups of women, it is often challenging to engage with 'kiwi' drinking cultures whilst upholding values related to their Māori or Pasifika cultural context. For Pasifika women, in particular, the 'kiwi' drinking culture is much more permissive, so they have to work hard at church and family gatherings to disguise their levels of intoxication (Hutton & Wright, 2015). Thus, their 'experiences of alcohol consumption develop within a contradictory framework in terms of both gender and ethnicity, further complicated by cultural practices' (Hutton & Wright, 2015, p. 13).

In the Nigerian context, Dumbili and Williams (2017, p. 6) draw attention to the convention that in the 'traditional era', pre-1949, adult men dominated drinking spaces. Alcohol consumption for adult women and young people was taboo, with beer, rum and spirits constructed as 'men only' drinks. Although this context has now changed after the aggressive marketing of alcohol to women and young people, Nigerian women avoid drinking and playing drinking games in public with alcoholic drinks positioned as 'male'. In doing so, they retain both respectability and femininity (Dumbili & Williams, 2017). Therefore the cultural conventions surrounding femininity and what the idea of femininity means will vary dependent on the social, cultural and historical norms that diverse groups of women are situated within. Femininity will also mean different things to women who are situated differently because of class, ethnicity, sexuality and other markers of identity. However, despite these differences, women still have to negotiate patriarchal constraints and values in order to enact their intoxications.

Therefore, femininities and the use of both legal and illegal substances have a complex and problematic relationship. Women are constrained by the social, cultural and patriarchal values of societies that urge them to conform to 'respectable' practices and ways of being, while, at the same time, in some westernised societies, they are exhorted to engage in the night-time economy (NTE), with its 'anything goes' atmosphere, happy hours and widening choice of venues in which to consume both alcohol and illicit substances. Intoxication for the purposes of this discussion is positioned as a set of diverse practices, ranging from drinking alcohol to injection drug use, and as affected by multiple, interrelated factors such as ethnicity, class, sexuality and age. Intoxication is defined for the purposes of this chapter as using legal or illegal drugs to alter one's state of consciousness, whether visible to others or not, in order to change the way that the person interacts with the world.

The social and cultural positions of women and whether their intoxication is perceived to be within acceptable social and cultural boundaries are important, alongside responses to women whose intoxication is viewed as 'inappropriate' or 'wrong'. Contemporary debates about intersectionality are also important in considering the diversity of intoxications that women engage with and are further discussed later in this chapter. In order to broaden out the debate, intoxication through alcohol and illicit drugs is considered to emphasise the diversity of both femininity and intoxication. This chapter focuses on how women negotiate the tensions and inconsistencies in the ways they are supposed to 'be'. The tensions and inconsistencies that are encountered in enacting intoxicated femininities are multiple, complex and entangled (Poulsen, 2015), and it is these complexities that this chapter seeks to explore.

Femininities and Intoxication

Although intoxication is often tolerated in contemporary westernised societies, it is still bounded by social norms, and there are limits to periods of 'time out'. Intoxicated women are still required to stay within culturally accepted parameters of femininity, albeit that these are often relaxed in contemporary cultures of intoxication. Therefore, women's engagement with drinking femininities must be viewed within the developments in contemporary drinking cultures—for some groups of women, gendered dimensions and acceptability of intoxication have altered in the current neo-liberal landscape (McEwan, Campbell, Lyons, & Swain 2013). Women's AOD takes place within particular social, cultural and historical settings that have changed significantly in the past 30 years or so. A 'distinct post-industrial pattern of drinking' is argued to have emerged, 'characterised by recurrent episodes in which an individual drinks to intoxication or past intoxication in one session' (Hutton, Wright, & Saunders, 2013, p. 452; Measham & Brain, 2005). Contemporary cultures of intoxication are often viewed with a strong moral undertone, highlighting the continued significance of Becker's assertion that 'the goal of artificially inducing change in one's consciousness is considered by many to be immoral' (Becker, 1967, p. 164, cited in Hunt & Antin, 2019).

Additionally, whilst there has been a lack of attention historically to women's AOD, feminist researchers have substantially developed this field of scholarship in recent years (Ettorre, 2007, 2015: Griffin, Szmigin, Bengry-Howell, Hackley, & Mistral, 2012; Hutton, 2006; Lyons & Willott, 2008; Measham, 2002). In counteracting this dearth of research about women's experiences, feminist research has often focused on the meanings of intoxication for women, as well as the patriarchal constraints that women operate under in their use of AOD. Key debates have been developed around exploring women's experiences, in particular, the way that feminine identities interact with the notion of intoxication via both legal and illegal drugs. Intoxication has always raised social anxieties over the conduct of women (Jackson & Tinkler, 2007; Kohn, 1992), although in recent decades, spaces and places for women to become intoxicated have developed as the NTE has grown. This development of nightlife in some countries also meant that alcohol companies actively marketed products to young women who were seen as an important group of consumers within the burgeoning NTE (Lindsay & Supski, 2017). For women, this meant that they could engage with alcohol and other drug cultures in ways not open to previous generations, although this enthusiastic engagement led to a number of 'moral panic'–type responses to young women's 'binge drinking'.[3] In recent times and with the advent of the recognised and well-documented culture of intoxication, the enactment of drinking femininities has come to the fore of both academic and public attention. Although the rise of binge drinking was an issue more broadly about all young people's drinking, young women, in particular, were singled out as problematic precisely because of their gender. Enactments of femininities were reviled in the popular press, with 'ladettes' (Jackson & Tinkler, 2007) and other kinds of behaviours such as shouting, staggering, fighting, vomiting labelled as 'unfeminine' and undesirable.

This view—that intoxication is unacceptable for women—can be seen at least as far back as Roman times where the drinking of un-watered wine by women was seen as 'unspeakably vulgar' (Walton, 2001, p. 19). In Roman society, women were 'absolutely forbidden to drink alcohol because drunkenness was held to be unbecoming to their sex' (Walton, 2001, p. 19). There appears to be a subtle distinction here between being *overly* intoxicated, perhaps by drinking un-watered wine, thus exhibiting drunkenness, and the notion of controlled intoxication by women. So, it may have been acceptable to be intoxicated to a certain degree, after which social norms were breached in terms of enacting 'proper' femininities. These subtle distinctions are still present in contemporary society. For example, *drinking* femininities are seen to be acceptable in 2019, but *drunken* femininities are still regarded as highly problematic (Hutton, Griffin, Lyons, Niland, & McCreanor, 2016).

Women who use alcohol and other drugs are often seen in terms of 'appropriate' social norms and values surrounding femininity. Women who become intoxicated are constructed as mad, bad or dangerous for contravening social and cultural norms related to 'good' feminine behaviour (Ettorre, 2007). There is a large disconnect between the rigid and narrowly defined female roles, and social norms surrounding femininity, and how in reality femininities are actually constructed and enacted. Although, as recent feminist scholarship has noted, traditional or dominant notions of gender and femininity are positioned as prescriptive and 'natural' (Campbell & Herzberg, 2017), affecting women's lived experiences to the extent that they are constantly alert about 'appropriate' presentations of self. Dominant constructions of femininity also present it as a fixed 'thing' that women must somehow fit themselves into. However, a much more useful and less restricting way of viewing femininities is that they are fluid, complex and changeable. Femininity can be seen as 'an interactive process that is adopted and resisted as it is encountered over time, context and space' (Hutton et al., 2013, p. 476). However, for women themselves, their drinking femininities have a range of risks, pleasures and benefits that are fluid, changing and require constant negotiation. For example, young women have strong attachments to particular spaces for particular kinds of drinking practices, with emotion playing a crucial role in intoxication practices in different social spaces. Across a variety of intoxications, women search for different emotions such as happiness, freedom, excitement, risk and pleasure, and these emotions affect and are affected by bodies, objects and spaces (Ahmed, 2004; Hutton et al., 2013). It is these tensions between acceptability, rigidity and complexity, agency and fluidity that women negotiate in enacting femininities whilst pursuing intoxication.

Female Sexuality, Post-feminism and Intoxication

One of the key tensions that women face in enacting femininities is the way that intoxicated practices are linked to female sexuality. Femininity is inextricably bound up with sexuality, and female sexuality has historically been seen as threatening to men and to society. Women's sexuality was seen as dangerous and as having power over men and therefore had to be strictly controlled (Barton, 2005). It is still the case in contemporary times that the 'double standard' related to male and female behaviour is evident. Women are censured for engaging in casual sex and are at pains to distance themselves from representations of femininity that show them in a 'bad light' or as 'tragic' (Hutton et al., 2016). Women's sexuality is policed and controlled in a way that most men's sexuality has never been, and this has consequences not only for women in their everyday lives but specifically for the enactment of intoxicating femininities. In westernised nations, gender and femininity cannot be disconnected from wider social structures. In relation to intoxication, femininities are entangled in discourses about consumption and neo-liberalism (McRobbie, 2007, 2009). Recent work has noted the post-feminist context of women's experiences of intoxication (Gill, 2007; Griffin et al., 2012), as well as developing key ideas such as hypersexuality in relation to women's use of alcohol in particular (Griffin et al., 2012; Hutton et al., 2016). Structural changes such as 'second-wave' feminism, which challenged the patriarchal order that had endured around alcohol and other drug use, alongside the rise of the NTE and post-industrial cultures of intoxication meant that women's intoxication was viewed differently compared to previous decades. Cultural symbols of agential, 'empowered' femininities, such as girl power, and 'ladette' culture, were reflected in the spaces and places for intoxication, as well as in women's intoxication practices (Jackson & Tinkler, 2007).

However, the promise of this post-feminist, neo-liberal social order and its challenge to dominant patriarchal constructions of how women should behave came at a price. As Griffin et al. (2012, p. 185) note the 'pornification of culture' and the 'hypersexualisation' of drinking femininities meant that as bold neo-liberal consumers making choices about consumption, women were often castigated for adopting post-feminist drinking identities involving heavy consumption of alcohol in public spaces. Women engaging with cultures of intoxication in contemporary society teeter on the knife edge of enacting 'up for it' agential femininities that are required to engage with the neo-liberal NTE, without transgressing acceptable boundaries of femininities through which they are still judged. As Griffin et al. (2012) argue, this has become the 'impossible space' in which femininities are enacted, and it could be added that this 'impossible space' of femininity is replicated, to a greater or lesser degree, whatever the means of intoxication, whether consuming alcohol or injecting heroin. Therefore, young women engaging with contemporary drinking cultures perform different ways of being feminine within patriarchal discourses (Lyons & Willott, 2008), and women are still constrained by historical notions of respectability and restraint. In the last decade or so, the rise of Facebook and other social networking sites (SNS) has intensified concerns over young women's intoxication practices and use of alcohol in particular. Research to date has focused on alcohol advertising on SNS (Carah, 2017; Carah & Shaul, 2016; Nicholls, 2012), as well as how women manage their identities online to stay within the parameters of 'acceptable' femininities (Hutton et al., 2016). It should also be acknowledged that SNS do not escape the structural constraints that are present in wider society, such as social class, ethnicity and gender (Bailey, Steeves, Burkell, & Regan, 2013; De Ridder & Van Bauwel, 2013; Lindsay & Supski, 2017). Women engaging with their drinking identities in these spaces also face the contradictions and tensions of post-feminism, hypersexuality, intoxication and respectability (Hutton et al., 2016).

Whilst feminist work in this area is important, it should also be acknowledged that ways of being feminine and engaging with the NTE are not open to all women. The hypersexual femininities that are often required to engage in drinking and other drug-using spaces are often based on white middle-class ideals and confined to westernised societies that have developed post-industrial NTEs in which cultures of intoxication have flourished. Post-feminist notions of 'empowerment' are also not open to all women; those who remain within structural constraints are open to more severe judgements about 'respectability', based on moral judgements about what 'femininity' is supposed to look like (Bailey, 2012; Griffin et al., 2012).

Femininities, Intersectionality and Intoxication

The concept of intersectionality becomes important in these debates about morality, structural constraints and intoxication. Intoxicated women are not all viewed equally and for some, who are viewed as stepping the furthest from acceptable boundaries of femininity, societal condemnation is intensified and stigmatising. Current literature exploring intersectionality urges the viewing of the masculine/feminine gender binary as a social construction (Hunt & Antin, 2019), and it argues that this socially constructed binary marginalises those, both men and women, who do not conform to particular roles. This is evident in the debates about intoxication and femininities, and whilst acknowledging gendered divisions as socially constructed, it must also be acknowledged that social constructions of gender and of masculine and feminine affect 'real-life' experiences of intoxication (Hunt & Antin, 2019, Hunt, Amusen Frank & Moloney, 2015). For women within the NTE, engaging in drinking femininities becomes problematic because the behaviours that are often linked to drinking are related to masculinities: heavy group drinking, enactments of violence, male bonding and sexual promiscuity. For women who become intoxicated, their behaviours are linked to gendered expressions which are viewed as unfeminine, that is, masculine, and this creates tensions that need to be carefully negotiated. Constructions of 'acceptable' femininities affect the experiences of women's intoxications, and how these intoxications are viewed often depends on *more than* gender, with social class, ethnicity and sexuality all affecting women's intoxication, alongside how it is perceived and responded to. Feminist critiques of 'doing gender'[4] (Miller & Carbone-Lopez, 2015) also highlight these issues, that gender can only be understood more fully when other categories such as inequality, ethnicity, age and sexuality are also considered alongside it.

In considering intoxication through the use of a variety of licit and illicit drugs, the assertion by Antin (2015) that intoxication itself is often stigmatised is an important one, alongside, that adherence to sobriety or moderation became an important marker of respectability during the industrialisation era (from the late 1800s to early 1900s). This legacy can still be seen in contemporary times, although entangled in neo-liberal, individualised narratives about both men's and women's drinking. As Ettorre (2007) notes, men and women suffer from the 'damaging effects of gender', but women more so as masculinist structures and epistemologies 'pervade all our theories and practices' (Ettorre, 2007, p. 22). Schippers' (2007, p. 95) concept of 'pariah femininities' becomes significant in these debates. For women who enact characteristics that are associated with men and masculinity such as acting with authority, they are stigmatised and excluded as unfeminine. 'Pariah femininities' enact the characteristics of hegemonic masculinity such as being authoritative, desiring the female body and so on, but these hegemonic masculine characteristics enacted by women are feminised and positioned in a negative light as *not masculine*. Thus 'when a woman is authoritative she is not masculine she is a bitch—both feminine and undesirable' (Schippers, 2007, p. 95). For drinking women, this means that 'up for it' expressions of intoxication that are traditionally 'masculine' (recognising that this binary is socially constructed) are viewed as feminine, subordinate and undesirable. 'Pariah femininities' enact characteristics that are seen as 'less than' and 'othered' when performed by women.

Discourse about drugs and intoxication are heavily entangled in discourses about morality, class, gender, ethnicity, sexuality and so on, and as such intoxication needs to be considered in the structural, social and cultural context in which it occurs. As authors like Bailey, Griffin, and Shankar (2015), Day, Gough, and McFadden (2003) and Dobson (2014) also note, the dilemmas, contradictions and tensions surrounding intoxication are exacerbated for working-class women who are often othered in societal discourses, as well as in the discourses of more privileged women (Watts, Linke, Murray, & Barker, 2015). For example, media discourses focusing on young women's so-called binge drinking—itself a problematic concept—raise the spectre of uncontrolled femininities and the 'figure of the ladette, the bedraggled and scantily clad young working-class woman who stumbles drunkenly through city centre streets' (Watts et al., 2015, p. 220), suggesting a moral outrage that still pervades some women's 'unfeminine' drinking practices. Feminist scholars have also noted that women often distance themselves from other women's drinking which they position as problematic, as in the construction of 'power femininity' where othered drinking practices by denigrated social groups are critiqued as 'skanky people drinking white lightening [cheap cider] at the bus stop' (Watts et al., 2015, p. 224). Through the use of 'positioned othering' (Hutton et al., 2016, p. 81), women distance themselves from problematic constructions of 'other' women's intoxications.

Intoxication or non-intoxication/sobriety is also viewed as a marker of respectability, and for women, this is accompanied by expectations that they will display appropriate markers of femininity such as being passive and pure. For example, recent research exploring media representations of women's drinking practices notes that women who are identified as 'binge drinking' are discussed in terms of their adherence to 'respectable' femininities (Patterson, Emslie, Mason, Fergie, & Hilton, 2016). Women in a sample of media articles were referred to in terms of physical appearance, for example, how drinking has 'wrecked' their physical appearance, as being a danger to themselves, as putting themselves at risk of sexual assault, as a burden to men who have to look after them, as well as being out of control and unfeminine. References to women's clothing as being inappropriate were also invested with a heavily moral tone, suggesting that

> representations of women's 'binge' drinking do not focus solely on the effects of binge drinking on women but also reflect broader social expectations about women's public behaviours. (Patterson et al., 2016, p. 7)

Therefore, engaging with intoxication in the spaces and places of the NTE is inherently risky for women who are judged severely if they deviate from particular forms of femininity, often those that are attractive to heterosexual men. These 'impossible spaces' (Griffin et al., 2012) for femininity are a particular risk environment for women, defined by Rhodes (2009, p. 193) as '…the space—whether social or physical—in which a variety of factors interact to increase the chances of harm occurring'. Despite this, women often engage in the NTE precisely because it allows them to step outside of their everyday selves, and engage with the pleasures intoxication offers for alternative expressions of identity (Day et al., 2003; Hutton, 2006; Hutton & Wright, 2015). It is when this 'stepping outside of the regulated self' is interpreted as also stepping outside of the boundaries of acceptable femininities that women are exposed to the risks inherent in this particular environment. Therefore, where women's risk environments are *social and culturally situated* is also important. Certain groups or populations are seen as more risky than others, and their pleasures are seen as more dangerous and contaminating. For women, who are viewed as *symbolically and dangerously intoxicated*, transgressing the social mores of femininity can be highly problematic, as there is *more to* pleasure and intoxication than the drug itself.

Illicit Drugs, Femininities and Intoxication

Intoxication particularly through the use of illicit drugs, despite many advances in drug law reform,[5] remains subject to objections based on moral arguments. Getting 'out of it' using illegal drugs, in particular, is viewed as unseemly and undesirable. Displaying *visible* signs of intoxication is also viewed with disgust, particularly for women who are perceived as contravening societal norms of femininity. As women who use illicit drugs are constructed as more deviant than their male counterparts, negotiating the spaces and places of intoxication carry risks but also pleasures for intoxicated women. Negotiating these conflicting issues becomes intensely problematic when stigma is associated with the ways in which women seek intoxication. Stigma is one of the key issues that affects the lives of those who take illicit drugs, and stigma is also related to intoxication via alcohol, dependent upon the drinking practices of particular groups. For women, who are more heavily stigmatised than their male counterparts (Boyd, 2015), becoming intoxicated is both risky and problematic in terms of societal expectations, although it may be pleasurable and exciting from the perspective of the women themselves. Stigma is also often related to the use of illicit drugs only and not to those prescribed by a medical practitioner, despite that the drugs may be used for the same purposes: to cope with pain. The way women who use illicit drugs are viewed is therefore heavily stigmatising

> …when women self-medicate they are constructed as irresponsible, immoral, capable of damaging the fetus, and incapable of parenting. When women take prescribed drugs they are constructed as compliant for

following medical advice and their drug use is viewed as therapeutic. (Boyd, 2015, p. xiii)

Thus, the embodied deviance of intoxication and illicit drug use is argued to be emphasised for women (Ettorre, 2015). A 'deviant's' body is marked in particular ways that are suggestive of drug use, lack of control and intoxication. Simply engaging in practices of intoxication leads women's bodies to be stigmatised and heavily marked as symbolically dangerous and defiled. For women enacting intoxication, avoidance of having one's body marked in this way is of paramount importance, not least due to the stigma that is attached to visible signs of illicit drug use and more broadly 'intoxication', on already 'deviant' bodies. However, women use drugs for experiencing pleasure and 'women do not necessarily need to view their actions as being deviant' (Ettorre, 2015, p. 799), emphasising that there is often more than these bodily inscriptions involved in women's pursuit of intoxication.

Research exploring women's experiences of enacting both intoxication and femininities speaks to this point that women engage in the NTE, in public and private licit and illicit drug use, for a wide variety of reasons—pleasure, trauma, fun, socialising—and in doing so engage with pleasure as well as with risks in the expression of intoxicated femininities. As noted in earlier research, risk and pleasure can be constructed on a continuum that women negotiate in their use of intoxicating substances (Hutton, 2006). One of the risks that women have to contend with is the 'cultural outrage' (Ettorre, 2015, p. 799) that surrounds their intoxication practices. Morality is also a highly gendered expression of this cultural outrage, and discourses around drugs refuse to 'shed their ancient moral weight' (Douglas, 1992 cited in Sparks, 2003 p. 159), although some kinds of intoxicated drug use have more moral weight attached to them than others. Here, the concept of entanglement becomes important. Within debates about femininity and AOD use 'the body is analysed as a site of cultural inscription and a nexus between gendered discourses and consumption practices' (Poulsen, 2015, p. 5). Thus, intoxication(s), femininities, the female body and sexualities are all entangled with each other in the presentation of the self. Intoxication for women (and men) cannot be divorced from dominant discourses of femininity and the social and cultural contexts in which AOD takes place. All of these factors are entangled and come together in the enactment of intoxicated femininities.

Women who inject drugs (WWID) are seen as the ultimate transgressors of femininity, they are seen as abject, lost and as having a spoilt, discredited feminine identity (Goffman, 1963). WWID are also perceived to be the victims of male injectors, despite that they often inject with other women or with men who are not their sexual partners (Gibson, 2016). As Bryant and Treloar (2007) note, WWID have agency and the view of them as passive victims of men or male partners is not necessarily accurate, as injecting relationships are more complex and nuanced. Rhodes, Rance, Fraser, and Treloar (2017) further note that intimate relationships where both parties are people who inject drugs (PWID) can be sites of protection and trust, based on care and affection as well as injecting drug use. Furthermore, intoxication via injecting drug use is often done in private, or as privately as the PWID's circumstances will allow. It is not often a public display as with alcohol intoxication, for example, and therefore WWID are identified via other markers of intoxication or past intoxications. WWID's bodies are marked by their drug use as inferior, so publicly visible signs of injecting such as 'track marks' make visible the private. This opens up WWID to stigma and critique based on their deviations from ascribed feminine roles, leading to their intoxications becoming more secret, hidden and risky.

Female drug users are seen as the antithesis of 'normal' womanhood (du Rose, 2015); thus, intoxication for WWID can be fraught with complex negotiations, as well as trying to manage their spoilt identity (Goffman, 1963) or 'gender failure' (Campbell as cited in Stengel, 2014, p. 38). This 'gender failure' can have extensive ramifications for WWID in terms of access to treatment, coerced treatment and through increased surveillance from the state and medical agencies. For women in the US who are mothers or pregnant, they can have their children removed from their care if they admit to using illicit drugs, and they can be prosecuted for homicide if their baby dies during birth (du Rose, 2015). However, WWID and PWID are a very small proportion of drug users overall, and not all women who use drugs are so heavily stigmatised or carry visible, long-lasting markers of intoxication. The majority of drug-using episodes cause users, their families and communities no harm, just like the majority of alcohol-using episodes. However, media and public discourses are filled with stigmatising images of PWID and other problematic drug users, thus painting an inaccurate and stereotypical picture of who drug users are (see Taylor and Ayres, Chap. 11 this volume; Alexandrescu, 2018). For intoxicated women, this means that they are placed in stereotypical categories of (un)femininity and 'othered'.

Femininities, Intoxication and Pleasure

There has also historically been a problematic relationship between intoxication, femininity, desire and pleasure. Pleasure and desire are often seen as inappropriate for female bodies that are inscribed instead with virtues of chastity, purity and morality. In fact, the use of licit and illicit drugs by women is seen as so abhorrent that even women who researched these transgressors of the feminine were 'viewed as contemptible' (Ettorre, 2017, p. 357). The idea of pleasure in relation to alcohol and other drugs is a troublesome concept in AOD research, with most public health campaigns related to intoxication focusing on harm and addiction. To acknowledge pleasure is problematic as the use of both legal and illegal substances does cause harms. However, only *some* drugs and drug users are constructed as dangerous and risky, only *some* drugs and drug users are seen to be in need of control and only *some* drugs and drug users are those whose *harm is anticipated from* (Rhodes, 2009). Those who harm is anticipated from are also excluded from debates about pleasure: practices labelled as harmful are negatively viewed and any pleasures gained through intoxication are denied. Similarly, O'Malley and Valverde (2004) argue that pleasure as an acceptable reason for using drugs fades from the picture, the more problematic a drug-using practice is *seen to be*. In relation to the enactment of intoxicated femininities, the more symbolically and dangerously intoxicating a substance is perceived to be, the more symbolically and dangerously intoxicating its female users are also perceived to be.

As a result, the intense pleasures that women also get from their involvement with alcohol and other drug use are often missing from debates about femininities and intoxication. As documented by Hutton

(2006), Pini (2001) and Measham (2002), although there were distinct ways of 'doing gender' within the dance scene of the 1990s and early 2000s, involvement in particular club spaces was immensely pleasurable, as was risk-taking and casual sex. Whilst harms were acknowledged by women in these studies, so was a sense of female agency and being 'up for it' (drug use, dancing and sex) in the context of ecstasy and polydrug drug use. In particular, female participants in studies about recreational drug use often noted illicit drug use as a way of negotiating different and more empowering forms of femininity, whilst not being naïve to the ways this could be exploited by drug-using men who also inhabited these clubbing and drug-use spaces.

However, pleasure is also problematic as it contradicts key aspects of neo-liberalism that 'good' citizens are supposed to adhere to: responsibility, rationality and reasonableness (O' Malley & Valverde, 2004, p. 27), so much so that

> Governmental discourses about drugs and alcohol, in particular, tend to remain silent about pleasure as a motive for consumption and raise instead visions of a consumption characterised by compulsion pain and pathology. (O' Malley & Valverde, 2004, p. 26)

So those who engage in intoxications that are pathologised in this way are more heavily censored through policy and public discourse, with moderate or 'sensible' consumers being characterised as the ideal. It could be argued though that this is what is pleasurable about intoxication, that these neo-liberal restraints are temporarily released and that for women, whose intoxications are over policed through social norms, they receive double the pleasures from escaping these pressures. Additionally, the idea of intoxications that are *sought after*, for example, 'controlled loss of control' or 'calculated hedonism' (Szmigin et al., 2008) are often seen as immoral and irresponsible. The reasons why women (and men) may pursue intoxications via mind-altering substances remain remarkably unacknowledged and warrant sustained research attention.

Intoxications occur across a variety of spaces and places both within and related to the NTE. For example, bars and clubs may become the endpoint for an evening of intoxication, with a range of femininities engaged with or displayed along the way (Hutton et al., 2013). Risk and pleasure therefore are also fluid and context specific. In exploring connections to the spaces and places of intoxication, scholars focusing on the relationships between emotion and bodies have argued that 'it is through emotion…that the links between the body and the social world can be clearly drawn' (Lyon & Barbalet, 1994, cited in Lupton, 1998, p. 4). Female drug users' bodies are often seen as damaged (Ettorre, 2007), so these damaged bodies have a different emotional link to the social world and elicit a different response than non-intoxicated female bodies. Enactments of intoxicated femininities through diverse bodies can be viewed with an equally diverse range of emotions. For example, 'liminality disgust' is related to the breaching of symbolic categories such as acceptable feminine traits. Lupton (2015, p. 9) further notes that 'practices considered morally wrong according to the accepted norms of behaviour in specific cultural or social groups may evoke disgust'. For intoxicated women, this has a range of implications. For those intoxicated in the public sphere of the NTE, disgust is evoked by the breaching of bodily boundaries, for example, through vomiting or urinating in public, or through breaching symbolic boundaries, by being loud and 'unfeminine' in public spaces. For those intoxicated via the injection use of heroin and other drugs, disgust related to markers of such drug-use position their female users as inferior, which also often intensifies stigma and marginalisation. Breaching the symbolic boundaries of acceptable femininities places WWID outside the boundaries of respectability and renders them blameworthy for a number of social ills. Those who evoke disgust, such as WWID are seen as 'less than' (Lupton, 2015), cementing their position as morally wrong towards whom moral outrage is often directed. However, the pleasures of transgression are the other side of the coin, the side that is often forgotten: to use licit and illicit drugs, to transgress, to escape from the bonds of the regulated self are intensely pleasurable experiences and to evoke disgust could be argued for some as a form of resistance against the constricting norms of conventional femininity. Even for those whose injection (and other) drug use has become problematic, used as a way to cope with trauma, there is pleasure (however fleeting) in soothing these pains.

Conclusion

In considering the debates about femininities and intoxication, it appears that there are serious tensions when femininities and intoxication come together. Across diverse intoxications, women have to (re)negotiate both femininities and intoxication practices, and they are disadvantaged on multiple levels whilst engaging in the use of AOD. Historically, women's engagement with 'drugs' has been framed within patriarchal discourse about 'good' women and, as such, has caused societal anxieties focused on 'unfeminine' expressions of intoxication. As some groups of women have inhabited the spaces and places of the NTE more freely, concerns about their practices of, and engagement with, a range of intoxications have intensified. For women themselves, the contemporary culture of intoxication that has developed in most westernised nations created new pleasures and freedoms but also, at times, intensified risks.

The social and cultural positions of intoxicated women are a crucial element in response to their intoxications. Women are viewed as *symbolically and dangerously* intoxicated, although this often varies, depending on how visible the markers or effects of intoxication are. 'Embodied deviance' (Ettorre, 2007) is ascribed to women's bodies and disorderly bodies, those that step outside the accepted boundaries of femininity, are heavily stigmatised. The context within which recent cultures of intoxication have developed is also significant, with westernised NTE based on values of consumption and leisure. For women, this post-feminist context means that they remain constrained within hypersexual expressions of femininity in order to engage with drinking and other drug cultures. The tensions inherent in drinking cultures in particular are evident in young women's use of SNS, with drinking stories precariously balanced between 'fun' and being 'tragic'. 'Power femininity' and 'positioned othering' remove women from 'other's' problematic intoxications, demonstrating that intoxication is often about *more than* the drug itself: class, ethnicity, age and sexuality, among other markers of identity, are all entangled (Poulsen, 2015) in expressions of intoxicated femininities.

Notes

1. Māori are the indigenous people of New Zealand. They are a diverse population affiliated to different Iwi (tribes/tribal group). Māori make up 14.9% of the New Zealand population (Statistics New Zealand, 2013).
2. The phrase 'Pacific' is commonly used in New Zealand to refer to people who self-affiliate with one or more of the Island nations in the Pacific: Samoa, Tonga, Fiji, Cook Islands, Niue, Tokelau, Tuvalu and Tahiti (Suaalii-Sauni, Samu, Dunbar, Pulford, & Wheeler, 2012, p. 2). Pacific peoples are a diverse population that make up 7.4% of the New Zealand population (Statistics New Zealand, 2013).
3. 'Binge drinking' is a term that refers to drinking often large amounts of alcohol in one sitting to reach a particular level of intoxication. The term is often seen as problematic as it means different things in different social, cultural and historical contexts. Further, units-based definitions of binge drinking often vary resulting in inaccuracies in measuring binge drinking among particular populations.
4. The concept of 'doing gender' was first coined by West and Zimmerman (1987) and was an important development in the field of feminist research and scholarship. The idea that gender is socially produced in response to embedded norms and values around masculinity and femininity continues to be an important concept. However, criticisms of this viewpoint often note that it sidelines other important categories such as ethnicity and class, and that it encourages bigenderism (Miller & Carbone-Lopez, 2015).
5. Some countries are stepping back from their 'war on drugs' stance. For example, several US states have legalised recreational cannabis, following Colorado in 2012. Canada also legalised cannabis for personal recreational use in 2018, following Uruguay who instigated a legal market in 2017. Portugal's often quoted decriminalisation of all drugs for personal possession is also a recognition that the 'war on drugs' approach itself creates harm and does not work to reduce drug use or drug-related harm.

References

Ahmed, S. (2004). *The cultural politics of emotion*. Edinburgh, UK: Edinburgh University Press.

Alexandrescu, L. (2018). Ethnobotanicals' and 'Spice zombies': New psychoactive substances in the mainstream media. *Drugs: Education, Prevention and Policy, 25*(4), 356–364.

Antin, T. (2015). Bodies and behaviors as Taboo – The gendered stigma of substance use, a commentary on Enefalk, Bailey, Griffin and Shankar and Harder and Demant. *Substance Use and Misuse, 50*(6), 768–770.

Bailey, J., Steeves, V., Burkell, J., & Regan, P. (2013). Negotiating with gender stereotypes in social networking sites: From "Bicycle Face" to Facebook. *Journal of Communication Inquiry, 37*(2), 91–112.

Bailey, L. (2012). *Young women and the culture of intoxication: Negotiating classed femininities in the postfeminist context.* PhD thesis, University of Bath, School of Management, England, pp. 1–238.

Bailey, L., Griffin, C., & Shankar, A. (2015). "Not a good look": Impossible dilemmas for young women negotiating the culture of intoxication in the United Kingdom. *Substance Use and Misuse, 50*(6), 747–758.

Barton, A. (2005). *Fragile moralities and dangerous sexualities: Two centuries of semi-penal institutionalisation for women.* Aldershot: Ashgate.

Bayley, M., & Hurcombe, R. (2010). Drinking patterns and alcohol service provision for different ethnic groups in the UK: A review of the literature. *Ethnicity and Inequalities in Health and Social Care, 3*, 6–17.

Becker, H. (1967). History culture and subjective experience: An exploration of the social bases of drug induced experiences. *Journal of Health and Social Behaviour, 8*(3), 163–176.

Boyd, S. (2015). *From witches to crack moms: Women, drug law and policy.* Durham, NC: Carolina Academic Press.

Bryant, J., & Treloar, C. (2007). The gendered context of initiation to injecting drug use: Evidence for women as active initiates. *Drug and Alcohol Review, 26*(3), 287–293.

Campbell, N., & Herzberg, D. (2017). Gender and critical drug studies: An introduction and an invitation. *Contemporary Drug Problems, 44*(4), 251–264.

Carah, N. (2017). Alcohol corporations and marketing in social media. In A. Lyons, T. McCreanor, I. Goodwin, & H. Moewaka Barnes (Eds.), *Youth drinking cultures in a digital world: Alcohol, social media and cultures of intoxication* (pp. 115–131). London: Routledge.

Carah, N., & Shaul, M. (2016). Brands and Instagram: Point, tap, swipe, glance. *Mobile Media and Communication, 4*(1), 69–84.

Day, K., Gough, B., & McFadden, M. (2003). Women who drink and fight: A discourse analysis of working-class women's talk. *Feminism and Psychology, 113*(2), 141–158.

De Ridder, S., & Van Bauwel, S. (2013). Commenting on pictures: Teens negotiating gender and sexualities on social networking sites. *Sexualities, 16*(5), 565–586.

Dobson, A. S. (2014). "Sexy" and "Laddish" girls: Unpacking complicity between two cultural imag(inations)es of young femininity. *Feminist Media Studies, 14*(2), 253–269.

Du Rose, N. (2015). *The governance of female drug users: Women's experiences of drug policy*. Bristol: Bristol University Press.

Dumbili, E., & Williams, C. (2017). Drinking game participation, gender performance and normalisation of intoxication among Nigerian university students. *Addictive Behaviors Reports, 5*, 1–8.

Ettorre, E. (2007). *Revisioning women and drug use: Gender, power and the body*. Basingstoke, UK: Palgrave Macmillan.

Ettorre, E. (2015). Embodied deviance, gender and epistemologies of ignorance: Re-visioning drug use in a neurochemical, unjust world. *Substance Use and Misuse, 50*(6), 794–805.

Ettorre, E. (2017). Feminist autoethnography, gender, and drug use: "Feeling About" empathy while "Storying the I". *Contemporary Drug Problems, 44*(4), 356–374.

Gibson, K. (2016). *Women who inject drugs: Barriers to their access of needle exchange services and gendered experiences*. MA Thesis, Institute of Criminology, Victoria University, Wellington, pp. 1–157.

Gill, R. (2007). Postfeminist media culture: Elements of a sensibility. *European Journal of Cultural Studies, 10*(2), 147–166.

Goffman, E. (1963). *Stigma; notes on the management of spoiled identity*. Englewood Cliffs, NJ: Prentice-Hall.

Gray, J., & Nosa, V. (2009). Tau Fifine Fiafia: The binge drinking behaviours of nine New Zealand born Niuen women living in Auckland. *Pacific Health Dialogue, 15*, 104–111.

Griffin, C., Szmigin, I., Bengry-Howell, A., Hackley, C., & Mistral, W. (2012). Inhabiting the contradictions: Hypersexual femininity and the culture of intoxication among young women in the UK. *Feminism and Psychology, 23*(2), 184–206.

Hunt, G., Aamusen Frank, V., & Moloney, M. (2015). Rethinking gender within alcohol and drug research. *Substance Use and Misuse, 50*(6), 685–692.

Hunt, G., & Antin, T. (2019). Gender and intoxication: From masculinity to intersectionality. *Drugs: Education, Prevention and Policy, 26*(1), 70–78.

Hutton, F. (2006). *Risky pleasures? Club cultures and feminine identities.* Aldershot: Ashgate.

Hutton, F., Griffin, C., Lyons, A., Niland, P., & McCreanor, T. (2016). "Tragic girls" and "crack whores": Alcohol femininity and Facebook. *Feminism and Psychology, 26*(1), 73–93.

Hutton, F., & Wright, S. (2015). 'You don't ditch your girls': Young Maori and Pacific women and the culture of intoxication. *Critical Public Health, 25*(1), 101–119.

Hutton, F., Wright, S., & Saunders, E. (2013). Cultures of intoxication: Young women, alcohol and harm reduction. *Contemporary Drug Problems, 40*, 451–480.

Jackson, C., & Tinkler, P. (2007). 'Ladettes' and 'modern girls': 'Troublesome' young femininities. *The Sociological Review, 55*(2), 251–272.

Kohn, M. (1992). *Dope Girls: The birth of the British drug underground.* London: Granta.

Lindsay, J., & Supski, S. (2017). Curating identity: Drinking, young women, femininities and social media practices. In A. Lyons, T. McCreanor, I. Goodwin, & H. Moewaka Barnes (Eds.), *Youth drinking cultures in a digital world: Alcohol, social media and cultures of intoxication* (pp. 49–65). London: Routledge.

Lupton, D. (1998). *The emotional self: A sociocultural exploration.* London: Sage.

Lupton, D. (2015). The pedagogy of disgust: The ethical, moral and political implications of using disgust in public health campaigns. *Critical Public Health, 25*(1), 4–14.

Lyons, A., & Willott, S. (2008). Alcohol consumption, gender identities and women's changing social positions. *Sex Roles, 59*, 694–792.

McEwan, B., Campbell, M., Lyons, A., & Swain, D. (2013). *Pleasure profit and pain: Alcohol in New Zealand and the contemporary culture of intoxication.* Hamilton, New Zealand: University of Waikato.

McRobbie, A. (2007). Top Girls? Young women and the post-feminist sexual contract. *Cultural Studies, 21*(4), 718–737.

McRobbie, A. (2009). *The aftermath of feminism: Gender, culture and social change.* London: Sage.

Measham, F. (2002). "Doing gender"-"doing drugs": Conceptualizing the gendering of drugs cultures. *Contemporary Drug Problems, 40*, 375–373.

Measham, F., & Brain, K. (2005). "Binge drinking", British alcohol policy and the new culture of intoxication. *Crime, Media and Culture: An International Journal, 1*(3), 262–283.

Miller, J., & Carbone-Lopez. (2015). Beyond 'doing gender': Incorporating race, class, place and life transitions into feminist drug research. *Substance Use and Misuse, 50*(6), 693–707.

Nicholls, J. (2012). Everyday, Everywhere: Alcohol marketing and social media – Current trends. *Alcohol and Alcoholism, 47*(4), 486–493.

O' Malley, P., & Valverde, M. (2004). Pleasure, freedom and drugs: The uses of 'pleasure' in liberal governance of drug and alcohol consumption. *Sociology, 38*, 25–42.

Park, J. (1995). New Zealand. In D. Heath (Ed.), *International handbook on alcohol and culture* (pp. 201–212). Westport: Greenwood Press.

Patterson, C., Emslie, C., Mason, O., Fergie, G., & Hilton, S. (2016). Content analysis of UK newspaper and online news representations of women's and men's 'binge' drinking: A challenge for communicating evidence-based messages about single-episodic drinking? *BMJ Open, 6*, 1–10.

Pini, M. (2001). *Club cultures and female subjectivity: The move from home to house*. Basingstoke: Palgrave.

Poulsen, M. (2015). Embodied subjectivities: Bodily subjectivity and changing boundaries in post-human alcohol practices. *Contemporary Drug Problems, 42*(1), 3–19.

Rhodes, T. (2009). Risk environments and drug harms: A social science for harm reduction approach. *International Journal of Drug Policy, 20*, 193–201.

Rhodes, T., Rance, J., Fraser, S., & Treloar, C. (2017). The intimate relationship as a site of social protection: Partnerships between people who inject drugs. *Social Science and Medicine, 180*, 125–134.

Schippers, M. (2007). Recovering the feminine other: Masculinity, femininity and gender hegemony. *Theory and Society, 36*(1), 85–102.

Sparks, R. (2003). States of insecurity: Punishment, populism and contemporary political culture. In S. McConville (Ed.), *The use of punishment.* Cullompton: Willan Publishing.

Statistics New Zealand. (2013). Population census. Retrieved from http://www.stats.govt.nz/Census/2013-census.aspx

Stengel, C. (2014). The risk of being 'too honest': Drug use stigma and pregnancy. *Health Risk and Society, 16*(1), 36–50.

Suaalii-Sauni, T., Samu, S. K., Dunbar, L., Pulford, J., & Wheeler, A. (2012). A qualitative investigation into key cultural factors that support abstinence or responsible drinking amongst some Pacific youth living in New Zealand. *Harm Reduction Journal, 9*(36), 1–12.

Szmigin, I., Griffin, C., Mistral, W., Bengry-Howell, A., Weale, L., & Hackley, C. (2008). Re-framing 'binge drinking' as calculated hedonism: Empirical evidence from the UK. *International Journal of Drug Policy, 19*(5), 359–366.

Walton, S. (2001). *Out of it: A cultural history of intoxication*. London: Hamish Hamilton.

Watts, R., Linke, S., Murray, E., & Barker, C. (2015). Calling the shots: Young professional women's relationship with alcohol. *Feminism & Psychology, 25*(2), 219–234.

West, C., & Zimmerman, D. H. (1987). Doing gender. *Gender & Society, 1*, 125–151.

10

Masculinities and Intoxication: Notes Towards a Co-constitutive Approach

David Moore

Introduction

In this chapter, I explore some of the theoretical resources available for developing ways of approaching masculinities and intoxication that go beyond social constructionist accounts. If these accounts have provided a valuable corrective to pharmacologically determinist accounts of drugs and their effects, they tend to privilege human subjectivity, agency and discourse, avoid questions of materiality (i.e., drugs as matter) and be less attentive to the agency of the non-human (e.g., objects, technologies, spatio-temporalities). In attempting to address the limitations of social constructionism, recent research on drugs, informed by wider developments in social theory, has begun to grapple with several key questions in highly original ways. How can drugs as matter be taken seriously without reintroducing the essentialist assumptions of pharmacology and biology that social constructionism worked so hard to overcome? How might the

D. Moore (✉)
Australian Research Centre in Sex, Health and Society, La Trobe University, Bundoora, VIC, Australia
e-mail: D.Moore4@latrobe.edu.au

F. Hutton (ed.), *Cultures of Intoxication*,
https://doi.org/10.1007/978-3-030-35284-4_10

agency of non-human forces and elements, generally neglected in social constructionism, be incorporated into accounts of the materialisation of drug effects such as intoxication? How do we move beyond the constructionist canon of 'drug, set and setting', in which each element of the triad is conceptualised rather simplistically as anterior to its interaction with the other two elements? A co-constitutive approach to masculinities and intoxication—in which diverse elements and forces are understood to co-produce one another in the course of their entanglement—might offer answers to these questions. Such an approach has the capacity to 'acknowledge the role of materiality in the production of [drug] realities without characterising that role as determining', and to identify the ways in which even those drug effects considered to be 'the most predictable [...] turn out to be very heavily dependent upon other factors and how all these factors encounter each other in specific situations' (Fraser & Moore, 2011, pp. 4–5).

To begin sketching the contours of a co-constitutive approach to masculinities and intoxication, I draw on selected resources from feminist theory, feminist science studies and science and technology studies, as well as recent empirical work on drugs that puts these resources to work. In the course of this enquiry, a number of issues come into view: the meanings of intoxication across a spectrum of masculinities; whether particular masculinities are associated with danger and risk; drug types and masculinities; and the relationships between intoxication, hegemonic masculinity and other kinds of masculinities. My aim is not to offer a comprehensive review of the relevant literatures or of these issues, but to draw out insights that could prove useful in developing a co-constitutive approach to masculinities and intoxication.[1] Because gender is relational (Davies, 2003; Fausto-Sterling, 2000), the processes that constitute masculinities necessarily also work to constitute femininities. Although the two are related, the primary focus of this chapter is masculinities and intoxication, with 'intoxication' defined as 'the use of substances to alter consciousness' (Hunt & Antin, 2019, p. 71).

Social Constructionist Accounts of Masculinities and Intoxication

An extensive social constructionist literature has addressed questions of masculinities and intoxication, especially in relation to alcohol. As Hunt and Antin (2019, p. 70) note: 'Within many cultures, to drink is to be masculine and to drink heavily and become intoxicated is to be even more masculine'. Drinking and intoxication have often been linked with socially constructed ideals of masculinity, such as autonomy, independence, bodily control, self-discipline and strength (Campbell, 2000; Dumbili & Williams, 2017; Peralta, 2007; Thurnell-Read, 2013). Many studies have focused on heavy drinking to intoxication as an expression of working-class masculinities, along with virility, toughness and male solidarity (e.g., Gough & Edwards, 1998; Hinote & Webber, 2012; Nayak, 2003; Roebuck & Murty, 1996; Tomsen, 1997). Research has also focused on violence as a central element of 'masculine' drinking (e.g., Burns, 1980; Graham & Wells, 2003; Lindsay, 2012; Marsh & Kibby, 1992; Marshall, 1979a; Moore, 1990; Wells, Speechley, Koval, & Graham, 2007), as well as on the relationship between masculinity, intoxication and sexual aggression (Graham et al., 2014), and that between intoxication and uncontrolled masculine embodiment and comportment (e.g., Thurnell-Read, 2011). Young men's drinking practices are also changing rapidly, with a range of masculine drinking identities now available (de Visser & Smith, 2007a, 2007b; Mullen, Watson, Swift, & Black, 2007; Törrönen & Roumeliotis, 2014). More recent research has focused on the emerging role of social media in the creation of new cultures and practices of masculinity and intoxication (Lyons & Gough, 2017).

Illicit drug use has also been linked with the social construction of masculinities. For example, Quintero (1998) examines how ideals of 'machismo' are internalised and re-created among Mexican men through heroin use and aggression in the context of urban street life. For Collison (1996), alongside drug dealing and 'normal' crime, illicit drug use provides cultural and emotional resources for masculine identity 'scripts' among marginalised young men in the UK. Ayres and Treadwell (2012) explore the functionality of cocaine and alcohol intoxication in the violently 'hypermasculine' subcultures of English football fans, while Nasir and Rosenthal (2009) examine the relationships between masculinity and marginalisation, violence, crime, heroin injecting and drug dealing in Indonesia. Writing about male heroin use in Sweden, Lalander (2003) describes it as a 'protracted ritual of masculinity' characterised by 'action, outsidership, strong character and material wellbeing' (p. 134).

Other research, although mainly focused on femininities, has explored the relationship between ecstasy intoxication and the emergence of new forms of masculinity in rave culture, which involve increased physical contact among young men, a less overtly sexualised orientation and greater interest in dancing (e.g., Henderson, 1999; Measham, Aldridge, & Parker, 2001). Club drugs (particularly methamphetamine but also ecstasy, cocaine, gamma hydroxybutyrate [GHB] and ketamine) are used among gay and bisexual men to reduce sexual inhibition, increase sexual performance, produce intimacy and foster a sense of 'community', and become more comfortable with the 'erotic repertoires revolving around impersonal sex' (Green, 2006, p. 72; see also Green & Halkitis, 2006; Hurley & Prestage, 2009). Bryant et al. (2018) critique the methamphetamine 'disinhibition' thesis to more fully explain the relationship between intoxication, sex and masculinity among gay men. Instead they offer the concept of 'sex-based sociality': that is, the ways in which gay and bisexual men draw on methamphetamine intoxication and sex as social resources for building masculine identities, establishing relationships, participating in gay communities and maximising pleasure while protecting themselves and others from harm.

In these accounts, masculinities and intoxication are shaped by the interaction between social class, ethnicity and sexuality, and the pharmacological properties of drugs. Two general observations can be made about this constructionist orientation—one concerning its theoretical underpinnings and the second its treatment of drug properties and effects, including intoxication. Each is dealt with in turn in the following discussion.

Theorising Masculinities

Many of the accounts of masculinities and intoxication cited above are framed by, or engage with, Connell's (1995) influential theory of 'hegemonic masculinity', in which gender is understood as socially produced in institutions and practices. Connell identified four configurations of masculinity: 'hegemonic masculinity' (culturally valorised masculinities with greatest access to power, status and resources); 'subordinated masculinity' (masculinities with least access to power, status and resources, e.g., gay men); 'complicit masculinity' (masculinities that benefit from gender inequality, but do not appear active in the maintenance of the gender order) and 'marginalised masculinity' (masculinities that share common ground with hegemonic forms, but are marginalised on the basis of race and class, e.g., Black or Asian men). In addition to the explicit or implicit application of Connell's theory in many of the studies cited above, this work also indirectly shaped Measham's (2002) influential statement that 'doing drugs' is 'doing gender'.

However, the widespread application of Connell's (1995) original and revised framework (Connell & Messerschmidt, 2005), useful though it has been and continues to be, may also have limited further theoretical development. Writing from within masculinity studies, Pascoe and Bridges (2016, p. 21), for example, argue that the 'dominance of the single approach [Connell's theory] has – we suggest – produced a field of inquiry that has become overly segregated from gender studies, writ large'. Similarly, Waling (2019, p. 90) argues that theorisation of masculinity has devolved into the categorisation of 'fixed and fluid "types" of masculinities': hegemonic, metrosexual, hybrid, inclusive and so on. This trend has led to 'stagnant theorizations of men and masculinity as being only either victim of or responsible to various models of masculin(ities) and masculine practices' (Waling, 2019, p. 90).

Similar calls for fresh approaches have come from within drug research. Hunt and Antin (2019), for example, argue that analyses of gender and drug use would benefit from greater engagement with feminist 'intersectionality' theory (Crenshaw, 1991) (even though discussions of class, ethnicity and sexuality have regularly appeared in recent accounts of masculinities and intoxication). While they note earlier calls to adopt such an approach from feminist drug researchers (e.g., Ettorre, 1992, 2004), they argue that only recently have researchers studying intoxication begun to consider intersectionality (Hunt & Antin, 2019, p. 74; see also Miller & Carbone-Lopez, 2015).

Although calls for greater engagement with feminist (and other) theory in drug research are welcome, such engagement need not be confined to intersectionality (e.g., Campbell & Herzberg, 2017).[2] Puar (2012), for example, identifies herself as a 'staunch advocate' of an intersectional approach, but also argues that it 'must be supplemented – if not complicated and reconceptualized – by a notion of assemblage' (p. 50). This is because:

> intersectional identities are the byproducts of attempts to still and quell the perpetual motion of assemblages, to capture and reduce them, to harness their threatening mobility [...] Subject positioning on a grid is never self-coinciding; positioning does not precede movement but rather it is induced by it; epistemological correctives cannot apprehend ontological becomings; the complexity of process is continually mistaken for a resultant product. (Puar, 2012, p. 50)

In this view, gender, race and social class do not simply 'interact' (there is no raceless femininity or masculinity to which 'race' might be added) but co-constitute one another in the 'perpetual motion of assemblages'. If concepts emphasising emergence and co-constitution, such as 'assemblage', have begun to influence the theorisation of gender (see also Campana, 2015; Fuller, 2015), they have also begun to inform theorising on drug effects.

Theorising Drug Effects

The second general observation that can be made about the social constructionist work on masculinities and intoxication cited above concerns its treatment of drug properties and effects, including intoxication. This work is, in the main, consistent with previous anthropological, sociological and historical understandings of intoxication as shaped by the historical, social and political contexts of consumption (e.g., Douglas, 1987; Gefou-Madianou, 1992; Heath, 1958; Levine, 1978; MacAndrew & Edgerton, 1969; Mandelbaum, 1965; Marshall, 1979b). In this framing, intoxication arises from the interactions between 'drug' (pharmacological properties), 'set' (individual characteristics) and 'setting' (sociocultural context) (Zinberg, 1984), and pharmacology is assumed to be anterior to its interaction with set and setting. In MacAndrew and Edgerton's classic work, 'drunken comportment' is culturally shaped, but alcohol's biological effects remain constant. Similarly, in Marshall's (1979b) review of anthropological literature, alcohol's effects (as well human biology) are also understood as constant. In these cases (and in Zinberg's 1984 formulation), pharmacology and biology are outside—that is, anterior to—culture: drugs have specific effects on the body and brain, which are then subject to cultural interpretation. However, as McDonald (1994) argues, there is no 'culture-free' substance called 'alcohol' (or any other drug) and no neutral, objective position from which to approach its properties and effects, including intoxication. Scientific disciplines such as pharmacology, biology and increasingly neuroscience claim a position external to culture in their assessment of drug properties and effects. Yet, a 'substance has no reality external to perceptions of it, or to the context of its use [...]. The substance is always the cultural values invested in it, and this applies whether the values be those of the police, the pharmacologist, or the user' (McDonald, 1994, p. 18).

Recent work has begun to articulate an alternative theorisation of drug properties and effects. Drawing on key social theorists (e.g., Barad, Deleuze, Haraway, Latour, Law, Mol), this research critiques the view that the properties and effects of drugs (and indeed of set and setting) are anterior to drug 'events'. Rather, drug effects emerge from—are co-constituted by—the multiple forces and elements assembled in consumption networks or events. These, of course, include drugs themselves, but also gender, bodies, affects, knowledge, spatio-temporalities and technologies. Sometimes labelled the 'ontological turn',[3] these studies have drawn on a range of theoretical frameworks in science and technology studies (e.g., Bøhling, 2015; Demant, 2009; Dilkes-Frayne, 2014; Duff, 2014; Farrugia, 2014; Fitzgerald, 1998; Fraser, Moore, & Keane, 2014;

Gomart, 2002; Keane, Moore, & Fraser, 2011; MacLean & Moore, 2014; Malins, 2004; McLeod, 2014; Pedersen, Tutenges, & Sandberg, 2017) and feminist science studies (e.g., Fraser & Moore, 2011; Fraser & valentine, 2008; Pienaar et al., 2017; Vitellone, 2017).

While the theoretical premises and commitments sometimes differ across this work, it shares an interest in drug effects as emergent and co-constituted. As Race (2011, p. 410) argues, drug effects are the:

> contingent outcome of the collective activity of a diverse range of actors, both human and non-human, including techniques, devices, objects, meanings, affects, environments, practices, prehensions, narratives, and desires. […] Crucially, the emphasis is on the performance of things in the world, as they come into encounter with various other elements in interaction so as to produce certain ontological effects.

In the next section, four empirical examples are considered, all of which illustrate the possibilities opened up by approaching masculinities and intoxication as co-constituted. All four attempt to acknowledge materiality in the production of drug realities without treating it as determining, and to analyse drug effects as the contingent outcome of the collective activity of diverse human and non-human elements.

Co-constituting Masculinities and Intoxication

In exploring some of the resources available for re-framing work on masculinities and intoxication, I first consider Gomart's (2002) actor-network analysis of methadone, and Fraser and valentine's (2008) feminist analysis of methadone maintenance treatment (MMT). Though neither account is specifically concerned with 'intoxication', both provide useful theoretical tools for thinking in terms of co-constitution. The former warrants attention as an early and compelling analysis of drug effects as co-constituted, while the latter is a lucid example of the kind of feminist analysis that could productively be applied to masculinities and intoxication. As Waling (2019) argues, theorisation of masculinities has become divorced from feminist work on gender to its detriment. For these reasons, I attend more closely to the theoretical elements of Gomart (2002) and Fraser and valentine's (2008) work than is the case with the work considered further below: Farrugia (2015) on new masculinities and ecstasy intoxication, and Race (2015) on drugs (especially methamphetamine), sex and masculinities among gay men.

Methadone as Un-finished Actant

Gomart (2002) analyses the effects of methadone as they arise in two experiments conducted in the US and France. She first re-analyses Becker's classic symbolic interactionist work on 'becoming a marihuana user' and its 'orthodox' theory of drug action (substance → predictable action → inter-subjective interpretation). Although acknowledging Becker's then-radical shift from pathology to a focus on the techniques and social practices from which drug effects and experiences emerge, she also notes that Becker remains wedded to 'traditional notions of how drugs act [...] where the drug is the *source* of action, and acts *first*, before [inter-subjective] interpretation' (Gomart, 2002, p. 101).[4] To develop an alternative theory of drug effects, Gomart supplants ontological assumptions about 'stable homogenous entities' (such as methadone) as possessing 'pre-given properties' that produce specific 'actions', with a focus on 'heterogenous networks' of (human and non-human) 'actants', 'performances' and 'mediation, emergence, effects' (2002, pp. 97–99).

Gomart then traces how the properties of methadone—and its 'effects'—emerge differently in the networks (the *dispositifs* or apparatuses) constituting the two experiments. In the US experiment, methadone materialises as a medication that successfully 'blocks' heroin craving. However, Gomart (2002) demonstrates how this conclusion emerges only at the end of the trial, and is made possible by foregrounding methadone as the 'source' of action and backgrounding other medical practices (e.g., increased dosing, record-keeping, patient care, institutional regulations and so on) that perform—that is, co-constitute—this effect. In the French trial, a different effect emerges from a different network of medical practices (e.g., the criteria for patient selection, conditions of treatment participation, decreased dosing, psychiatric assessment). Methadone materialises as a diagnostic tool for distinguishing 'pure addicts' (i.e., those without underlying psychopathologies) from those with pre-existing psychiatric illnesses 'who happened to be addicted'. Here, it is not the main source of action but 'an usher for *other* techniques' such as psychiatric treatment with other substances. For Gomart, methadone's action is not 'autonomous' but 'emerges' from the activity of the treatment *dispositif.* In contrast to the orthodox theory of drug action:

> What methadone does varies with the *dispositif.* If we ignore these *particulars,* we would ignore the most important and concrete evidence that 'methadone' is not at the start of these trials an object standing alone, already there but an 'in-between', an *un*-finished actant coextensive (for the time being) with the rest of the *dispositif.* (Gomart, 2002, p. 119)

Methadone as Phenomenon

Whereas Gomart (2002) focuses specifically on methadone's effects, Fraser and valentine (2008) focus on the material/semiotic subjects, objects and practices that co-produce, and are co-produced by, methadone maintenance treatment. To frame their analysis, they draw on the work of physicist and feminist science studies scholar Karen Barad (see also Fraser & Moore, 2011; Pienaar et al., 2017). They do this because Barad provides the conceptual tools for taking into account both the 'social/cultural/discursive' and 'materiality' of methadone as substance, without characterising either as determining (Fraser & valentine, 2008, p. 21). In particular, they draw on Barad's (2003) concept of the 'phenomenon', which comprises 'ontologically primitive relations – [i.e.] relations without pre-existing relata [or components]' (Fraser & valentine, 2008, p. 23). The phenomenon replaces the 'notion of the independent object which possesses inherent boundaries and properties' as well as conventional notions of agency as a 'quality or characteristic of humans' (Fraser & valentine, 2008, p. 23). It destabilises conventional formulations of causality: a pre-formed object (with inherent attributes) enters into subsequent relations with other pre-formed objects, and together they produce predictable, stable effects and meanings. Instead of assuming *inter-action* between pre-existing objects, subjects or entities (as is the case in intersectionality theory), Barad proposes the '"intra-action" of phenomena which themselves are produced through the inseparability of object and observer' (Fraser & valentine, 2008, p. 23). This framing:

> opens up ways of understanding the co-construction – the intermingling and fluid intra-action – of all kinds of material/semiotic subjects, objects and practices, for example, that of methadone as substance, media representations of methadone, treatment regulation, the dosing point, client identities and prevailing social and political values. (Fraser & valentine, 2008, pp. 24–25)

Fraser and valentine apply this frame to MMT and, in one chapter of their book, explore how 'MMT materialises differently for men and women, how the practices enacted with it rely upon and co-produce certain forms of femininity and masculinity, and equally, how notions of femininity and masculinity shape how treatment is understood' (Fraser & valentine, 2008, p. 142). They do this through a close analysis of MMT client and practitioner constructions of gender, and of the ways in which heterosexual relationships, power and gender violence influence treatment practices. They focus on how a set of 'related concepts – addiction, repetition, femininity and passivity or lack of agency – operate intra-actively to materialise treatment in different ways for male and female clients' (Fraser & valentine, 2008, p. 166). Addiction itself is feminised, as is repetition. Treatment is experienced by clients as repetitive and constraining (with onsite daily dosing being characterised as similar to daily heroin use), and leads to perceptions of clients, both male and female, as lacking agency, albeit in different ways for male and female clients. For example, female clients are conceptualised relationally, as doubly subject to the power of male partners (e.g., through violence) and service providers (e.g., through the provision or withdrawal of treatment). While male clients are similarly subject to the power of service providers, they are conceptualised in more autonomous terms: not subject to the same levels of surveillance around their female partners or seen as responsible for, or subject to, them. In turn, gender and treatment co-produce one another in specific and different ways for men and women, by shaping client access and referral to service providers, as well as treatment delivery.

There are notable similarities between the *dispositif* of Gomart's (2002) work and Fraser and valentine's (2008) formulation (via Barad) of the phenomenon: because drugs do not have inherent attributes separate from the processes of observation or of intra-action with other objects, it makes little sense to see them as acting independently or consistently on other objects, or as 'determining' reality in predictable ways. So, for example, we might question the orthodox causal chain that drug A (e.g., crystalline methamphetamine) has B inherent properties (e.g., it is a powerful stimulant), affects people in C specific way (e.g., it induces psychosis, paranoia and violence) and should be responded to in D way (e.g., prevent people from consuming it). What drugs *do*, what they *are*, is dependent on their circumstances, and blanket assumptions about the physical and pharmacological properties of drugs, their actions and their intoxicating effects cannot be assumed. Gomart's (2002) account also introduces the idea of the 'in-between' or '*un*-finished actant'. In other words, actants such as drugs have a set of potentialities, possibilities or eventualities, which have been capacitated by previous intra-actions and by their materiality. Which, if any, of these potentialities are realised—are 'finished'—depends on intra-action with other objects.

Affective Assemblages

If Gomart (2002) provides a compelling account of the materialisation of methadone, and Fraser and valentine (2008) of the co-constitution of treatment and gender, a more empirically relevant example of work addressing the co-constitution of masculinities and intoxication is provided by Farrugia's (2015) analysis of young men and ecstasy use. He first notes the reliance on simplistic notions of 'peer pressure' and common deployment of 'hegemonic masculinity' frameworks in existing research on youth drug use (and, we might add, in the accounts of masculinity and intoxication outlined above). For Farrugia (2015, p. 243), such research fails to address the 'specific dynamics, relations, and practices making up events in which [non-hegemonic] masculinity is assembled', and cannot account for the human and non-human bodies, or the potential pleasure and sociality, enacted within them. As a result, it tends to reiterate established, and often negative, accounts of young men's drug use. His aim, instead, is to understand how pleasures, desires, communication, intimacy and friendship emerge and are co-constituted in the ecstasy event. To achieve this, he draws not on the language of '*dispositif*' or 'phenomenon' but on Deleuzian ontology, in which '[a]ll bodies, be they human or non-human, are thought of as relational and emergent phenomena or assemblages' (Farrugia, 2015, p. 244). As the 'minimum unit of reality', assemblages are temporary sets of relations that 'constitute bodies, objects, substances, expressions, qualities, practices, and affects' (Farrugia, 2015, p. 244). In this formulation, 'drugs, spaces, and indeed young men, are not "interacting" with each other; instead, bodies are ontologically implicated in the constitution of each other' (Farrugia, 2015, pp. 244–245).

Having established the tools for his theoretical interest in co-constitution, Farrugia (2015) provides an analysis of three themes in the accounts of the pleasures of ecstasy intoxication offered by the young men he interviewed: honest, open communication, spatio-temporality and intimacy, and shared experience. With respect to the first theme, Farrugia (2015) argues that male sociality is disrupted and reconstituted 'beyond the limits imposed by hegemonic norms and values'. This reconstitution includes valuing more open, honest and profound verbal communication and physical contact. Farrugia highlights the pleasures of participation in assemblages that allow such 'communicative affective capacities, usually denied to young men in hegemonic understandings of their lives, to emerge' (2015, p. 247).

Taking up the second theme identified in the interviews, spatio-temporal arrangements and intimacy, Farrugia (2015) expands his analysis to include non-human bodies and forces. Here, he focuses on the 'very specific assembling of relations' co-constituting the ecstasy events described in his interviews. One example of the importance of spatio-temporality in 'co-constituting affective capacities' focuses on ecstasy intoxication in a small garage measuring three by five metres. According to one of the interviewees, there were 'seven or eight of us just in there [...] sitting very, very close. When we were talking to people, we were talking *to* them' (Farrugia, 2015, p. 249). Farrugia draws out the constitutive role of time together in this small space by showing how spatial-temporal arrangements are implicated in the co-constitution of bodies possessing particular 'affective capacities' (2015, p. 249). In this event, specific assemblages constituted a physical intimacy that enabled 'pleasurable affective experiences' (2015, p. 249).

In addressing the third theme identified in the interviews, the importance of sharing experiences with others, Farrugia (2015) highlights participant accounts of 'sharing corporeal sensations with friends'. Importantly, drugs and intoxication have been enacted within a specific assemblage and could be enacted differently in future assemblages. Taken together, the 'ontological separation of bodies felt outside of these events again becomes fluid and an assemblage of their own bodies, the bodies of their friends, the song, the space and time, and the drugs emerges [in] its place' (2015, p. 251). Furthermore, disruptions to the 'ontological boundaries between bodies [...] perhaps leads [the participants] to consistently refer to weird sensations, connections, and experiences' (2015, p. 251). In Farrugia's account, far from being an explanation for practices, 'hegemonic masculinity' is a property that may emerge from some 'complex consumption assemblages' but not others.

Farrugia's (2015) insightful account focuses on the co-production of new masculinities and intoxication but also of bodies, sociality, affective capacities, objects and space time. Nevertheless, there remains a lingering sense in this account that ecstasy takes part in the assemblage's constellation of relations more fully formed, less 'un-finished', than other bodies, objects and forces. The feelings of emotional intimacy, desire for honesty and enjoyment of shared experience described by the young men in Farrugia's (2015) article echo earlier accounts of ecstasy intoxication. Although this might be read as suggesting ambiguity in Farrugia's account about whether ecstasy's properties are anterior or emergent, such effects may have come to be associated with ecstasy—been capacitated by previous intra-actions and by their materiality—because earlier research has tended to focus on settings (e.g., rave culture) that are similarly conducive to their emergence. Indeed, research on ecstasy conducted in a very different setting—among 'mainstream' (i.e., not associated with the 'countercultural rave scene') 18- to 25-year-olds in Atlanta, Georgia (Reid, Elifson, & Sterk, 2007)—explores aggression and violence as effects of ecstasy use.[5] Following Gomart (2002), could ecstasy's reported effects have emerged from various *dispositifs* (e.g., rave culture) and only *later* attributed to the drug's pharmacology? Whatever the reason, that such questions come into view highlights the immense challenges in formulating emergent theories of drug action.

Intimate Infrastructures

The final example of empirical work emphasising co-constitution is provided by Race (2015). His article is concerned with drugs, sex and masculinity among gay men in the context of what he calls 'intimate infrastructures': the 'material technologies, objects and environments that facilitate erotic encounters'. In particular, his focus is the new forms of sexual encounter afforded and mediated by online hook-up devices: the 'cluster of practices' known as 'PNP, or Party 'n' Play', which involves crystal methamphetamine use and sex with multiple partners in private homes. Rather than echoing the depiction of such practices in the HIV prevention literature as 'pathogenic', or in gay community discourse and queer critical literature as 'contemptible', Race (2015) approaches them as having 'their own organizing logics and relative coherence' and as a 'significant source of pleasure, connection, eroticism and intimacy – notwithstanding the known dangers' (p. 256).

Three features of the 'sociotechnical environment' of online hook-up culture are explored in Race's (2015) work. First, members are free to communicate their preferred sexual practices, desires and HIV identities, using a range of 'abbreviations, acronyms, and loaded terms' (Race, 2015, p. 263), prior to meeting offline. The relative anonymity afforded by online devices is important here. Second, this 'textual and material space' allows the co-construction of sexual activities and desires as a 'prelude to – or irrespective of – a sexual encounter', although they may also 'constitute an erotic practice in themselves' (Race, 2015, p. 266). Third, sexual encounters are 'enacted through specific practices, objects, devices and arrangements' (Race, 2015, p. 267), which include having sex with multiple partners, using drugs, talking, watching pornography, browsing online profiles, and locating and inviting new participants. In this formation, crystal methamphetamine is 'used' to 'effectuate certain capacities: it enhances sexual sensation, but also keeps consumers awake and alert [...]. The drug also delays ejaculation, sometimes indefinitely [...]' (Race, 2015, p. 268). Most valued is the 'capacity to maintain focus on various sexual possibilities and activities, and the staying power or stamina required to sustain these erotic engagements' (Race, 2015, p. 268). Other drugs 'used' in these sessions include gamma hydroxybutyrate (GHB) and Viagra or Cialis.[6]

These sex sessions can be viewed as a specific 'instantiation of a more general mode of experimentality (or play) that characterizes participation in this context' (Race, 2015, p. 268). Here participants play in order to explore 'what men can do with each other, bodily and relationally, [...] so as to produce more expansive experiences of pleasure and masculinity' (Race, 2015, p. 269). This is a 'specific sphere of sociability and amiable acquaintance among men in urban centres that prioritizes sex as a principle mechanism for connection and sociability' (Race, 2015, p. 271).

Race's incisive analysis, like Farrugia's, draws out the co-production of gay masculinities and drug intoxication, and their intra-action with bodies, practices, social relations and material technologies. Interestingly, it also offers glimpses of possible ontological ambiguity with respect to anteriority/emergence. The phrase 'effectuate certain capacities' (which is unreferenced but presumably inspired by Deleuze) does considerable conceptual heavy-lifting in the treatment of drug effects. We might, therefore, take Race to mean that crystal methamphetamine (alongside other drugs) is implicated in PNP infrastructures as an un-finished actant, as having potentialities (rather than stable, anterior properties) realised only in the intra-action of bodies, technology, objects and environments. On the other hand, crystal methamphetamine is also described as being 'used' to 'enhance sexual sensation', to keep consumers 'awake and alert' and to delay ejaculation. In these passages, the ontological status of the drug shares more with conventional accounts. That said, his account stands in stark contrast to the literature on methamphetamine and violence (e.g., Boles & Miotto, 2003; Maxwell, 2005; McKetin et al., 2014).

Conclusion

In this chapter, I first explored a subset of the many valuable social constructionist studies of masculinities and intoxication. These included studies of the relationship between alcohol and other drug intoxication and masculine ideals (e.g., autonomy, independence, bodily comportment, control, self-discipline and strength), working-class masculinities, violence and sexual aggression, masculine embodiment and comportment, changing masculine identities, (including those shaped by the emerging role of social media), ethnicity, marginalisation, 'hypermasculinity', new forms of masculinity and sexuality. In general, these accounts conceptualised masculinities and intoxication as shaped by the interaction between pharmacology and social context. The influential theory of 'hegemonic masculinity' shaped much of this work, but may also have limited further theoretical development, leading to the segregation of masculinity studies (including those focused on intoxication) from the broader field of gender studies, and to an emphasis on the development of masculine typologies. While there have been calls for greater engagement with feminist intersectionality theory in analyses of gender and drugs, other theoretical frameworks are also available (e.g., feminist science studies, science and technology studies, new materialism). In addition to their capacity to illuminate issues of gender, these theoretical frameworks also offer new ways of thinking about drug effects, including intoxication, that go beyond social constructionist accounts of drunken comportment or drug, set and setting, and beyond 'intersection'. In the research influenced by these theoretical developments, drug effects emerge from, or are co-constituted by, the 'collective activity of a diverse range of actors, both human and non-human, including techniques, devices, objects, meanings, affects, environments, practices, prehensions, narratives, and desires' (Race, 2011, p. 410).

To explore some of the resources available for re-framing work on masculinities and intoxication, four empirical accounts have been considered. All four attempt to acknowledge materiality in the production of drug realities without treating it as determining, and to analyse drug effects as the contingent outcome of the collective activity of diverse human and non-human elements. Although the first two accounts do not deal directly with intoxication, they provide useful theoretical tools for thinking in terms of co-constitution. Methadone as material substance is central to Gomart's (2002) compelling account of how the drug's effects emerge differently in two networks of medical practices: as a medication that successfully 'blocks' heroin craving in one network, and as a diagnostic tool for distinguishing between categories of patient in the other. Fraser and valentine's (2008) feminist analysis draws on Barad's (2003) related concepts of 'phenomenon' and 'intra-action' to trace how understandings of addiction, repetition, femininity and passivity co-produce gender and methadone maintenance treatment. This co-production occurs in specific and different ways for men and women, and it shapes client access and referral to treatment providers, as well as treatment delivery. In both analyses, drugs do not have inherent attributes separate from the processes of observation or of intra-action with other objects, and it makes little sense to see them as acting independently or consistently on other objects, or as 'determining' reality in predictable ways. These issues are also central to the analyses of affective assemblages and intimate infrastructures offered by Farrugia (2015) and Race (2015), respectively. Both emphasise the co-production of masculinities and intoxication but also of bodies, social relations, affective capacities, practices, objects, spatio-temporalities and technologies. That it remains possible to glimpse ambiguity about the ontological status of drugs in such incisive accounts merely underlines the immense challenges in formulating theories of drug effects that emphasise emergence and contingency. These studies provide excellent resources for developing a co-constitutive approach to masculinities and intoxication, and chart promising directions for future research.

Acknowledgements This chapter draws on the intellectual work associated with a project funded by the Australian Research Council (DP18010036). The project has been based in two institutions over time: the National Drug Research Institute, Curtin University, and the Australian Research Centre in Sex, Health and Society, La Trobe University. The National Drug Research Institute is supported by core funding from the Australian government under the Drug and Alcohol Program and also receives significant funding from Curtin University. I am extremely grateful to Adrian Farrugia, Suzanne Fraser, Helen Keane, Kane Race and Fiona Hutton for helpful comments on an earlier version.

Notes

1. For recent comprehensive reviews of the literature on gender, alcohol and other drug use, and intoxication, see Hunt and Antin (2019), Hunt, Antin, Bjønness, and Ettorre (2016), and Hunt and Asmussen Frank (2016).
2. Reviewing the extensive feminist literature debating the merits of intersectionality is beyond the scope of this chapter (for recent examples, see Carastathis, 2014; Cooper, 2016 and Nash, 2017). The intention here is to draw a parallel between some recent developments in feminist work and those occurring in the drug field (see below).
3. See Keane (2017, p. 10) on the limitations of the 'turn' metaphor.
4. Gomart's analysis of Becker could also be applied to the theorising of drug action in MacAndrew and Edgerton (1969), Marshall (1979b) and a range of other social constructionist accounts.
5. It is worth noting that Reid et al. (2007) endorse an orthodox theory of drug action. A positive linear relationship between levels of ecstasy use and levels of aggressive and violent behaviour, 'levels of serotonin' and 'alcohol-induced aggression', mediated by 'low self-control', are all central to their account.
6. In conventional medical usage, Viagra and Cialis are drugs for the treatment of erectile dysfunction in men.

References

Ayres, T. C., & Treadwell, J. (2012). Bars, drugs and football thugs: Alcohol, cocaine use and violence in the night time economy among English football firms. *Criminology and Criminal Justice, 12*(1), 83–100.

Barad, K. (2003). Posthumanist performativity: Toward an understanding of how matter comes to matter. *Signs: Journal of Women in Culture and Society, 28*(3), 801–831.

Bøhling, F. (2015). Alcoholic assemblages: Exploring fluid subjects in the night-time economy. *Geoforum, 58*, 132–142.

Boles, S. M., & Miotto, K. (2003). Substance abuse and violence: A review of the literature. *Aggression and Violent Behavior, 8*, 155–174.
Bryant, J., Hopwood, M., Dowsett, G. W., Aggleton, P., Holt, M., Lea, T., … Treloar, C. (2018). The rush to risk when interrogating the relationship between methamphetamine use and sexual practice among gay and bisexual men. *International Journal of Drug Policy, 55*, 242–248.
Burns, T. F. (1980). Getting rowdy with the boys. *Journal of Drug Issues, 10*(2), 273–286.
Campana, J. (2015). Distribution, assemblage, capacity: New keywords for masculinity? *European Review of History: Revue européenne d'histoire, 22*(4), 691–697.
Campbell, H. (2000). The glass phallus: Pub(lic) masculinity and drinking in rural New Zealand. *Rural Sociology, 65*(4), 562–581.
Campbell, N., & Herzberg, D. (2017). Gender and critical drug studies: An introduction and an invitation. *Contemporary Drug Problems, 44*(4), 251–264.
Carastathis, A. (2014). The concept of intersectionality in feminist theory. *Philosophy Compass, 9*(5), 304–314.
Collison, M. (1996). In search of the high life: Drugs, crime, masculinities and consumption. *British Journal of Criminology, 36*(3), 428–444.
Connell, R. (1995). *Masculinities*. Berkeley: University of California Press.
Connell, R., & Messerschmidt, J. W. (2005). Hegemonic masculinity: Rethinking the concept. *Gender & Society, 19*(6), 829–859.
Cooper, B. (2016). Intersectionality. In L. Disch & M. Hawkesworth (Eds.), *The Oxford handbook of feminist theory* (pp. 1–22). Oxford: Oxford University Press.
Crenshaw, K. (1991). Mapping the margins: Intersectionality, identity politics, and violence against women of color. *Stanford Law Review, 43*(6), 1241–1299.
Davies, B. (2003). *Frogs and snails and feminist tales: Preschool children and gender*. Cresskill: Hampton Press.
de Visser, R. O., & Smith, J. A. (2007a). Alcohol consumption and masculine identity among young men. *Psychology & Health, 22*(5), 595–614.
de Visser, R. O., & Smith, J. A. (2007b). Young men's ambivalence toward alcohol. *Social Science & Medicine, 64*(2), 350–362.
Demant, J. (2009). When alcohol acts: An actor-network approach to teenagers, alcohol and parties. *Body & Society, 15*(1), 25–46.
Dilkes-Frayne, E. (2014). Tracing the 'event' of drug use: 'Context' and the co-production of a night out on MDMA. *Contemporary Drug Problems, 41*(3), 445–479.

Douglas, M. (Ed.). (1987). *Constructive drinking: Perspectives on drink from anthropology*. Cambridge: Cambridge University Press.

Duff, C. (2014). *Assemblages of health: Deleuze's empiricism and the ethology of life*. Dordrecht: Springer.

Dumbili, E., & Williams, C. (2017). Drinking game participation, gender performance and normalization of intoxication among Nigerian university students. *Addictive Behaviors Reports, 5*, 1–8.

Ettorre, E. M. (1992). *Women and substance use*. Houndsmill: Macmillan.

Ettorre, E. M. (2004). Revisioning women and drug use: Gender sensitivity, gendered bodies and reducing harm. *International Journal of Drug Policy, 15*, 327–335.

Farrugia, A. (2014). Assembling the dominant accounts of youth drug use in Australian harm reduction drug education. *International Journal of Drug Policy, 24*(4), 663–672.

Farrugia, A. (2015). 'You can't just give your best mate a massive hug every day': Young men, play and MDMA. *Contemporary Drug Problems, 42*(3), 240–256.

Fausto-Sterling, A. (2000). *Sexing the body: Gender politics and the construction of sexuality*. New York: Basic Books.

Fitzgerald, J. L. (1998). An assemblage of desire, drugs and techno. *Angelaki, 3*(2), 41–57.

Fraser, S., & Moore, D. (2011). The drug effect: Constructing drugs and addiction. In S. Fraser & D. Moore (Eds.), *The drug effect: Health, crime and society* (pp. 1–16). Melbourne: Cambridge University Press.

Fraser, S., Moore, D., & Keane, H. (2014). *Habits: Remaking addiction*. Basingstoke: Palgrave Macmillan.

Fraser, S., & valentine, K. (2008). *Substance and substitution: Methadone subjects in liberal societies*. Basingstoke: Palgrave Macmillan.

Fuller, G. (2015). In the garage: Assemblage, opportunity and techno-aesthetics. *Angelaki, 20*(1), 125–136.

Gefou-Madianou, D. (Ed.). (1992). *Alcohol, gender and culture*. London: Routledge.

Gomart, E. (2002). Methadone: Six effects in search of a substance. *Social Studies of Science, 32*(1), 93–135.

Gough, B., & Edwards, G. (1998). The beer talking: Four lads, a carry out and the reproduction of masculinities. *Sociological Review, 46*, 409–435.

Graham, K., Bernards, S., Osgood, D. W., Abbey, A., Parks, M., Flynn, A., ... Wells, S. (2014). 'Blurred lines?' Sexual aggression and barroom culture. *Alcoholism: Clinical and Experimental Research, 38*(5), 1416–1424.

Graham, K., & Wells, S. (2003). 'Somebody's gonna get their head kicked in tonight!' Aggression among young males in bars – A question of values? *British Journal of Criminology, 43*(3), 546–566.
Green, A. I. (2006). 'Chem friendly': The institutional basis of 'club drug' use in a sample of urban gay men. In B. Sanders (Ed.), *Drugs, clubs and young people: Sociological and public health perspectives* (pp. 67–76). Farnham: Ashgate.
Green, A. I., & Halkitis, P. N. (2006). Crystal methamphetamine and sexual sociality in an urban gay subculture: An elective affinity. *Culture, Health & Sexuality, 8*(4), 317–333.
Heath, D. B. (1958). Drinking patterns of the Bolivian Camba. *Quarterly Journal of Studies on Alcohol, 19*, 491–508.
Henderson, S. (1999). Drugs and culture: The question of gender. In N. South (Ed.), *Drugs: Cultures, controls and everyday life* (pp. 36–48). London: Sage Publications.
Hinote, B. P., & Webber, G. R. (2012). Drinking toward manhood: Masculinity and alcohol in the former USSR. *Men and Masculinities, 15*(3), 292–310.
Hunt, G., & Antin, T. (2019). Gender and intoxication: From masculinity to intersectionality. *Drugs: Education, Prevention and Policy, 26*(1), 70–78.
Hunt, G., Antin, T., Bjønness, J., & Ettorre, E. (2016). The increasing visibility of gender in the alcohol and drug fields. In T. Kolind, G. Hunt, & B. Thom (Eds.), *The SAGE handbook of drug and alcohol studies: Social science approaches* (pp. 396–417). London: SAGE Publications.
Hunt, G., & Asmussen Frank, V. (2016). Reflecting on intoxication. In T. Kolind, G. Hunt, & B. Thom (Eds.), *The SAGE handbook of drug and alcohol studies: Social science approaches* (pp. 322–336). London: SAGE Publications.
Hurley, M., & Prestage, G. (2009). Intensive sex partying amongst gay men in Sydney. *Culture, Health and Sexuality, 11*(6), 597–610.
Keane, H. (2017). Drug use assemblages: Substances, subjects, and the city. *Contemporary Drug Problems, 44*(1), 3–11.
Keane, H., Moore, D., & Fraser, S. (2011). Addiction and dependence: Making realities in the DSM. *Addiction, 106*(5), 875–877.
Lalander, P. (2003). *Hooked on heroin: Drugs and drifters in a globalized world.* Oxford: Berg.
Levine, H. G. (1978). The discovery of addiction. Changing conceptions of habitual drunkenness in America. *Journal of Studies on Alcohol, 39*(1), 143–174.
Lindsay, J. (2012). The gendered trouble with alcohol: Young people managing alcohol related violence. *International Journal of Drug Policy, 23*, 236–241.

Lyons, A. C., & Gough, B. (2017). Masculinities, alcohol consumption and social networking. In A. C. Lyons, T. McCreanor, I. Goodwin, & H. M. Barnes (Eds.), *Youth drinking cultures in a digital world: Alcohol, social media and cultures of intoxication* (pp. 66–79). London: Routledge.

MacAndrew, C., & Edgerton, R. B. (1969). *Drunken comportment: A social explanation*. London: Nelson.

MacLean, S., & Moore, D. (2014). 'Hyped up': Assemblages of alcohol, excitement and violence for outer-suburban young adults in the inner city at night. *International Journal of Drug Policy, 25*(3), 378–385.

Malins, P. (2004). Body-space assemblages and folds: Theorizing the relationship between injecting drug user bodies and urban space. *Continuum, 18*(4), 483–495.

Mandelbaum, D. G. (1965). Alcohol and culture. *Current Anthropology, 6*(3), 281–293.

Marsh, P., & Kibby, K. (1992). *Drinking and public disorder: A report on research conducted for the Portman Group by MCM Research*. London: Portman.

Marshall, M. (1979a). *Weekend warriors: Alcohol in a Micronesian culture*. Palo Alto: Mayfield.

Marshall, M. (1979b). Introduction. In M. Marshall (Ed.), *Beliefs, behaviors, and alcoholic beverages: A cross-cultural survey* (pp. 1–11). Ann Arbor: University of Michigan Press.

Maxwell, J. (2005). Emerging research on methamphetamine. *Current Opinion in Psychiatry, 18*, 235–242.

McDonald, M. (1994). Introduction: A social-anthropological view of gender, drink and drugs. In M. McDonald (Ed.), *Gender, drink and drugs* (pp. 1–31). Oxford: Berg.

McKetin, R., Lubman, D. I., Najman, J. M., Dawe, S., Butterworth, P., & Baker, A. L. (2014). Does methamphetamine use increase violent behaviour? Evidence from a prospective longitudinal study. *Addiction, 109*(5), 798–806.

McLeod, K. (2014). The missing work of collaboration: Using assemblages to rethink antidepressant action. *Contemporary Drug Problems, 41*(1), 109–142.

Measham, F. (2002). 'Doing gender' – 'Doing drugs': Conceptualizing the gendering of drugs cultures. *Contemporary Drug Problems, 29*(2), 335–373.

Measham, F., Aldridge, J., & Parker, H. (2001). *Dancing on drugs: Risk, health and hedonism in the British club scene*. London: Free Association Books.

Miller, J., & Carbone-Lopez, K. (2015). Beyond 'doing gender': Incorporating race, class, place, and life transitions into feminist drug research. *Substance Use & Misuse, 50*(6), 693–707.

Moore, D. (1990). Drinking, the construction of ethnic identity, and social process in a Western Australian youth subculture. *British Journal of Addiction, 85*, 1265–1278.

Mullen, K., Watson, J., Swift, J., & Black, D. (2007). Young men, masculinity and alcohol. *Drugs: Education, Prevention and Policy, 14*(2), 151–165.

Nash, J. C. (2017). Intersectionality and its discontents. *American Quarterly, 69*(1), 117–129.

Nasir, S., & Rosenthal, D. (2009). The social context of initiation into injecting drugs in the slums of Makassar, Indonesia. *International Journal of Drug Policy, 20*(3), 237–243.

Nayak, A. (2003). Last of the 'Real Geordies'? White masculinities and the subcultural response to deindustrialisation. *Environment and Planning D: Society and Space, 21*, 7–25.

Pascoe, C. J., & Bridges, T. (2016). *Exploring masculinities: Identity, inequality, continuity, and change*. New York: Oxford University Press.

Pedersen, W., Tutenges, S., & Sandberg, S. (2017). The pleasures of drunken one-night stands: Assemblage theory and narrative environments. *International Journal of Drug Policy, 49*, 160–167.

Peralta, R. (2007). College alcohol use and the embodiment of hegemonic masculinity among European college men. *Sex Roles, 56*(11), 741–756.

Pienaar, K., Moore, D., Fraser, S., Kokanovic, R., Treloar, C., & Dilkes-Frayne, E. (2017). Diffracting addicting binaries: An analysis of personal accounts of alcohol and other drug 'addiction'. *Health, 21*(5), 519–537.

Puar, J. K. (2012). 'I would rather be a cyborg than a goddess': Becoming-intersectional in assemblage theory. *philoSophia, 2*(1), 49–66.

Quintero, G. (1998). Cultural models of masculinity and drug use: 'Machismo', heroin, and street survival on the U.S.-Mexico border. *Contemporary Drug Problems, 25*(1), 147–168.

Race, K. (2011). Drug effects, performativity and the law. *International Journal of Drug Policy, 22*, 410–412.

Race, K. (2015). 'Party and Play': Online hook-up devices and the emergence of PNP practices among gay men. *Sexualities, 18*(3), 253–275.

Reid, L. W., Elifson, K. W., & Sterk, C. E. (2007). Hug drug or thug drug? Ecstasy use and aggressive behavior. *Violence and Victims, 22*(1), 104–119.

Roebuck, J. B., & Murty, K. S. (1996). *The Southern subculture of drinking and driving: A generalized model for the Southern White male*. New York: Garland.

Thurnell-Read, T. (2011). 'Off the leash and out of control': Masculinities and embodiment in Eastern European stag tourism. *Sociology, 45*(6), 977–991.

Thurnell-Read, T. (2013). 'Yobs' and 'snobs': Embodying drink and the problematic male drinking body. *Sociological Research Online, 18*(2), 1–10.
Tomsen, S. (1997). A TOP NIGHT: Social protest, masculinity and the culture of drinking violence. *British Journal of Criminology, 37*(1), 90–102.
Törrönen, J., & Roumeliotis, F. (2014). Masculinities of drinking as described by Swedish and Finnish age-based focus groups. *Addiction Research & Theory, 22*(2), 126–136.
Vitellone, N. (2017). *Social science of the syringe: A sociology of injecting drug use.* London: Routledge.
Waling, A. (2019). Rethinking masculinity studies: Feminism, masculinity, and poststructural accounts of agency and emotional reflexivity. *Journal of Men's Studies, 27*(1), 89–107.
Wells, S., Speechley, M., Koval, J. J., & Graham, K. (2007). Gender differences in the relationship between heavy episodic drinking, social roles, and alcohol-related aggression in a U.S. sample of late adolescent and young adult drinkers. *American Journal of Drug and Alcohol Abuse, 33*(1), 21–29.
Zinberg, N. E. (1984). *Drug, set, and setting.* New Haven: Yale University Press.

Part III

Representations of Intoxication

11

Media and Intoxication: Media Representations of the Intoxicated

Tammy Ayres and Stuart Taylor

Introduction

The neoliberal era of consumer capitalism sees engagement with consumer markets and the consumption of goods mediating all aspects of social life. Resultantly, the health, economic, environmental and, indeed, moral good of society are entwined with who consumes what, how they consume it and the resultant ends of such practices. Consumers are provided with the freedom to choose from an array of products and as responsible agents of choice are left to navigate their own consumption. Such liberty, however, proves problematic when consumers make the *wrong* choices (Bauman, 1997). For example, a Friday night takeaway is a gastronomic treat, yet those who continually eat fatty or sugary foods causing obesity and tooth decay prompt concern. A Cuban cigar at a

T. Ayres
University of Leicester, Leicester, UK
e-mail: tca2@leicester.ac.uk

S. Taylor (✉)
Liverpool John Moores University, Liverpool, UK
e-mail: s.taylor2@ljmu.ac.uk

F. Hutton (ed.), *Cultures of Intoxication*,
https://doi.org/10.1007/978-3-030-35284-4_11

wedding distinguishes the occasion as a special celebration, yet smoking 40 cigarettes a day causing lung cancer evokes worry. Taking opioid painkillers as a form of treatment can be a medical necessity, while injecting illegal heroin warrants arrest.

Whilst consumer-based lifestyle choices offer us apparent freedom, this freedom is illusionary. Instead, the entrepreneurial self is held accountable for our consumption choices, ergo our own fate. Freedom to choose, therefore, is only given 'on condition that you make the right choices; you are given freedom on the condition that you will not really use it' (Žižek, 2008, p. 129). Thus construed, freedom represents 'a formal gesture of consent to our own oppression and exploitation' (Žižek, 2008, p. 147), as both desire and choice are structured and controlled by capitalism and its effectual mass media. In true neoliberal ethos, those who step outside the accepted parameters of freedom become socially excluded, flawed consumers who 'deserve everything they get' for failing to adhere to the socio-cultural norms that sublimate the systemic violence[1] of consumer capitalism (Ayres, 2019; Raymen & Smith, 2016; Žižek, 2008).

Intoxication by its very nature centres upon consumption. Whilst the consumption of drugs has been constant within every civilisation throughout history, the social reaction to such use has been open to fluctuation; fluctuations tied to the exigencies and advancement of capitalism (Chambliss, 1977; Pryce, 2012). Hence, at certain times, certain intoxication practices are embraced, whilst others arouse alarm and denunciation (Bancroft, 2009). In this chapter, we seek to explore the socio-cultural framing of intoxication through the lens of news media representations. In doing so, we contemplate how intoxication relates to neoliberal notions of (ir)responsibility and (im)morality in the context of capital consumerism and how the media representation of intoxication constitutes a form of objective violence (Žižek, 2008).

We employ a straightforward definition of intoxication here—a state of non-sobriety purposely achieved through the consumption of any drug—which enables us to consider intoxication that relates to both legal and illegal substance uses. Importantly, rather than concentrating on intoxication per se, the focus of this chapter is on the media emphasised social object of *the intoxicated*. We argue that media representations of the intoxicated fit within a wider individualistic consumer responsibilisation agenda, which serves to camouflage the underpinning tensions and contradictions of capitalism. Simultaneously, these media representations reinforce the apartheid between acceptable and unacceptable intoxication practices (Taylor, Buchanan, & Ayres, 2016), constructing substance use as both socially embedded, even desirable, and concurrently problematic. This agenda allows the identification of the purposeful consumer majority whose right to engage in appropriate intoxication is a marker of cultural competence, whilst simultaneously framing the intoxicated minority as consumers who lack rational judgement and warrant concern.

Through drawing primarily on news media representations of intoxication, this chapter concludes that the objective violence of the media serves to marginalise and criminalise flawed consumption practices; responsibilise *the intoxicated* for a plethora of social ills and disavow the harmful practices of consumer capitalism. Whilst the chapter predominantly draws upon research and experiences from the UK, the key points have relevance to all Westernised consumer states.

Media Representations of the Intoxicated

Substance use is framed through a narrow reductionist drugs discourse whereby governmental rhetoric, empirical research, public knowledge and media representations revolve around the same, tapered array of issues (Taylor, 2016). Understanding the dominant media themes representing substance use is therefore crucial as they mirror the themes evident in wider political/public dialogue (Taylor, 2008). Both discursive and visual news media representations of substance use predominantly focus on detrimental anti-social, criminal, economic and health-related outcomes (Ayres & Jewkes, 2012; Hilton, Wood, Patterson, & Katikireddi, 2014). Interestingly, whilst depictions of illicit drug users centre upon notions of addiction (Alexandrescu, 2018; UKDPC, 2010), media portrayals of alcohol have moved away from primarily being concerned with dependence towards a series of pathologised problematic modes of alcohol consumption (Nicholls, 2011)—all of which emphasise the dangers associated with a failure to self-regulate one's freedoms (e.g.

alcohol-related disease, anti-social behaviour, physical and mental ill-health). Significantly, rather than media representations considering the diversity of populations engaged in such risky practices, problematic consumption is disproportionately embodied within a generic typology—that of the irresponsibly intoxicated (binge drinking) consumer. For example, each New Year's Day, the UK's most popular newspaper, the Daily Mail, greets readers with a familiar headline:

New year, same old binge Britain: Arctic weather fails to stop drunken revellers causing chaos on streets of UK. (Levy, 2010)
Welcome to 2013: Shameful scenes of booze-fuelled New Year's chaos in cities across Britain. (O'Hare, 2013)
New Year... depressingly familiar scenes: Festivities are marred by drunken revellers causing chaos in towns and cities across Britain. (Robinson, 2014)
New Year, but the same old shocking scenes: Mayhem in streets across Britain as drunken revellers lose their senses. (Tomkin, 2016)
Some people won't be having a happy new year! Carnage on the streets of Britain as revellers see in 2017 with a night of fighting, vomiting and a LOT of flesh on show. (Burrows, 2017)
Happy SPEW Year! Britons see in 2018 with a night of drunken revelry and plenty of flesh on show—followed by violence and lashings of regret as celebrations turn to carnage. (Tahir, 2018a)

Such representations provide a fetishistic insight to armchair readers of the ubiquitous nightlife landscape that appears after dark in most Western nations. In the UK, this is a landscape worth nearly 6% of gross domestic product (NTIA, 2015), the majority of which comes from consumers drinking at risky levels (Bhattacharya et al., 2018; Sheron & Gilmore, 2016). Central to these media depictions is intoxication, in the form of binge drinking and drunken revelry, which is presented as both a given and as problematic (Patterson, Emslie, Mason, Fergie, & Hilton, 2016). Written into these scripts are concerns around violence, crime, vulnerability, health and economic consequences. Following the moral panic tradition, *the intoxicated* are framed as a symbolic social *other* with a breakdown of moral virtue posing a risk to the normative social order (Critcher, 2011)—a process which sees the UK news media preoccupied by an irresponsible minority of uncivilised binge drinkers whose behaviours 'are blamed for a range of both intentional and unintentional harms to "others" through their "alcohol-fuelled" anti-social behaviour' (Wood, Patterson, Katikireddi, & Hilton, 2014, p. 580).

Here *the intoxicated* binge drinkers are framed as representing a risk to *us* (Taylor, 2016) through their 'chaos' and 'carnage' in the orderly society of 'normal' consumers who make the 'right' choices (Bauman, 2007). However, alongside the normative set of harmful risks presented to us by this group (e.g. physical violence, anti-social behaviour, burdens on health and emergency services), we see a new paradigm of risk subtlety emerging—that of a threat to our consumer freedoms. Irresponsible drinkers who cross the divide between acceptable and unacceptable consumption are seen as lacking restraint. As a potential risk to *our* consumer experience, not only in a direct physical sense but also in terms of prospective restrictions on the consumer marketplace itself which spoil the fun of non-flawed consumers (Bauman, 2007). For example, policies of minimum unit alcohol pricing in the UK are framed as punishing 'the vast majority of responsible drinkers of cheap alcohol for the actions of problem drinkers' (Bourne, 2012, p. 1) as there is 'no such thing as problem drinks, only problem drinkers' (McArdle, 2018, p. 2).

Consequently, there is a framing of *the intoxicated* as bad apples who are unable to engage with consumer markets in an appropriate fashion. For example, Hilton et al. (2014, p. 3) indicate that the legislative decision to ban smoking in cars with children present in the UK was framed by the media as necessary due to 'thoughtless', 'seriously bad' and 'selfish' parental consumption practices. Meanwhile, the role of commercial enterprise is side-lined, such as the aggressive marketing of alcohol or the sexist promotional practices of night-time leisure venues (Gunby, Carline, & Taylor, 2017). Consequently, the intoxication practices and individual choices of consumers, rather than the nature of the consumer market that encourages hedonism and excess, attracts condemnation (Smith, 2014; Winlow & Hall, 2016).

Importantly, media representations of *the intoxicated* cluster around common demographical profiles regardless of what substance they consume. Measham and Moore (2008, p. 280) observe that problematic drinking 'may be less of a question of intoxication, than of <u>who</u> is drunk and where they are drunk'. Hence, the media use the *who* and *where* as indicators of concerning, dysfunctional consumption. Consequently, alcohol-intoxicated women are framed as acting outside of the prescribed boundaries of femininity (Day, Gough, & McFadden, 2004; Griffin, Szmigin, Bengry-Howell, Hackley, & Mistral, 2013; Hutton, Griffin, Lyons, Niland, & McCreanor, 2016), whilst intoxicated working-class females are viewed with 'visceral disgust' (Lennox, Emslie, Sweeting, & Lyons, 2018, p. 19). Similarly, intoxicated working-class male drinkers are seen as a dysfunctional element of 'rough youth' (Measham & Moore, 2008, p. 284) whose 'living for the weekend' philosophy and violent tendencies appear at odds with the work hard, keep your nose clean mentality of conservative life (Tomsen, 1997; Winlow & Hall, 2006). Additionally, whilst bar-going male and female binge drinkers are essential to the night-time economy (NTE), intoxicated street drinkers are actively excluded from these spaces (Measham & Brain, 2005).

Such depictions of the legally intoxicated integrate with the media's characterising of illegal drug users with the media differentiating between recreational middle-class drug users risking their productive, pro-social status and working-class 'addicts' whose use represents one of a number of ingrained characteristics relating to non-productivity (Alexandrescu, 2018). Here, dysfunctionality is emphasised around classed notions of an inability (or unwillingness) to work, a lack of education, links to criminality and addiction (Taylor, 2008). Indeed, within a neoliberal context, the illegally intoxicated are framed as a redundant population (Alexandrescu, 2018) within a contemptive scrounger narrative (Wincup & Monaghan, 2016) that questions their societal worth and place (Monaghan & Yeomans, 2016). A narrative is often associated with dependence (on welfare, on substances, on housing, healthcare and other state institutions) that has no place in a neoliberal society (Bauman, 2001). Grounded in their analysis of a UK-based reality TV show, Atkinson and Sumnall (2018, p. 1) argue that this application of neoliberal rhetoric frames working-class drug users as failing 'to meet the neoliberal notion of the productive citizen' whilst the 'structural causes of substance use and inequality were silenced, and an emphasis on individual responsibility prioritised'.

Consequently, the only *responsible* choice in relation to illegal drugs is to 'just say no' with attempts to encourage more informed choices amongst those who say 'yes' responded to in the media with contempt and ridicule (Taylor, 2016). Instead, the media blames the flawed intoxication practices of marginalised populations for ruining people's lives, communities, town centres and businesses (e.g. Cooper, 2018; Doward, 2017; ITV News, 2015). Intoxicated users of illegal substances are framed in media discourses as dehumanised agents of irresponsibility, but also as the zombies, monsters and demons plaguing, corrupting and causing fear in contemporary society (e.g. Alexandrescu, 2019; Cooper, 2018; Gregory, 2018; Thornton, 2018). Simultaneously, the systemic causes underpinning these ills are disavowed and the ideological emphasis on self-governance is reiterated and reinforced.

As such, the flawed choices of *the intoxicated* are constructed as *falling* 'outside of righteous and respectable consumption' (Measham & Moore, 2008, p. 276). Hence, they need to be 'blamed and shamed...scapegoated and stigmatised for their behaviours in public, media and political discourse' (Atkinson & Sumnall, 2018, p. 2). This process serves two purposes. Firstly, it ascribes cultural boundaries to (licit and illicit) intoxication (Presdee, 2000). These boundaries align with the arbitrary drug apartheid (Taylor et al., 2016), hence, certain cultures of intoxication enjoy the privileged impunity of laissez-faire consumption practices, whilst others become the target of policy advancements which seek to control and change, or failing that exclude and criminalise, such behaviour. Secondly, it legitimises the socio-legal and economic status quo. For whilst the media unfavourably depict those who consume legal substances inappropriately (to excess, within incorrect places), the corporate respectability and profitability of the alcohol industry legitimises legal regulation. Illegal substances lack such credentials and perhaps, more importantly, their consumers lack any such respectability (Measham & Moore, 2008). Consequently, the media deflect attention away from the destructive practices of legitimate industry whilst simultaneously framing drug prohibition as essentialism (Taylor, 2016). This legitimises the continued marginalisation and criminalisation of the irresponsibly intoxicated consumer (regardless of the legality of the substance used).

The Irresponsibly Intoxicated Consumer

In the hyper-masculine Western or action movie genres, intoxication is something rarely experienced by the lead (male) character—they drink whisky and vodka martinis galore, but never fall from their horse or out of their Aston Martin. Their alcohol use is instead an indicator of their social identity—they are so tough that they are impervious to intoxication (and indeed its potentially harmful effects). In the same way, an epoch of conspicuous consumption sees individuals seek out social recognition through engaging with alcohol (and the NTE more widely) to assist them in their construction of social identity (Ayres & Treadwell, 2012; Smith, 2014). Gone are the days of walking into a bar and asking for a generic beer, wine or gin. Instead those inhabiting the NTE choose from a plethora of options; requesting a Peroni, Marlborough Sauvignon or Hendricks gin with Fevertree tonic. Preferred brands which are asked for by name, say as much about the persona of the user as they do their taste buds. Increased consumption of Prosecco in the UK (UHY, 2018) has been accompanied by promotional events such as 'Fizzy Fridays' the essence of which is to provide (a diluted version of) the celebrity champagne lifestyle to the masses as people seek out their own piece of luxury.

Yet engagement with such consumables is only cool if one remains in control and does not show the lack of responsibility which characterises *the intoxicated*. So, whilst amassing impressive bar bills is presented in the news media as aspirational (e.g. Binns, 2013; Byrne & Boyle, 2012; Sporn, 2018; The Telegraph, 2013), being openly intoxicated to the point of embarrassing oneself represents the antithesis of this, even if you are a celebrity (Atkinson, Elliott, Bellis, & Sumnall, 2011), and particularly if you are female (Nicholls, 2011). Ironically, whilst such behaviour is posited as undesirable in official discourse and policy (Home Office, 2012), it actually demonstrates a hyperconformity to consumerism (Ayres, 2019; Raymen & Smith, 2016) as excessive intoxication is integral to leisure, pleasure and 'man-ing up' in contemporary consumer society (Ayres & Treadwell, 2012; Iwamoto, Cheng, Lee, Takamatsu, & Gordon, 2011; Smith, 2014). The contradiction being that we are encouraged to want 'more, more, more' (Winlow & Hall, 2016; Žižek,

1997), whilst simultaneously demonstrating restraint and control in the face of such consumer forces and their paradoxical control mechanisms. Hence, the need for people to enact an individualised controlled loss of control (Measham, 2004) when engaging with intoxication. Those unwilling to exercise such restraint and regulate their behaviour are publicly branded and vilified in the media (e.g. Burrows, 2017; Couzens, 2018; Tahir, 2018b).

These paradoxical messages reflect the wider contradictions of capitalism (Ayres, 2019). For example, whilst the UK government's alcohol policy encourages the continued availability/expansion of products for the responsible consumer/business, it simultaneously associates such products with the very themes of problematic consumption and (ir) responsibility which predominate media representations (e.g. disease, risk, crime, violence and disorder) (Hackley, Bengry-Howell, Griffin, Mistral, & Szmigin, 2008; Haydock, 2014a). Hence, policy cuts red tape for responsible business whilst restricting the liberty of the intoxicated other. Resultantly, whilst pop-up Prosecco and craft beer bars are permitted to appear in city centres, those same locations are subject to Public Space Protection Orders restricting the use of alcohol amongst street drinkers. Simultaneously whilst purveyors of alcohol have been encouraged to remove high strength varieties of cheap lager and cider from their shelves due to their association with problematic populations (Sumpter et al., 2016), those same shops have expanded the available range of higher-end alcohol products they stock that cater for the 'right' clientele (Hancock, 2017; Riley, 2016). Here, the responsible consumer is encouraged to engage with the newest consumer trends whilst the freedoms of *the intoxicated* are restricted. Similarly, whilst city centre nightscapes continue to see new venues appearing for the discerning consumer to enjoy, the use of drunk tanks for those who go too far, become intoxicated and, in doing so, add to the statistics of disorderly conduct is being piloted (Evans & Whitehead, 2013; NHS, 2017).

This repression and demonisation is perhaps most explicit to those who either refuse or are unable to engage in regulated drug markets. The irresponsibility of these users—who after all needs to engage with illicit intoxication cultures in the face of such a glittering array of legal choices—is focussed upon via a multi-pronged strategy of control, criminalisation and incarceration. Yet, demographical distinctions are again evident here. For example, whilst the Chief Constable of London's Metropolitan Police attempts to simply shame (the otherwise responsible) middle-class cocaine user into ethical sobriety (Siddique, 2018), the criminal justice system proactively coerces working-class drug users towards abstinence. Here, the 'problematic behaviours of problematic populations...who exist somewhere outside of the societal mainstream' (Monaghan & Yeomans, 2016, p. 126) remain the focus of policy. Indeed, Alexandrescu (2018, p. 363) observes that media representations of drug users act as 'symbolic frames' which 'mark collective identities and shape hierarchies of moral worth' with certain drug-using populations presented as 'threat and pollution'. A process that serves to reinforce the established parameters of freedom, reflecting neoliberal governance and control through individual freedom and choice.

Objective Violence, Civilised Consumption and the Drug Apartheid

To further understand the significance of the media's framing of the (ir) responsible citizen and intoxicated other, we now consider how this represents an integral role in neoliberalism, consumerism and individualisation, ultimately serving three interlinking key purposes. Firstly, it enables the media to establish a clear demarcation of normality providing a platform for the repression of liberty and the implementation of harm via what Žižek (2008) terms objective violence. Secondly, media representations underline the juxtaposition between civilised and barbaric consumption with the former celebrated and the latter leading to condemnation and criminalisation. Thirdly, media reporting serves to camouflage the contradictory practices of consumer capitalism reinforcing the exclusionary drug apartheid, which simultaneously embeds and forbids alternative cultures of intoxication, legitimising the capitalist status quo. As such, these three issues require further consideration.

Demarcation of the Normal

Media representation of intoxication is a 'sublime object of ideology' (Žižek, 1989) that 'act as the cultural wallpaper in our lives' (Taylor, 2010, p. 97). Such representation is an ideological bluff ignoring reality in subtly conflated ways that are consumed and treated as if they were real by the general population; who know but pretend not to know (Žižek, 1989). In fact, the media representation of drugs and their resultant intoxication has become more real than the reality itself creating a 'simulacrum' of acceptable and unacceptable intoxication that feeds into a media-created hyper-reality surrounding the phenomenon (Baudrillard, 1994). It is this media-created hyper-reality that generates much of the misinformation, misunderstanding and ambiguity outlined above, while also serving to direct attention away from the contradictions of neoliberalism and its systemic violence. Thus, the media plays a key role in the symbolisation of normality, portraying acceptable intoxication in a positive, healthy light (e.g. Bosely, 2018; Dodgson, 2018; Jennings, 2018), while anything that deviates from this normality is portrayed in a distorted and manipulated misrepresentation (Cohen, 1972).

The media representation engenders social conformity by illustrating the consequences for those unwilling to abide by the rules of the societies and refrain from flawed consuming. Therefore, media simplification, complicit within a wider reductionist discourse espoused by politicians, commercial enterprise, researchers and the public alike, ignores the underlying structural causes of intoxication in favour of blaming individuals. The media attributes many of society's ills to the intoxicated other, the flawed consumer who has lost control, while disavowing the systemic violence arising from consumer capitalism, which is imperceptible and in turn explains much of the subjective violence focused on by the media (Taylor, 2010; Žižek, 2008).

Media representation of *the intoxicated* not only supports subjective violence but should also be seen as a form of objective violence. The symbolic violence of the media is embodied in its discourse and representation, while the systemic 'structural' violence arising from consumer capitalism and its ever-expanding market is hidden and negated (Žižek,

2002). The onus on individuals to regulate their behaviour, monitor their own freedoms and to guard against risk is emulated in the micro-control mechanisms implemented to regulate and prevent flawed intoxication. From the no drinking signs on the streets of town centres reinforced by the on-the-spot penalty fines and the creation of zones of exclusion, to the criminalisation of certain forms of intoxication, these controls, although justified on the grounds of 'chaos' and 'carnage' as depicted in the media, are discriminatory. They disproportionately discriminate along the lines of gender, race, ethnicity and social class, inflicting structurally embedded harms on already disadvantaged groups as control mechanisms and are increasingly, but 'surreptitiously woven into the very fabric of the city' (Hayward, 2004, p. 138), differentiating the civilised from the barbaric.

Civilised and Barbaric Consumption

Media representation ignores the barbarism of consumer capitalism and its ability to produce 'cultural forms and identities that are closed, intolerant and violent, and, as such, constitute a threat to civilised life' (Hall & Winlow, 2004, p. 277). The persuasive power of the media ignores these harmful subjectivities, whilst portraying the 'visceral and occasionally violent' way, excluded people are attempting to conform to the values of pseudo-pacified consumer capitalism (Hall & Winlow, 2004) as problematic, unwanted and undesirable. Resultantly, the media demarcates civilised consumption of intoxicating substances and civilised consumers along demographical lines. However, the substance use of the bourgeoise is preserved and promoted since they can be trusted to act like responsible citizens and implement the necessary controlled loss of control demanded by neoliberal consumerism. Wealthier customers are not only a better class of clientele that represent the 'ideal drinking style', but they have a 'civilising effect' while also increasing profits. Not only do they attract the right kind of people, but they encourage or shame the uncivilised into buying expensive and civilised intoxicants as everyone competes to stand out, fit in and elicit envy (Haydock, 2014b; Smith, 2014; Winlow & Hall, 2016). Meanwhile, the substance use of the uber wealthy remains hidden both from plain sight, but also from the media's gaze, as the market offers access to exclusive private members clubs and chauffeur-driven cars accessed through underground car parks, ensuring a blanket of public invisibility for their (excessive) intoxication practices.

Consumer capitalism therefore demands that we must consume excessively, although only in a civilised and non-risky way, from the array of commodified substances offered, or risk being labelled as flawed and intoxicated consumers (Bauman, 2007). Scapegoating hides the fact that many of society's ills are not a consequence of the intoxicated other but the intensification of neoliberal consumer capitalism, its consequential disintegration of the underlying order (Hall & Winlow, 2015; Winlow & Hall, 2016) and its ideological thuggery (Angell, 2000). The depiction of flawed consumers and intoxication in the media as the uncivilised other means these intoxicated 'savages' deserve everything they get and have no place in a civilised society, creating a clear demarcation between us (the civilised) and them (the barbarians) which feeds into the existing system of drug apartheid.

Drug Apartheid

The media clearly segregates between what constitutes illegitimate and legitimate, barbaric and civilised intoxication, ascribing to the dominant philosophy based on legal status (illegal drugs are bad and thus criminal, while legal drugs are acceptable and thus civilised), method and level of use (extreme intoxication, problematic and dependent patterns of substance use regardless of legal status is bad and should be prohibited). However, this demarcation is not premised on science or harm, instead as Ayres (2017, 2019) has argued, it is about prioritising the exigencies of capitalism and corporate profits as many of the benefits ascribed to legitimate substances permitted for civilised intoxication are erroneous and their harmfulness denied and concealed, partly by the media's ideological function.

Alcohol is a good example—we see the symbolic framing of alcohol according to social class and age, social grouping of users and types of drink. Media representations of unacceptable (binge drinking induced) intoxication sit on par with the framing of illegal drugs and their users, as dependent drinkers face coerced sobriety, enforced by surveillance technology (Agerholm, 2017; BBC, 2016), mimicking sanctions already imposed on illicit drug-using offenders. Meanwhile, the civilised consumption of the respectable middle classes, who drink wine or craft beer, is portrayed as healthy, even medicinal, and yet they are most likely to engage in harmful drinking practices (Brierley-Jones et al., 2014; Iparraguirre, 2015). Here, the drug apartheid allows us to differentiate between appropriate and inappropriate drug consumption and to develop a system of control that results in the exclusion of flawed consumers.

The excommunication of flawed consumers, the 'collateral casualties' of these inherent contradictions, offers a solution to the social ills identified in the media's reductionist discourse as *the other* becomes an 'object of ethical responsibility and moral concern' (Bauman, 2007, p. 92). Thus, the drug apartheid is constructed along the lines of vested economic interest and moralistic virtue rather than scientific evidence of harm, resulting in the oppression of ostracised consumers. Concurrently, the media sustains the political, economic and moral status quo underpinning the consumer market and its drive for profit. It is this culmination which results in an arbitrary system that allows commercial interests to flourish, the causes of harm to be camouflaged and the intoxicated other to be excluded and criminalised as, for example, alcohol-related problems are ascribed to 'drinkers themselves and not to the availability of alcohol' (Mercille, 2016, p. 62). Thus, the drug apartheid allows for both the cultural inclusion and accommodation of intoxication, whilst simultaneously ensuring the exclusion and stigmatisation of *the intoxicated*. Similar to Linnemann's (2016) concept of 'governing through meth', the media depiction of intoxication has created an imaginary that is then substituted for the truth. Consequently, this hyper-reality is used to justify control mechanisms that govern individual consumption and criminalise unacceptable modes of intoxication that supposedly cause harm to others, while the systemic harms of consumer capitalism are disavowed.

Conclusion

Media representations transcend the boundaries of legality, with the predominant focus on the irresponsible outcome of intoxication rather than the legal status of the substance consumed. Flawed consumers, drawn from a lower order of drug-using bodies (Alexandrescu, 2018), warrant media condemnation and vilification. The media depicts forms of subjective violence as caused by the intoxicated other, rather than acknowledging the systemic harm that underpins much of the subjective violence in the media. According to the media, the intoxicated other needs to be controlled or excluded since they ruin it for everyone and threaten civilised ways of life.

A clear demarcation is established between acceptable and unacceptable intoxication. On one side, sensible, pro-social and desirable. On the other, reckless, anti-social and threatening. Whilst the majority therefore enjoy a good time through responsible drug use, the minority are a risk to the creative consumerist experience that the rest of society depends on for pleasure, leisure and indeed social distinction. The majority are able to responsibly navigate consumerism, and *the intoxicated* cannot be allowed to ruin it for us all. Yet, framing these problematic outcomes as personal failings takes attention away from those industries who manufacture these harms therefore legitimising consumer capitalism and reinforcing the arbitrary nature of contemporary drug regulation and prohibition; an illusion perpetuated by the media as the intoxicated other is merely obeying the 'siren calls of commodified hedonism' (Smith, 2014, p. 159).

Whilst heroin users have consistently maintained a position as fallen and flawed individuals, they have been joined by binge drinkers and pregnant mothers who smoke as irresponsible social pariahs. This process of framing those who use certain substances in certain ways as flawed consumers serves a functional Durkeimian purpose as it constructs those who enjoy the good life in a restraining and reasonable manner as viable members of society, whilst those who are unable to demonstrate such restraint are othered and warrant control attracting state intervention. The media therefore dutifully reinforce the dominant status quo and rhetoric espoused by politicians, as they partake in a 'sublime object of ideology' (Žižek, 1989). As such, it detracts from the contradictions and systemic violence of neoliberal consumer capitalism and its inherent paradoxes, which feed into the fantasy that to fix these contradictions, the intoxicated other that 'wants to steal our enjoyment (by ruining our way of life)' (Žižek, 1993, p. 203) must be excluded. Resultantly, we *all* partake in what Mark Fisher (2009) terms 'Capital Realism' and the perpetuation of an innately violent system that prioritises profit over its people (Chomsky, 1999).

Note

1. Inspired by the works of Slavoj Žižek, this chapter applies the label of violence to a number of different social behaviours. As such, a brief definition of Žižek's interpretation of these terms is useful as this juncture. Žižek (2008, pp. 9–11) refers to systemic violence as that arising from capitalism and its smooth functioning and alongside symbolic violence, which is embodied in language, constitutes what he refers to as objective violence. Alongside this sits subjective violence which is 'enacted by social agents' and is the most visible form of violence.

References

Agerholm, H. (2017, October 12). Criminals could be banned from drinking after they are released from prison. *The Independent*. Retrieved from https://www.independent.co.uk/news/uk/home-news/criminals-banned-drinking-release-prison-probation-officers-gambling-online-content-a7997126.html

Alexandrescu, L. (2018). Ethnobotanicals' and 'Spice zombies': New psychoactive substances in the mainstream media. *Drugs: Education, Prevention and Policy, 25*(4), 356–364.

Alexandrescu, L. (2019). Streets of the 'spice zombies': Dependence and poverty stigma in times of austerity. *Crime Media Culture*, 1–17. https://doi.org/10.1177/1741659019835274

Angell, I. (2000). *The new barbarian manifesto*. London: Kogan Page.

Atkinson, A., Elliott, G., Bellis, M., & Sumnall, H. (2011). *Young people, alcohol and the media*. York: Joseph Rowntree Foundation.
Atkinson, A., & Sumnall, H. (2018). Neo-liberal discourse of substance use in the UK reality TV show. *The Jeremy Kyle Show Drugs: Education, Prevention and Policy*. https://doi.org/10.1080/09687637.2018.1498456
Ayres, T. C. (2017). Drugs, leisure, consumption and harm. *BSC Newsletter* (Winter Edition), pp. 20–26.
Ayres, T. C. (2019). Substance use in the night-time economy: Deviant leisure? In O. Smith & T. Raymen (Eds.), *Deviant leisure and social harm* (pp. 135–160). Cambridge: Policy Press.
Ayres, T. C., & Jewkes, Y. (2012). The haunting spectacle of crystal meth: A media-created mythology. *Crime, Media, Culture, 8*(3), 315–332.
Ayres, T. C., & Treadwell, J. (2012). Bars, drugs and football thugs: Cocaine use amongst English Football Firms. *Criminology and Criminal Justice, 12*(1), 83–100.
Bancroft, A. (2009). *Drugs, intoxication and society*. Cambridge: Polity Press.
Baudrillard, J. (1994). *Simulcra and simulation*. Michigan: University of Michigan Press.
Bauman, Z. (1997). *Postmodernity and its discontents*. Cambridge: Polity.
Bauman, Z. (2001). Consuming life. *Journal of Consumer Culture, 1*(1), 9–29.
Bauman, Z. (2007). *Consuming life*. Cambridge: Polity.
BBC. (2016, February 25). 'Sobriety tags' rollout as 92% comply in pilot scheme. *BBC*. Retrieved from https://www.bbc.co.uk/news/uk-england-london-35660946
Bhattacharya, A., Angus, C., Pryce, R., Holmes, J., Bennan, A., & Mier, P. S. (2018). How dependent is the alcohol industry on heavy drinking in England? *Addiction, 113*(2), 2225–2232.
Binns, D. (2013, October 10). Champagne 'war' in bar leaves tycoons with £131,000 bill. *The Metro*. Retrieved from https://metro.co.uk/2013/10/10/champagne-war-in-bar-leaves-tycoons-with-131000-bill-4142369/
Bosely, S. (2018, February 6). E-cigarettes should be on sale in hospital shops, health body says. *The Guardian*. Retrieved from https://www.theguardian.com/society/2018/feb/06/vaping-is-safe-way-to-quit-smoking-says-health-body
Bourne, R. (2012). Minimum alcohol pricing: Illogical, illiberal, unfair. Retrieved from https://www.cps.org.uk/blog/q/date/2012/03/23/minimum-alcohol-pricing-illogical-illiberal-unfair/
Brierley-Jones, L., Ling, J., McCabe, K. E., Wilson, G. B., Crosland, A., Kaner, E. F., & Haighton, C. A. (2014). Habitus of home and traditional drinking:

A qualitative analysis of reported middle-class alcohol use. *Sociology of Health and Fitness, 36*(7), 1054–1076.

Burrows, T. (2017, January 1). Some people won't be having a happy new year! Carnage on the streets of Britain as revellers see in 2017 with a night of fighting, vomiting and a LOT of flesh on show. *Daily Mail*. Retrieved from https://www.dailymail.co.uk/news/article-4079616/Some-people-won-t-having-happy-new-year-Carnage-streets-Britain-revellers-2017-boozy-night-no-one-s-wrapping-warm.html

Byrne, P., & Boyle, S. (2012, March 6). Revealed: The big-spending businessman who ran up £203,948 bar bill was 23-year-old City whizkid. *The Mirror*, 6. Retrieved from https://www.mirror.co.uk/news/uk-news/the-businessman-who-ran-up-203-752576

Chambliss, W. J. (1977). Markets, profits, labor, smack. *Contemporary Crises, 1*(1), 53–75.

Chomsky, N. (1999). *Profit over people*. New York, NY: Seven Stories Press.

Cohen, S. (1972). *Folk devils and moral panics: The creation of the Mods and Rockers*. Oxford: Basil Blackwood.

Cooper, S. (2018, August 7). Worker fears spice users are making Sheffield city centre unsafe. *The Star*. Retrieved from https://www.thestar.co.uk/news/worker-fears-spice-users-are-making-sheffield-city-centre-unsafe-1-9288379

Couzens, G. (2018, January 11). 'Adios!' Passengers cheer as 'drunk and aggressive' Irish couple are escorted off Ryanair flight after they forced it divert to northern Spain. *Daily Mail*. Retrieved from https://www.dailymail.co.uk/news/article-5257577/Ryanair-flight-diverted-remove-drunk-Irish-couple.html

Critcher, C. (2011). Drunken antics: The gin craze, binge drinking and the political economy of moral regulation. In S. Heir (Ed.), *Moral panics and the politics of anxiety* (pp. 171–189). New York, NY: Routledge.

Day, K., Gough, B., & McFadden, M. (2004). "Warning! alcohol can seriously damage your feminine health" a discourse analysis of recent British newspaper coverage of women and drinking. *Feminist Media Studies, 4*(2), 165–183.

Dodgson, L. (2018, September 17). An anti-inflammatory diet, including coffee, chocolate, and red wine, could reduce your chances of dying early, according to new research. *The Independent*. Retrieved from https://www.independent.co.uk/life-style/health-and-families/diet-live-longer-weight-loss-chocolate-wine-beer-anti-inflammatory-a8541816.html

Doward, J. (2017, November 12). The killer on Britain's streets – Super-strength alcohol. *The Observer*. Retrieved from https://www.theguardian.com/soci-

ety/2017/nov/12/super-strength-cider-lager-killer-on-britain-streets-homelessness-rough-sleepers
Evans, M., & Whitehead, T. (2013, September 13). Sober up in drunk tank and pay £400 to leave. *The Telegraph*. Retrieved from https://www.telegraph.co.uk/news/uknews/law-and-order/10316456/Sober-up-in-drunk-tank-and-pay-400-to-leave.html
Fisher, M. (2009). *Capitalist realism*. Ropley: Zero-books.
Gregory, A. (2018, September 12). Save us from this zombie drug hell, pleads MP calling for "decisive action" on spice drug epidemic. *The Mirror*. Retrieved from https://www.mirror.co.uk/news/politics/theresa-told-must-take-decisive-13233818
Griffin, C., Szmigin, I., Bengry-Howell, A., Hackley, C., & Mistral, W. (2013). Inhabiting the contradictions: Hypersexual femininity and the culture of intoxication among young women in the UK. *Feminism and Psychology, 23*(2), 184–206.
Gunby, C., Carline, A., & Taylor, S. (2017). Location, libation and leisure: An examination of the use of licensed venues to help challenge sexual violence. *Crime, Media, Culture, 13*(3), 315–333.
Hackley, C., Bengry-Howell, A., Griffin, C., Mistral, W., & Szmigin, I. (2008). The discursive constitution of the UK alcohol problem in safe, sensible, social: A discussion of policy implications. *Drugs: Education, Prevention and Policy, 15*(1), 61–74.
Hall, S., & Winlow, S. (2004). Crime and violence in the breakdown of the pseudo-pacification process. In J. Ferrell, K. Hayward, W. Morrison, & M. Presdee (Eds.), *Cultural criminology unleashed* (pp. 275–286). London: Glasshouse Press.
Hall, S., & Winlow, S. (2015). *Revitilizing criminological theory*. London: Routledge.
Hancock, E. (2017). Supermarket sales soar despite price rises. Retrieved from https://www.thedrinksbusiness.com/2017/11/alcohol-sales-soar-despite-supermarket-prices-rising-at-their-highest-rate-in-4-years
Haydock, W. (2014a). The rise and fall of the 'nudge' of minimum unit pricing: The continuity of neoliberalism in alcohol policy in England. *Critical Social Policy, 34*(2), 260–279.
Haydock, W. (2014b). The 'civilising' effect of a 'balanced' night-time economy for 'better people': Class and the cosmopolitan limit in the consumption and regulation of alcohol in Bournemouth. *Journal of Policy Research in Tourism, Leisure and Events, 6*(2), 172–185.

Hayward, K. (2004). *City limits: Crime, consumer culture and the urban experience*. London: Glasshouse.

Hilton, S., Wood, K., Patterson, C., & Katikireddi, S. (2014). Implications for alcohol minimum unit pricing advocacy: What can we learn for public health from UK newsprint coverage of key claim-makers in the policy debate? *Social Science & Medicine, 102*, 157–164.

Home Office. (2012). *The government's alcohol strategy*. London: Home Office.

Hutton, F., Griffin, C., Lyons, A., Niland, P., & McCreanor, T. (2016). "Tragic girls" and "crack whores": Alcohol, femininity and Facebook. *Feminism and Psychology, 26*(1), 73–93.

Iparraguirre, J. (2015). Socioeconomic determinants of risk of harmful alcohol drinking among people aged 50 or over in England. *BMJ, Open, 5*, e007684.

ITV News. (2015, February 19). Grieving father of homeless man calls for crack-down on cheap alcohol which ruined his life. *ITV News*. Retrieved from https://www.itv.com/news/central/2015-02-19/grieving-father-of-homeless-man-calls-for-crack-down-on-cheap-alcohol-which-ruined-his-life/

Iwamoto, D. K., Cheng, A., Lee, C. S., Takamatsu, S., & Gordon, D. (2011). "Man-ing" up and getting drunk: The role of masculine norms, alcohol intoxication and alcohol-related problems among college men. *Addictive Behaviors, 36*(9), 906–911.

Jennings, K. (2018, August 17). British MPs push e-cigarettes as health benefit. *POLITICO*. Retrieved from https://www.politico.eu/article/e-cigarettes-for-get-big-tobacco-back-vaping-for-health-benefits-say-mps/

Lennox, J., Emslie, E., Sweeting, H., & Lyons, A. (2018). The role of alcohol in constructing gender & class identities among young women in the age of social media. *International Journal of Drug Policy, 58*, 13–21.

Levy, A. (2010, January 1). New year, same old binge Britain: Arctic weather fails to stop drunken revellers causing chaos on streets of UK. *Daily Mail*. Retrieved from https://www.dailymail.co.uk/news/article-1239836/New-Year-celebrations-turn-ugly-revellers-drink-excess.html

Linnemann, T. (2016). *Meth wars: Police, media, power*. New York, NY: New York University Press.

McArdle, H. (2018, November 13). Surge in Buckfast sales blamed on minimum pricing 'trade off' from ciders. *Herald Scotland*. Retrieved from https://www.heraldscotland.com/news/17218694.surge-in-buckfast-sales-blamed-on-minimum-pricing-trade-off-from-ciders/

Measham, F. (2004). Play space: Historical and socio-cultural reflections on drugs, licensed leisure locations, commercialisation and control. *International Journal of Drug Policy, 15*, 337–345.

Measham, F., & Brain, K. (2005). "Binge" drinking, British alcohol policy and the new culture of intoxication. *Crime, Media, Culture, 1*(3), 262–283.

Measham, F., & Moore, K. (2008). The criminalisation of intoxication. In P. Squires (Ed.), *ASBO Nation: The criminalisation of nuisance* (pp. 273–288). Bristol: The Policy Press.

Mercille, J. (2016). Neoliberalism and the alcohol industry in Ireland. *Space and Polity, 20*(1), 59–74.

Monaghan, M., & Yeomans, H. (2016). Mixing drink and drugs: 'Underclass' politics, the recovery agenda and the partial convergence of English alcohol and drugs policy. *International Journal of Drug Policy, 37*, 122–128.

NHS. (2017). *NHS to consider routine use of 'drunk tanks' to ease pressure on A&Es*. Retrieved from https://www.england.nhs.uk/2017/12/drunk-tanks/

Nicholls, J. (2011). UK news reporting of alcohol: An analysis of television and newspaper coverage. *Drugs: Education, Prevention and Policy, 18*(3), 200–206.

NTIA. (2015). *Forward into the night*. London: NTIA.

O'Hare, S. (2013, January 1). Welcome to 2013: Shameful scenes of booze-fuelled New Year's chaos in cities across Britain. *Daily Mail*. Retrieved from https://www.dailymail.co.uk/news/article-2255587/New-Years-Eve-2012-Shameful-scenes-booze-fuelled-chaos-cities-Britain.html

Patterson, C., Emslie, C., Mason, O., Fergie, G., & Hilton, S. (2016). Content analysis of UK newspaper and online news representations of women's and men's 'binge' drinking: A challenge for communicating evidence-based messages about single-episodic drinking? *BMJ, 6*, e013124. https://doi.org/10.1136/bmjopen-2016-013124

Presdee, M. (2000). *Cultural criminology and the carnival of crime*. London: Routledge.

Pryce, S. (2012). *Fixing drugs: The politics of drug prohibition*. Basingstoke: Palgrave Macmillan.

Raymen, T., & Smith, O. (2016). What's deviance got to do with it? Black friday sales, violence and hyper-conformity. *The British Journal of Criminology, 56*(2), 389–405.

Riley, L. (2016). *Tesco extends craft beer offering at Express stores*. Retrieved from https://www.thegrocer.co.uk/stores/ranging-and-merchandising/tesco-extends-craft-beer-offering-at-express-stores/543682.article

Robinson, M. (2014, January 1). New Year… depressingly familiar scenes: Festivities are marred by drunken revellers causing chaos in towns and cities across Britain. *Daily Mail*. Retrieved from https://www.dailymail.co.uk/

news/article-2532094/Welcome-Britain-2014-Shameful-scenes-alcohol-fuelled-New-Years-chaos-spills-towns-cities-Britain.html
Sheron, N., & Gilmore, I. (2016). Effect of policy, economics, and the changing alcohol marketplace on alcohol related deaths in England and Wales. *British Medical Journal, 353*, 1–7.
Siddique, H. (2018, July 31). Middle-class cocaine users are hypocrites, says Met chief. *The Guardian*. Retrieved from https://www.theguardian.com/society/2018/jul/31/middle-class-cocaine-users-are-hypocrites-says-met-chief-cressida-dick
Smith, O. (2014). *Contemporary adulthood and the night time economy*. Basingstoke: Palgrave.
Sporn, N. (2018, February 20). Jay-Z 'racks up impressive $91,000 bar bill with $11,000 tip'. *Evening Standard*. Retrieved from https://www.standard.co.uk/showbiz/celebrity-news/jayz-racks-up-impressive-91000-bar-bill-with-11000-tip-a3771586.html
Sumpter, C., McGill, E., Dickie, E., Champo, E., Romeri, E., & Egan, M. (2016). Reducing the strength: A mixed methods evaluation of alcohol retailers' willingness to voluntarily reduce the availability of low cost, high strength beers and ciders in two UK local authorities. *BMC Public Health, 16*, 448.
Tahir, T. (2018a, January 3). Happy SPEW Year! Britons see in 2018 with a night of drunken revelry and plenty of flesh on show - followed by violence and lashings of regret as celebrations turn to carnage. *Daily Mail*. Retrieved from https://www.dailymail.co.uk/news/article-5225397/Revellers-hit-streets-best-party-outfits-New-Year.html
Tahir, T. (2018b, June 11). 'Deplorable' passenger forces Jet2 flight to Ibiza to land in France following 'disgraceful' behaviour with blow-up doll in front of children. *Daily Mail*. Retrieved from https://www.dailymail.co.uk/news/article-5828807/Passenger-forces-Jet2-flight-divert-following-disgraceful-behaviour-blow-doll-in.html
Taylor, P. (2010). *Žižek and the media*. Cambridge: Polity.
Taylor, S. (2008). Outside the outsiders: Drugs, drug use and the media. *Probation Journal, 55*(4), 369–388.
Taylor, S. (2016). Moving beyond the other: A critique of the reductionist drugs discourse. *Tijdschrift over Cultuur and Criminaliteit, 6*, 100–118.
Taylor, S., Buchanan, J., & Ayres, T. C. (2016). Prohibition, privilege and the drug apartheid: The failure of drug policy reform to address the underlying fallacies of drug prohibition. *Criminology and Criminal Justice, 16*(4), 452–469.
The Telegraph. (2013, January 31). Tamara Ecclestone blows £30,000 on nightclub champagne bar bill. *The Telegraph*. Retrieved from https://www.

telegraph.co.uk/news/celebritynews/9838424/Tamara-Ecclestone-blows-30000-on-nightclub-champagne-bar-bill.html

Thornton, L. (2018, September 11). Zombie nation: Britain in grip of spice epidemic as addicts resembling monsters plague streets, scaring children. *The Mirror*. Retrieved from https://www.mirror.co.uk/news/uk-news/zombie-nation-britain-grip-spice-13229735

Tomkin, S. (2016, January 1). New Year, but the same old shocking scenes: Mayhem in streets across Britain as drunken revellers lose their senses. *Daily Mail*. Retrieved from https://www.dailymail.co.uk/news/article-3380899/Where-streets-no-shame-New-Year-revellers-spill-pubs-clubs-night-drunken-excess-Britain.html

Tomsen, S. (1997). A top night: Social protest, masculinity and the culture of drinking violence. *British Journal of Criminology, 37*(1), 90–102.

UHY. (2018). Increase in UK's sparkling wine market reaches new high – But does slowdown in growth mean we are reaching 'peak Prosecco'? Retrieved from https://www.uhy-uk.com/news-events/news/increase-in-uks-sparkling-wine-market-reaches-new-high-but-does-slowdown-in-growth-mean-we-are-reaching-peak-prosecco/

UKDPC. (2010). *Representations of drug use and drug users in the British Press*. London: UKDPC.

Wincup, E., & Monaghan, M. (2016). Scrounger narratives and dependent drug users: Welfare, workfare and warfare. *Journal of Poverty and Social Justice, 2*(3), 261–275.

Winlow, S., & Hall, S. (2006). *Violent Night: Urban leisure and contemporary culture*. Oxford: Berg.

Winlow, S., & Hall, S. (2016). Criminology and consumerism. In P. Carlen (Ed.), *Criminologias Alternativas*. Buernos Aries: IEA.

Wood, K., Patterson, C., Katikireddi, S. V., & Hilton, S. (2014). Harms to 'others' from alcohol consumption in the minimum unit pricing policy debate: A qualitative content analysis of UK newspapers (2005–12). *Addiction, 109*(4), 578–584.

Žižek, S. (1989). *The sublime object of ideology*. London: Verso.

Žižek, S. (1993). *Tarrying with the negative*. Duke: Duke University Press.

Žižek, S. (1997). *The plague of fantasies*. London: Verso.

Žižek, S. (2002). *Welcome to the desert of the real*. London: Verso.

Žižek, S. (2008). *Violence*. New York, NY: Picador.

12

Social Media and Intoxication: 'Tweaker Nation': Celebrating Drug Use on Tumblr

Andy Ruddock

Introduction

On 4 July 2018, an Australian methamphetamine user made a *Breaking Bad* smoking device, and then posted a picture of it on Tumblr (My Breaking Bad pipe holder, 2018). The post was one of many images published on their *I'm Methed Up* blog, a celebration of the pleasures of methamphetamine intoxication that boasts 26,000 followers (wow, just hit the 26k mark, 2018). The blog is a part of a digital gathering called *Tweaker Nation. Tweaker Nation* is a Tumblr community congregated around that platform's capacity to provide a 'safe space' for those who use the drug (Christian, 2015). *I'm Methed Up* features stylized pictures of rocks, smoke, smoking devices and poems, and is part of a loose Tumblr genre, devoted to telling taboo stories about methamphetamine experiences. *Tweaker Nation* is not a naked celebration of intoxication; some of

A. Ruddock (✉)
Communications and Media Studies, Monash University,
Melbourne, VIC, Australia
e-mail: andy.ruddock@monash.edu

F. Hutton (ed.), *Cultures of Intoxication*,
https://doi.org/10.1007/978-3-030-35284-4_12

its participants are in recovery (Christian, 2015). However, its conversations about methamphetamine include talk about why people enjoy the lifestyle, demonstrated through Aussie Tweaker's[1] verse *This may bring us all together, it could be our drug salvation, so show your dedication, smoke your medication and join the congregation, all hail the Tweaker Nation* (All Hail the Tweaker Nation, 2018). Hence, also the decision to make and share a smoking pipe dedicated to a TV show about the destructive force of drug culture; an evocative symbol of a drug that is so dangerous precisely because users love using it so much.

We cannot know how far *Aussie Tweaker* reflected on that irony as she or he made the artefact, then blogged about it. Ironically, that is what makes the post a rich symbol of social media's place in cultures of intoxication. It would be difficult, if not impossible to find 'Aussie Tweaker', thanks to Tumblr's layers of anonymity. That is partly why counter cultures and publics find the platform more attractive than Facebook, for example. However, the reference to a globally adored TV show also reminds us that Tumblr's distinct contribution to framing intoxication sits within a longer history of how culture and media narrate drug use. So, the post is also evocative because it invites reflection on how an image that many may find confronting or bizarre makes sense within a longer timeline of media narration of 'deviance'. More significantly, the post also materialises enduring ambiguities in how drugs are viewed through media.

Taking all of this into account, this chapter posits that social media's role in directing experiences and perceptions of intoxication *is not* solely a social media phenomenon. American archaeological historian James Deetz inspires this hypothesis. Deetz's *In Small Things Forgotten* (1996) elegantly displays how mundane unearthed artefacts, things as simple as eating bowls, can profitably confound common sense views of antiquity. The remnants of everyday objects, literally dug from the ground, show us, for example, that early modern American race relations were more complex than is usually imagined. Deetz's (1996) point is that unearthed physical artefacts are enduring media for those wishing to scrutinise common sense.

Today's social media posts are tomorrow's *small forgotten things*. They are clues to how the people in history arranged their life. Tumblr posts are manufactured objects, buried deep in the digital detritus. In fact, today's posts are today's *small things forgotten*. It does not take centuries for a commonplace digital artefact to attain an air of mystery. There is no doubt that social media generate vast, invaluable evidence banks. Yet, excavating and construing this evidence is a tricky business. Who was *Aussie Tweaker*? Why does she or he merit attention? How to make sense of their blog? By looking at particular posts, because they connect with clear scholarly questions? Or by looking at overall patterns across every post? This chapter pursues these puzzles via simpler questions. Why bother gathering social media data in the first place? What might this data say, regarding intoxication's existence as a cultural reality?

One way to answer this question is to explain how an Australian meth smoker's decision to post a picture of TV-inspired drug paraphernalia to his or her 26,000 followers *makes sense* in a story of drugs, culture and the media. The task, here, is to reflect not so much on how social media change perceptions of intoxication, but how they steer existing conflicts over drug meanings in particular directions, by following social media affordances. That is, social media allow certain ways of representing intoxication that are not amenable to the conventions of other platforms. The fact that someone would celebrate his or her criminality, in an era of acute anxiety over social media privacy, is not that puzzling when taking the following points into account. First, intoxication has significantly informed understandings of culture as a process where politicised meanings are created, shared, contested and altered (Becker, 2008; Carey, 1989). Second, media's monopolisation of this *meaning making* amplified popular ambiguities towards intoxication. Although the capacity to share user-generated alternative perceptions of intoxication appears, prima facie, as a social media phenomenon, analyses of mid-twentieth-century comics, TV and film discovered celebrations of intoxication, which complimented the commercial ambitions of media industries (Gerbner, 1978). Third, social media normalisation of intoxication echoes the already *networked* nature of the addiction experience, which is significantly related to the social pleasures of drug culture. Intoxication reflects the pleasures of company, respect and power; this has been an enduring feature of drug and audience cultures before the dawn of social media (Linneman, 2016). Hence, the task is not to analyse the *Aussie Tweaker's Breaking Bad* pipe post, but to explain why the notion that the post materialised intersecting histories of drug and media cultures is at least conceivable. We start then, with drug cultures, move to television, and then to a discussion of how social media has harnessed both in its role as an articulator of intoxication.

Crystal Meth, Media and Drug Culture

Deetz (1996) viewed quotidian objects as incontestable truths in worlds of political myths. If Deetz (1996) turned his attention to social media, he might argue that when a meth user creates a smoking device inspired by *Breaking Bad*, then celebrates her or his ingenuity on Tumblr, it speaks to a real confluence between the deviant lair of the drug user and the norms of popular culture.

Breaking Bad is a much-loved and critically acclaimed TV show about a terminally ill high school teacher who goes into the methamphetamine business. Critics think the show is not really about drugs; intoxicants are but the landscape for a story about character, change, masculinity, race and class. Consequently, if it represents anything, it is quality television's agility in complicating common-sense assumptions about 'bad' people and taboo behaviours (Faucette, 2014; Johnson, 2017; Lewis, 2013; Mittell, 2013, 2015; Pierson, 2013; Ruiz, 2015; Smith, 2013; Wakeman, 2017). Over the last couple of decades, television has made audiences look at the world through the eyes of unlikely 'heroes'. *Dexter*, for instance, got its fans to empathise with a serial killer, and in the process to reflect on thorny issues in morality, justice and redemption. *Breaking Bad* was of the same ilk. At the same time, precisely because it was admired for its canny social commentary, the show does, according to some scholars, whisper seldom-heard ideas about intoxication as a social condition. It is conceivable that these features make *Breaking Bad* a vehicle for meth users like *Aussie Tweaker* to disclose and enact their habit online.

Writing in *Time* magazine, criminal lawyer Blake Ewing wrote: *while Breaking Bad may not glorify meth in the sense of making it attractive to the average viewer, it does normalise the idea of meth for a broad segment of society that might otherwise not know that dark and dangerous world* (2013, no page). Citing Ewing, tech blogger Brian Braiker (2013) wrote about another material artefact; toy company Citizen Brick's *Superlab Playset*. This *Lego Style* gift allowed users to build their own *Breaking Bad* meth lab. This stood as yet more evidence that the enormously successful TV hit about a meek chemistry teacher's transformation into a drugs kingpin had made meth culture a global source of fascination.

Critics thought it unlikely that *Breaking Bad* might encourage use; one would hardly wish to live in a world where everyone who touches the drug meets a grisly end. A fan Wiki calculates the series featured 269 deaths across its seasons, where major characters were regularly shot, stabbed, garrotted poisoned or left to die of overdoses (List of Deaths on *Breaking Bad*, n.d., no page). Set against this view, the decision to celebrate one's status as a meth user through symbolically referencing the show seems a spectacular misreading of popular culture. The people who made and loved the show were at pains to point out that *Breaking Bad* was a tragic drama about the human condition. Fans of the show—like those who find friendship, community and intellectual stimulation through their love of online games that just look violent to people who do not play them, or others who find a political voice through their appreciation of TV science fiction—would passionately argue that *Breaking Bad* does not glamorise drugs. Moreover, the question of whether or not the show does encourage drug use simply ignores decades of evidence on (a) the complexity of media-related behavioural effects and (b) the sophisticated and innovative ways that audiences interpret popular culture content (see Ruddock, 2017).

Media scholars know that audiences have always enjoyed the pleasures of community. In the 1930s, sociologists and psychologists were paid to find out if 1930s gangster movies seduced American teenagers into lives of crime. They quickly discovered that the main draw of Cagney et al. was the chance to hang out with other kids in dark theatres; what was on screen was barely relevant (Pietilä, 2005). Along the same lines, when television and radio prompted studies of how people coped with a new flood of dazzling commercial and political messages, they discovered viewers, readers and listeners who were adept at turning these messages into social capital.

Popular wisdom equates immersion in the fantasy worlds of advertising and the movies with the desire to escape reality. Evidence says otherwise. From the 1940s, scholars discovered that knowing about the latest film or advertisement was a way of finding company and esteem. Social networks developed around media content and knowing about that content was a way of winning leadership and respect (Katz & Lazarsfeld, 1955). Research on fan cultures has found similar results; immersing oneself in *cult media* is not about withdrawing from the social world; it is about making a better one for yourself (Hills, 2002; Jenkins, 1992; Sandvoss, 2005; Gray, Sandvoss, & Harrington, 2007).

Sociologies of meth users have found compelling parallels between media and drug intoxication. Like fan researchers, drug scholars who talk to meth users learn that intoxication is social as well as physical. Preparing, distributing and earning from the drug is as intoxicating as using. Dealers 'get high' from being the centre of user community life (Shukla, 2016). Fans and meth users have something in common; they know they live in a world of social pleasures that is opaque to outsiders, but which is entirely logical to those *in the know*. Hence, sharing the pleasures of meth intoxication via social media is a practice that synthesises complementary logics; we live in a world that usually equates media and drug use with a puzzling individual desire to escape something or other. Users know better. While the desire for escape and physical pleasure cannot be ignored, studies of drug cultures have found that users are often conscious of being part of networks that have rules, conventions and social gratifications (Linneman, 2016). Online social networks like Tumblr provide spaces where this knowledge can be articulated, shared and validated.

All of this is to say that we can locate concrete ways in which social media might affect the experience of intoxication, through histories of thought on drugs, culture and media that end with 'Aussie Tweaker's' Tumblr post. Literature on these topics casts media influence in terms of understanding, rather than behaviour. The idea that *Breaking Bad* somehow inspired meth use might seem preposterous to its makers and audiences, and unlikely within the history of media effects research (see, for example, Gunter, 2008). The contention that the show became part of a cultural repertoire that lent meth and drug culture *meaning* is less far-fetched. We can place our unearthed material artefact, *Aussie Tweaker's* post, in a real history of talk and media engagement with drug culture that explains how social media afford the space to celebrate meth intoxication.

Intoxication: From Culture to Digital Media

Social media have become part of the intoxication experience, because narrating drugs has been a significant political and intellectual concern for some time. This narration of intoxication is amply demonstrated through the popularity of Facebook and other social media sites as places where photos and narratives of nights out are extensively posted (Barnes et al., 2016: Carah, Brodmerkel, & Hernandez, 2014), extending the pleasures and pains of an evening's intoxicating practices (Niland, Lyons, Goodwin, & Hutton, 2014). The task, in this regard, is to pinpoint how social media make a distinct contribution to social conversations about intoxication. Today, Tumblr users' capacity to direct this conversation is guided by the architectures through which societies have told *drug stories* over the last century or so. Looking at our *unearthed object*, we might ask why *Aussie Tweaker* chose *Breaking Bad* to symbolise her or his appreciation of intoxication's pleasures. It is worth observing, then, that the show represents a noteworthy *destination* in a journey where television assumed a crucial role in determining the meanings that societies attribute to drug intoxication. To tell *this* story—how popular culture assumed a primary role in deciding what narcotics mean—it is necessary to examine how societies have narrated drug use. To understand why social media users started referencing a specific television show to celebrate intoxication, we must understand why stories about drugs matter, how television emerged as a primary teller of tales and how this emergence created the ambiguities that make it possible to publicly celebrate intoxication, in societies where such actions are ostensibly taboo.

Drug Stories: Howard Becker

The journey begins with famed sociologist Howard Becker. Among his many interests, Becker wrote extensively about the production of deviance. Social control of those who transgressed societal norms was achieved through the active production and policing of criminal activity (Becker, 1995, 2008).

The history of intoxication was a valuable case in point. Becker argued that intoxication is a learned state, requiring complex cultural frameworks (Becker, 1953, 1955, 1967, 1968, 1974). He spent time studying how and why people became intoxicated, and how they understood that condition. Becker made this effort because he believed doctors, lawyers and sociologists had done a poor job of imagining, understanding and explaining the pleasures and drivers of drug use (Becker, 1998).

Becker regarded intoxication as a synecdoche for the failings of mid-twentieth century sociology. These failings exacerbated drug problems, and Becker was frustrated with colleagues who would not reflect on their role in criminalising and stigmatising drug users. He considered that his peers too readily accepted the *outlaw* status of some groups, without questioning how crimes became crimes. Drug intoxication was a prime example. Intoxication was a *produced* form of criminality for a simple reason; for centuries, it was not a crime. Societies only worried about drug use when it spread beyond the confines of affluent, polite society, and passed on to the working classes. When this happened, Becker complained that sociologists rarely *explained* intoxication beyond vague gestures towards the desire for escape. Moreover, the *escape* narrative usually had more to do with literature than data. Unimaginative and asocial, sociologists had ignored weighty social issues, such as the reasons why poor neighbourhoods suddenly became the centre of drug industries (Becker, 1998).

Becker's *drug problems* were the assumptions that intoxication is exclusively physiological and naturally illegal. Beginning with studies of marijuana use, he showed that people had to learn to get high. This insight was a gateway to understanding that drug culture was precisely that; a set of values and practices that are less about individuals and failings, and more about how meanings are created and shared within groups. Seen from his point of view, 'Aussie Tweaker' was notable because she or he showed how social media provide a new way to do what drug-using communities have always done; provide people with the meanings and language that they must learn to find pleasure in drug consumption.

Becker defined intoxication as a cultural practice with complex meanings, which only an engagement with the intricacies and anomalies of knowledge production could decipher. It was, as he began his career, a state of being that was experientially susceptible to storytelling, and this is where media entered the equation.

Television Takes Over: George Gerbner

Just as Howard Becker was using drugs to reinvent sociology, an American-Hungarian scholar called George Gerbner became interested television's storytelling power over public thought and policy. By the 1970s, after years of content analysis, surveys and discussions with industry insiders, Gerbner was convinced that television had monopolised public storytelling, and had used this power to reduce democracy to the matter of consumer choice. Primetime drama, in particular, had done this by simplifying the principles of life; the world was an ultra-violent place ruled by men, and the only path to safety and happiness was to trust authoritarian consumer capital (Gerbner, 1973; Gerbner, Gross, Morgan, & Signorielli, 1980). Television taught people to be obedient and to consume. When media told drug stories, however, the flaws in this logic, that consumption was at one with good citizenship, became most apparent (Gerbner, 1998).

Like Becker, Gerbner was interested in how stories created reality. Like Becker, Gerbner was concerned about a lack of diversity in accounts of how the world came to be as it was. Unlike Becker, Gerbner believed that the problem was not unwitting, and that media violence, one of his key concerns, was prevalent because it was a globally readable, digestible narrative that guaranteed audiences and advertising revenues. Although survey evidence suggested that these stories scared audiences into believing that the world was far more dangerous than it really was, this was a by-product of corporate storytelling's bottom line; the desire to promote the idea that consumption was the most meaningful course of social action available to the viewer (Gerbner, 1994, 1998).

Although Gerbner is best known for his work on violence, it is also true that images of intoxication played a crucial role in his thinking on media, power and consumption. As a result, he added a media component to Becker's work on intoxication discourses. Gerbner (1978) expounded his thoughts on drugs in *Deviance and power; symbolic functions of drug abuse*. The essay is a crucial account of how media started doing the definitional labour that Becker had observed earlier around the causes and consequences of intoxication.

Media highlighted the arbitrary nature of drug discourses, since prohibitive approaches that sat quite comfortably in sociology and jurisprudence fell apart when presented by pleasure-centred media that often told stories where problems were solved by consuming things (Gerbner, 1978). Like Becker, Gerbner thought that anti-drug messages were caught up in many other issues such as poverty and foreign policy, for example, that hampered efforts to understand what was really at stake in complex arena of *drug problems*. What Gerbner added to the debate was the insight that hedonistic popular culture, which spent most of its time encouraging people to consume things that made them feel good, was ill-equipped to mount a nuanced discussion on intoxication. In illustration, Gerbner pointed to superheroes. For decades, societies had been entertained by tales of weaklings, instantly transformed by injecting or ingesting mysterious potions. Intoxication was bound to be a temptation in capitalist societies that insisted consumption solves problems. For Gerbner (1978, p. 28), the intoxicated person was not a deviant in popular culture, but a *tragic hero…the dutiful consumer chained to his purchasing habits, including the ultimate delusion of liberation through potent potions for pleasure, power, and profit.*

These words remain a compelling statement on how media create the reality of drug cultures through systems of knowledge production that have remained significantly consistent over the last 40 years. Gerbner suggested that post-war popular culture carried mixed messages about the pleasures and perils of intoxication. Where polite society viewed intoxication with disdain, simple consumer-friendly stories about instant gratification could hardly afford such morals. That Gerbner could have predicted a *tragic hero* driven by *delusions of liberation* via *potions and profit* speaks to the idea that digital media still make it possible to frame drug use and intoxication as something other than entirely deviant. Gerbner was arguing that there would always be contradictions in appeals to sobriety within media cultures that promoted and depended on conspicuous consumption, as well as highlighting the sentiment that any problem or desire could quickly be alleviated by using the right product. This argument is no less applicable to the digital world than it was the broadcast age.

Recall, we are trying to explain how *Aussie Tweaker* operated in a symbolic environment where it makes sense to use popular culture imagery to celebrate methamphetamine use. The story of the chapter so far is that such an action is not that transgressive, for the following reasons. First, intoxication is an ambiguous state that is open to alternative framing. Sociologists have told us that intoxication has its logics and carries significant social rewards. Thus, the decision to discuss intoxication on social media is a contemporary example of a drug practice that sociologists noticed in the 1950s. Second, popular media have made this *truth* visible for some time, as for example, superheroes become superheroes by taking the right pill or injection. Third, the celebration of intoxication fits smoothly in the business logic of commercial media. It is possible to argue, then, that *Breaking Bad* became *Aussie Tweaker*'s raw material, partly because popular stories have long voiced the contradictions in prohibitive discourses as noted by Becker and Gerbner.

The scholarship we have encountered so far has argued that intoxication is a social state that has no meaning absent of social, cultural and legal contexts. Intoxication is social because it has to be learned, and users tell us that the intoxications of methamphetamine are about lifestyle as well as drug use (Becker, 2008). The consumption-based discourse of television has always implied an ambiguous position on drug taking, and this has come to the fore in *Breaking Bad*, perhaps unsurprisingly, as media are prime drivers in generating stories that fix and dissemble conventional wisdom. Media scholars lauded *Breaking Bad* as a screen landmark, and part of the acclaim came down to the thinking it made possible about intoxication drivers. Pierson (2013) praised the series for doing the *framing* work that Becker felt sociologists so often failed to deliver, and argued that a key *Breaking Bad* theme is that meth use is neo-liberal; a response to 'gig economies' exposing the poor to extortionate working hours in service industries (Pierson, 2013). Meth's *high* is clearly articulated to economic conditions that create the thirst for this particular form of intoxication. All in all, there is a social and media history that charts the genesis of *Breaking Bad*'s apparently transgressive story, tied significantly to the affordances of commercial television. This notion of the affordance also explains how the show's potential meanings passed over into the sphere of social media blogging.

Tumblr, Social Media and Participatory Culture

We can locate a three-stage narrative in how social media have become involved in drug cultures. First, Becker outlined how the realities of drug experiences were shaped by stories about substances and the people who use them. Second, Gerbner noted how media monopolised this function. In our last development, we can point to *Aussie Tweaker* as a symbol of the role that social media users now play in framing drugs by creating and sharing their own stories in the age of 'mass self-communication' (Castells, 2007). This new 'age' does not imply a public free-for-all where anyone can create and consume any tale they please about the pleasures and perils of intoxication. Gerbner argued that comic books, films and television were all message systems, with unique grammars that shaped how stories were told. The *I'm Methed Up* blog illustrates that this argument remains true in digital media.

I'm Methed Up reflects the notion that intrinsic qualities of *disembodied* communication and the tightening grip of corporate media on social expression in the digital world explains the apparent chaos of social media (Murdock, 2017). *Aussie Tweaker* speaks because she or he can, but he or she can because businesses, bodies and technologies have drifted into alignment since the mid-nineteenth century. Her/his *freedom* comes from two things that have nothing to do with her/him. First, the expressive possibilities that emerged when electronic communication separated messages from the movement of the body (Peters, 1999). Second, the anonymity of a platform that is structured and promoted in particular ways.

This is sometimes hard to appreciate since Tumblr is often regarded as a unique part of the social media world. Founded in 2007 (Wargo, 2017), Tumblr is especially attractive to groups whose values do not fall within the mainstream (Renninger, 2015). Tumblr attracts *outlaw* identities by promising greater anonymity and protection from harassment than do Facebook, Twitter and Instagram. Tumblr *handles* are difficult to trace to *embedded* social identities. Trolling is discouraged, since interaction is largely confined to liking and reblogging (Milner, 2013; Reninger, 2015; Ringrose & Lawrence, 2018). Tumblr seems a *safe space*, then, for behaviours and communities that are less welcomed on other platforms; for example, sharing of "not safe for work" material, or the expression of Lesbian, Gay, Bisexual, Transgender, Queer or Questioning and Intersex (LGBTQI) identities (Dame, 2016; Fink & Miller, 2014; Oakley, 2016; Tiidenberg, 2016; Wargo, 2017). It is perhaps unsurprising, then, that Tumblr has also attracted those who wish to explore suicidal ideation, self-harm and pro-anorexia with like-minded others (Cavazos-Rehg et al., 2016; Schott & Langan, 2015; Seko & Lewis, 2018). Alongside these topics, Tumblr's capacity to circulate celebratory images of intoxication has also been noted (Primack, Carroll, Shensa, Davis, & Levine, 2016).

When we add in the popularity of drawing from pop culture images and ideas in Tumblr shares, then *My Breaking Bad Holder* appears entirely conventional. Since some enactments of intoxication became a mass outlaw practice in the early- to mid-twentieth century, societies have struggled with the notion that intoxication is a learned condition that makes sense to drug users engaging in these practices. Stories about intoxication thus assumed profound policy implications, at around the same time that mass media attained an unprecedented storytelling power. As this storytelling power principally involved the celebration of consumption, the approach to drug taking was always equivocal, because of the value placed on instant gratification. That is, where law and public common sense could unequivocally dismiss the notion that intoxication had its logic, television could never quite manage the same trick, because advertising in particular relied on the idea that consumer culture provides instant relief from social problems. We add to this, two things: *Breaking Bad*'s capacity to articulate the intoxicating lifestyle associated with methamphetamine, and the emergence of Tumblr, with its particular affordances to express counter-cultural ideas. These historical forces intersect in a picture of a smoking pipe. It is nothing less than the expression of a history where telling stories about intoxication encapsulates the notion that storytelling makes reality. None of this is to suggest that Tumblr is, or is seen as an *entirely* untrammelled space. Users know that the platform is tied to the corporate monopolisation of symbolic storytelling that concerned Gerbner so. Yahoo's acquisition of the company was met with dismay by many bloggers. Some feared that whatever using Tumblr felt like, it was now part of a corporate pincer movement, articulating all public expression to the monetisation of user labour (Renninger, 2015). It is just possible that future historians who discover this artefact of a homemade meth pipe will read it just as Gerbner interpreted earlier drug stories; a reflection of the structures and values that produced early twenty-first-century social media. That is, our descendants may view 'Aussie Tweaker' as the embodiment of how drug cultural practices migrated to social media, because of Tumblr's unique capacity to offer creativity, reward and security.

Conclusion

I'm Methed Up's homage to *Breaking Bad* is a small object with a rich history. This simple post demonstrated how the pedagogic function that Becker had observed in drug-taking communities had moved online. Intoxication has always been a learned state, and Tumblr is now one of the places where users can be schooled. Nonetheless, as we have seen, it would be a mistake to see this transition as a natural evolution, driven solely by users; it is just as plausible to see a history where the proclivities of drug users have been lured online by the designs of commercial media storytelling, online and offline.

The celebration of methamphetamine use on Tumblr reflects a history of media affordances, where the technical capacities, business models and user conventions of first mass culture and then social media, have affected the production of knowledge about intoxication; what it is, what it represents and why people do it. This Tumblr post can be used to reflect on how media became involved in turning intoxication into a social fact. It may be tempting to see 'My Breaking Bad Pipe holder' as signalling the democratisation of drug discourse. Where Becker once complained of the interlocking, staid ideas about intoxication that emanated from sociology and the law, it is now possible for thousands of people to create widely shared alternative knowledges about how intoxication works and why it appeals. However, this turn reflects commercial media's growing monopolisation of social thought and expression, tied to metanarratives of consumption. The notion that these conflicting discourses are reflected in social media practices has been established in Facebook studies. Hutton, Griffin, Lyons, Niland, and McCreanor (2016) discovered the discomfort that young women experience when representing their own drunkenness on the platform. Naturally, such unease can only exist in societies where we feel obliged to perform ordinary life online, including our interactions with substances viewed as both dangerous and fun. However, Brown and Gregg (2012) made a different argument. Their study found women dealt with contradictory conditions, such as the unavoidability of excessive drinking in alcohol-reliant night-time economies, combined with constant injunctions to regret excessive drinking, by refusing shame. Their participants grasped the chance to discuss the cultural, economic and moral pressures women face in neo-liberal societies. While each study maps out different realities, both are consistent with the core arguments that media narrative and media use are integral to the meanings we attribute to intoxication. If the intoxication problem is inherently ironic, the best way to deal with destructive habits is to recognise that there are rational reasons for abusing one's body, then narrative forms that have traditionally focussed on the promise of instant gratification are a logical home for outlaw discourse. Expressing a love of methamphetamine by sharing images of a TV show about the dangers of drugs, via social media, is not contradictory. It is in keeping with media industries where positive drug stories have always been 'on message'. That is, where many developed societies unequivocally condemn drugs that have been prohibited since the mid-twentieth century, Gerbner's work on film and TV showed that intoxication continued to be celebrated as a solution to social problems. While that was not the message that most saw in *Breaking Bad*, Walt Whitman did demonstrate that drug stories also suited a new entertainment trend that thrilled audiences with tales of moral ambiguities among criminalised communities (think *Dexter, The Sopranos, Peaky Blinders* and *Killing Eve*). More recent scholarship has shown that the celebration of drunkenness is a staple of youthful social media use (e.g., Barnes et al., 2016; Niland et al., 2014). Tumblr's anonymity makes it less than surprising, then, that a meth user would perform the same type of celebration. She or he had the history of research on drugs and media on their side.

Note

1. This is a pseudonym used by a contributor to the *I'm methed up* blog.

References

Barnes, H. M., McCreanor, T., Goodwin, I., Lyons, A., Griffin, C., & Hutton, F. (2016). Alcohol and social media: Drinking and drunkenness while online. *Critical Public Health, 26*(1), 62–76.

Becker, H. S. (1953). Becoming a marijuana user. *American Journal of Sociology, 59*(3), 235–242.

Becker, H. S. (1955). Marihuana use and social control. *Social Problems, 3*(1), 35–44.

Becker, H. S. (1967). History, culture and subjective experience: An exploration of the social bases of drug-induced experiences. *Journal of Health and Social Behavior*, 163–176.

Becker, H. S. (1968). Ending campus drug incidents. *Society, 5*(5), 4–5.

Becker, H. S. (1974). Consciousness, power and drug effects. *Journal of Psychedelic Drugs, 6*(1), 67–76.

Becker, H. S. (1995). Moral entrepreneurs: The creation and enforcement of deviant categories. In N. J. Herman (Ed.), *Deviance: A symbolic interactionist approach* (pp. 169–178). Dix Hills, NY: General Hall.

Becker, H. S. (1998). *Tricks of the trade*. Chicago, IL: University of Chicago Press.

Becker, H. S. (2008). *Outsiders*. New York: Simon and Schuster.

Braiker, B. (2013). Was 'Breaking Bad' good for the meth business? *Digiday*. Retrieved from Digiday website: https://digiday.com/marketing/breaking-bad-marketing-meth/

Brown, R., & Gregg, M. (2012). The pedagogy of regret: Facebook, binge drinking and young women. *Continuum: Journal of Media & Cultural Studies, 26*(3), 357–369.

Carah, N., Brodmerkel, S., & Hernandez, L. (2014). Brands and sociality: Alcohol branding, drinking culture and Facebook. *Convergence: The Journal of Research into New Media Technologies, 20*(3), 259–275. https://doi.org/10.1177/1354856514531531

Carey, J. (1989). *Communication as culture*. Boston: Unwin Hyman.

Castells, M. (2007). Communication, power and counter-power in the network society. *International Journal of Communication, 1*(1), 238–266.

Cavazos-Rehg, P. A., Krauss, M. J., Sowles, S. J., Connolly, S., Rosas, C., Bharadwaj, M., & Bierut, L. J. (2016). An analysis of depression, self-harm, and suicidal ideation content on Tumblr. *Crisis: The Journal of Crisis Intervention and Suicide Prevention, 38*(1), 44–52.

Christian, J. (2015). Tumblr has a hardcore meth scene *Motherboard*. Retrieved from Motherboard website: https://motherboard.vice.com/en_us/article/3dke7v/tumblr-has-a-hardcore-meth-scene

Dame, A. (2016). Making a name for yourself: Tagging as transgender ontological practice on Tumblr. *Critical Studies in Media Communication, 33*(1), 23–37.

Deetz, J. (1996). *In Small things forgotten: An archaeology of early American life*. New York: Random House.

Ewing, B. (2013). Breaking Bad normalizes meth., Argues Prosecutor. *Time*. Retrieved from Time.com website: http://ideas.time.com/2013/09/20/breaking-bad-promotes-meth-use-argues-prosecutor/

Faucette, B. (2014). Taking control: Male angst and the re-emergence of hegemonic masculinity in Breaking Bad. In*Breaking Bad: Critical essays on the contexts, politics, style, and reception of the television series*. Plymouth: Lexington Books.

Fink, M., & Miller, Q. (2014). Transmedia moments: Tumblr, 2011–2013. *Television & New Media, 15*(7), 611–626.

Gerbner, G. (1973). Cultural indicators: The third voice. In G. Gerbner, L. Gross, & W. Melody (Eds.), *Communications technology and social policy* (pp. 555–573). New York: John Wiley.

Gerbner, G. (1978). Deviance and power – Symbolic functions of "Drug Abuse". In C. Winick (Ed.), *Deviance and mass media* (pp. 13–230). Beverly Hills: Sage.

Gerbner, G. (1994). The· politics of media violence: Some reflections. In C. Hamelink & O. Linne (Eds.), *Mass communication research: On problems and policies* (pp. 133–146). Norwood, NJ: Ablex.

Gerbner, G. (1998). Cultivation analysis: An overview. *Mass Communication and Society, 1*(3–4), 175–195.

Gerbner, G., Gross, L., Morgan, M., & Signorelli, N. (1980). The mainstreaming of America: Violence profile #11. *Journal of Communication, 30*, 10–29.

Gray, J., Sandvoss, C., & Harrington, C. L. (Eds.). (2007). *Fandom: Identities and communities in a mediated world*. London: Routledge.

Gunter, B. (2008). Media violence is there a case for causality? *American Behavioral Scientist, 51*(8), 1061–1122.

Hills, M. (2002). *Fan cultures*. London: Routledge.

Hutton, F., Griffin, C., Lyons, A., Niland, P., & McCreanor, T. (2016). "Tragic girls" and "crack whores": Alcohol, femininity and Facebook. *Feminism & Psychology, 26*(1), 73–93.

Jenkins, H. (1992). *Textual poachers: Television fans & participatory culture*. London: Routledge.

Johnson, P. E. (2017). Walter White (ness) lashes out: Breaking Bad and male victimage. *Critical Studies in Media Communication, 34*(1), 14–28.

Katz, E., & Lazarsfeld, P. (1955). *Personal influence: The part played by people in the flow of mass communications*. New York: The Free Press.

Lewis, M. A. (2013). From victim to victor: "Breaking Bad" and the dark potential of the terminally empowered. *Culture, Medicine, and Psychiatry, 37*(4), 656–669.

Linnemann, T. (2016). *Meth wars: Police, media, power. New York*: NYU Press.

List of Deaths on Breaking Bad. (n.d.). *Breaking Bad Wiki*. Retrieved from https://breakingbad.fandom.com/wiki/List_of_deaths_on_Breaking_Bad

Milner, R. (2013). Pop polyvocality: Internet memes, public participation, and the occupy wall street movement. *International Journal of Communication, 7*, 2357–2390.

Mittell, J. (2013). The qualities of complexity: Vast versus dense seriality in contemporary television. In J. Jacobs & S. Peacock (Eds.), *Television aesthetics and style* (pp. 45–56). London: Bloomsbury.

Mittell, J. (2015). Lengthy interactions with hideous men: Walter white and the serial poetics of television anti-heroes. In*Storytelling in the media convergence age* (pp. 74–92). Springer.

Murdock, G. (2017). Mediatisation and the transformation of capitalism: The elephant in the room. *Javnost-The Public, 24*(2), 119–135.

My Breaking Bad pipe holder. (2018). Retrieved from http://methed-up.tumblr.com/post/175518895936/my-breaking-bad-pipe-holder can you put the date of retrieval? I can't remember offhand what APA convention is, but I think it requires retrieval dates for websites – Ok, cool with your research on APA here and no need to put date of retrieval!

Niland, P., Lyons, A. C., Goodwin, I., & Hutton, F. (2014). "See it doesn't look pretty does it?": Young adults' airbrushed drinking practices on Facebook. *Psychology and Health, 29*(8), 877–895.
Oakley, A. (2016). Disturbing hegemonic discourse: Nonbinary gender and sexual orientation labeling on Tumblr. *Social Media + Society, 2*(3). https://doi.org/10.1177/2056305116664217
Peters, J. D. (1999). *Speaking into the air: A history of the idea of communication.* Chicago: University of Chicago Press.
Pierson, D. P. (2013). *Breaking Bad: Critical essays on the contexts, politics, style, and reception of the television series.* Lexington Books.
Pietilä, V. (2005). *On the highway of mass communication studies.* New York: Hampton Press.
Primack, B. A., Carroll, M. V., Shensa, A., Davis, W., & Levine, M. D. (2016). Sex differences in hookah-related images poste Tumblr: A content analysis. *Journal of Health Communication, 21*(3), 366–375.
Renninger, B. J. (2015). "Where I can be myself ... where I can speak my mind": Networked counterpublics in a polymedia environment. *New Media & Society, 17*(9), 1513–1529.
Ruddock, A. (2017). *Exploring media research.* London: Sage.
Ruiz, J. (2015). Dark matters: Vince Gilligan's Breaking Bad, suburban crime dramas and Latinidad in the golden age of cable television. *Aztlan: A Journal of Chicano Studies, 40*(1), 37–62.
Sandvoss, C. (2005). *Fans: The mirror of consumption.* London: Polity.
Schott, N. D., & Langan, D. (2015). Pro-anorexia/bulimia censorship and public service announcements: The price of controlling women. *Media, Culture & Society, 37*(8), 1158–1175.
Seko, Y., & Lewis, S. P. (2018). The self – Harmed, visualized, and reblogged: Remaking of self-injury narratives on Tumblr. *New Media & Society, 20*(1), 180–198.
Shukla, R. (2016). *Methamphetamine: A love story.* Berkley: University of California Press.
Smith, A. N. (2013). Putting the premium into basic: Slow-burn narratives and the loss-leader function of AMC's original drama series. *Television & New Media, 14*(2), 150–166.
Tiidenberg, K. (2016). Boundaries and conflict in a NSFW community on Tumblr: The meanings and uses of selfies. *New Media & Society, 18*(8), 1563–1578.

Wakeman, S. (2017). The 'one who knocks' and the 'one who waits': Gendered violence in Breaking Bad. *Crime, Media, Culture*. https://doi.org/10.1177/1741659016684897

Wargo, J. (2017). "Every selfie tells a story …": LGBTQ youth lifestreams and new media narratives as connective identity texts. *New Media & Society, 19*(4), 560–578. mid-20th-century.

Part IV

Responses to Intoxication

13

Societal Responses to Intoxication

Robin Room

Responding to the Effects of Intoxication

With alcohol and many other psychoactive substances, consumption produces intoxication, affecting the mental and physical capabilities of the consumer. In everyday language, and often in law, the distinction between sobriety and intoxication is often seen as a dichotomy, but, in reality, there is a great deal of variation in the extent and manifestations of intoxication. This is dependent not only on the nature and amount of the substance consumed but also on sociocultural constructions and expectations of the meaning and implications of intoxication (Paton-Simpson, 1996). The associations and implications of intoxication may

R. Room (✉)
Centre for Alcohol Policy Research, La Trobe University,
Melbourne, VIC, Australia

Department of Public Health Sciences, Centre for Social Research on Alcohol and Drugs, Stockholm University, Stockholm, Sweden
e-mail: R.Room@latrobe.edu.au

F. Hutton (ed.), *Cultures of Intoxication*,
https://doi.org/10.1007/978-3-030-35284-4_13

be positive or negative or both. On the positive side, drinking or using drugs together is often a signal of commensality and equality of status, and may be seen as a means and signal of lowering social and personal boundaries. Potentially on the negative side, intoxication reduces predictability for others who interact with the intoxicated person. The intoxicated person's physical coordination may be impaired; reasoning and judgement may be affected and emotions may become more labile. The mental effects are often characterised in terms of disinhibition (Room & Collins, 1983). Most forms of intoxication impair the person's performance in working, parenting and other major social roles in everyday life. While those involved may feel a special bond where the intoxication is shared and social, on the other hand, their commensality has boundaries, and is defined in contrast to those outside the ring (Room, 2005); getting drunk together excludes as well as includes.

Such considerations and expectations about intoxication form the basis for societal and interactional responses to it. Since it interferes with carrying out the normal responsibilities of life and is commonly seen as resulting in irrational and unpredictable behaviour, intoxication tends to be heavily moralised, and often subject to legal prohibitions; there are many occasions and situations where intoxication is regarded as wrong and often is legally prohibited. While the ethnographic literature on alcohol intoxication shows enormous variation between cultures in expectations about and forms of comportment when intoxicated, MacAndrew and Edgerton (1969) observed that there is always a *within limits clause*, restricting not only the nature of the acceptable intoxicated behaviour but also the circumstances of its occurrence.

In European and many other societies, conclusions about and reactions to intoxication were primarily initially formed in terms of alcohol. However, in the last two centuries, responses to intoxication have also been extended to other psychoactive substances, often without much specific attention to differences in psychoactive effects between substances. Thus, much Australian criminal law about "intoxication", originally adopted concerning alcohol, has been legislatively extended without adaptation to cover other drugs (Quilter, McNamara, Seear, & Room, 2016). Although reflecting the different cultural and legal position of other drugs, "intoxication" is often interpreted for illicit drugs as synonymous with "use". Except as noted, the discussion in this chapter is primarily in terms of alcohol intoxication, but often applies also to intoxication in relation to other substances.

Normative Acceptance of Intoxication

Even where intoxication is encouraged or tolerated, it tends to be confined to specific circumstances and occasions. In population surveys of the collaborative Gender, Alcohol and Culture: An International Study (GENACIS) project in the early 2000s, surveying drinking practices and problems in the general population in a wide variety of countries (Wilsnack, Wilsnack, Kristjanson, Vogeltanz-Holm, & Gmel, 2009), respondents were asked to describe the injunctive norms on drinking in a series of ten situations and roles. These situations and roles were chosen to cover a wide range of variation in the acceptability of drinking at all, and of intoxication. For each situation, respondents were asked "how much a person in that situation should feel free to drink", with response alternatives of "no drinking; 1 or 2 drinks; enough to feel the effects, but not drunk; or getting drunk is sometimes all right". There was indeed wide variation between societies, and between situations in the acceptability of drinking at all and of drinking "enough to feel the effects", though there was considerable agreement across societies in the *ordering* of the situations in terms of the degree of acceptability (Room et al., 2019). Extending that analysis to the issue of intoxication—that is, responses that "getting drunk is sometimes all right"—Table 13.1 shows the percentage of respondents agreeing with this answer in each country for each of the ten situations and roles.

It will be seen that only for the four items at the right-hand side of the table was there agreement by 5% or more in any of the countries that getting drunk in that situation was sometimes all right. Furthermore, in only 3 of the 13 countries—in Uganda, Sweden and Australia—did more than 10% of the respondents accept intoxication in one or more of the four situations. Table 13.2 shows the rates of acceptance of intoxication in a subsample of each population: those who at least occasionally them-

Table 13.1 Percentage answering "getting drunk is sometimes all right" to "How much drinking is all right [in each situation]? Would you say no drinking, 1 or 2 drinks, enough to feel the effects, or getting drunk is sometimes all right?"

How much drinking is all right … —Getting drunk is sometimes all right Country (sample *N*)	j. when going to drive a car	b. as a parent, spending time with small children	g. for a couple of co-workers out for lunch	d. for a wife having dinner out with her husband	c. For a husband having dinner out with his wife	i. when getting together with friends after work before going home	f. for a woman out at a bar with friends	a. At a party, at someone else's home	e. for a man out at a bar with friends	h. when with friends at home
Argentina (*N* = 1000)	0.0	0.0	0.2	0.7	0.8	1.2	2.4	3.1	4.7	3.4
Uruguay (*N* = 1000)	0.1	0.0	0.3	0.2	0.2	0.4	1.5	1.8	3.4	1.5
Brazil (*N* = 1244)	0.0	0.0	0.4	0.0	0.0	0.0	0.0	1.0	0.8	1.5
Peru (*N* = 1531)	0.0	0.2	0.2	0.8	0.9	0.5	1.0	2.0	9.1	3.3
Costa Rica (*N* = 1273)	0.0	0.0	0.0	0.1	0.1	0.5	2.2	0.8	4.3	2.6
Nicaragua (*N* = 2030)	0.3	0.3	0.3	0.3	0.4	0.6	0.9	1.2	3.3	0.9
Nigeria (*N* = 2070)	0.8	0.1	1.2	0.7	0.2	2.8	1.2	4.0	4.0	2.5
Uganda (*N* = 1479)	0.7	0.7	2.4	3.3	4.1	4.1	2.5	8.7	13.5	7.1
Sri Lanka (*N* = 1201)	0.2	0.0	0.0	0.0	0.0	0.2	0.0	1.5	0.3	1.4

(continued)

Table 13.1 (continued)

How much drinking is all right ... —Getting drunk is sometimes all right Country (sample *N*)	j. when going to drive a car	b. as a parent, spending time with small children	g. for a couple of co-workers out for lunch	d. for a wife having dinner out with her husband	c. For a husband having dinner out with his wife	i. when getting together with friends after work before going home	f. for a woman out at a bar with friends	a. At a party, at someone else's home	e. for a man out at a bar with friends	h. when with friends at home
India (*N* = 2597)	0.1	0.0	0.7	0.0	0.1	3.2	0.3	2.9	4.7	0.3
Sweden (*N* = 1765)	0.0	0.7	0.1	2.2	2.4	1.0	13.6	22.2	15.2	15.3
Australia (*N* = 1210)	0.0	0.4	1.4	4.9	4.5	4.3	16.2	18.1	20.0	20.6
USA (*N* = 1126)	0.0	0.0	0.1	NA	0.4	0.6	2.6	2.8	4.4	5.1

The items are arranged in rough order of the acceptability of drinking at all or enough to feel the effects in the situation (see Room et al., 2019), but were asked in the order indicated by the leading letter (a, b, c...)

NA: not asked

Table 13.2 Percentage of Occasional Heavy Drinkers (5+ drinks on an occasion at least once in the last year) answering "getting drunk is sometimes all right" to "How much drinking is all right [in each situation]?"

How much drinking is all right ... —Getting drunk is sometimes all right Country	j. when going to drive a car	b. as a parent, spending time with small children	g. for a couple of co-workers out for lunch	d. for a wife having dinner out with her husband	c. For a husband having dinner out with his wife	i. when getting together with friends after work before going home	f. for a woman out at a bar with friends	a. At a party, at someone else's home	e. for a man out at a bar with friends	h. when with friends at home
Argentina	0.0	0.0	0.8	2.6	3.2	2.0	6.7	9.5	11.5	8.6
Uruguay	0.0	0.0	0.7	0.7	0.7	2.0	7.4	8.1	8.7	7.0
Brazil	0.0	0.0	2.3	0.0	0.0	0.0	0.0	4.7	2.3	4.7
Peru	0.0	0.2	0.0	0.8	0.8	1.0	1.4	4.5	17.3	5.3
Costa Rica	0.0	0.0	0.0	0.0	0.0	2.6	10.8	3.8	17.0	9.9
Nicaragua	1.5	1.5	1.9	1.9	2.2	2.8	4.0	5.0	10.5	4.4
Nigeria	1.9	0.0	2.5	1.1	0.3	4.6	2.7	5.9	7.0	6.2
Uganda	1.8	1.8	4.5	10.6	12.9	12.5	5.7	20.8	37.1	15.9
Sri Lanka	0.0	0.0	0.0	0.0	0.0	2.2	0.0	12.2	2.2	6.7
India	0.6	0.0	3.5	0.0	0.0	12.6	1.3	16.9	21.4	1.6
Sweden	0.0	1.2	0.3	3.9	3.9	2.0	25.4	38.0	28.1	29.5
Australia	0.0	0.4	5.0	9.4	9.8	9.5	27.4	35.4	31.4	41.1
USA	0.0	0.0	0.3	NA	0.3	1.5	7.4	7.3	11.9	15.7

The items are arranged in rough order of the acceptability of drinking at all or enough to feel the effects in the situation (see Room et al., 2019), but were asked in the order indicated by the leading letter (a, b, c...)

NA: not asked

selves drink five or more drinks on an occasion (i.e., about 60 gm or more of ethanol).

These respondents had thus acknowledged that they at least now and then had consumed enough alcohol to feel some effects, though they may not consider that they had become intoxicated. Among these occasional heavy drinkers (OHDs), at least 10% in one or more societies agree that "getting drunk is sometimes all right" in each of the seven situations on the right-hand side in the table. Still, there is a minority of OHDs agreeing that getting drunk in any of these situations is all right, even in the three societies (Uganda, Sweden and Australia) where the acceptance is greatest.

These data illustrate that, at the level of whole populations, and even at the level of those in the population who at least occasionally drink fairly heavily, intoxication is not normative, in the sense of there being substantial consensus on its acceptability, even in situations where it more commonly occurs. Qualitative studies among groups who engage in heavy drinking have found that even in these groups, there is uncertainty about intoxication as constituting a "time out" when normal rules of behaviour are relaxed (Cavan, 1966), and ambivalence about the "excuse value" of intoxication by which otherwise unacceptable behaviour becomes acceptable (Trygvesson, 2005). At the same time, it needs to be acknowledged that intoxication is not a rare phenomenon in many societies. In the European School Survey Project on Alcohol and Other Drugs (ESPAD) studies of 15- to 16-year-old schoolchildren in European countries in 2003, 34% of those in northern Europe (Baltics, Nordic countries except Denmark, Poland) reported having been drunk in the last 30 days, versus 17% in the wine cultures of Southern Europe and 44% in the beer cultures in between (Denmark, Czech Republic, Ireland, UK, Germany). The percentages were closer together (40%, 36%, 55%, respectively) for having drunk 5+ drinks at a time in the last 30 days, suggesting there are cultural differences in what it means to be "drunk" (Room, 2007). A recent analysis of Swiss data found that, for five harms due to drinking which might have occurred on a weekend drinking night, the threshold of amount of drinking which was the best predictor of any harm was 4+ drinks for women and 5+ drinks for men. For more serious harms—injury or involvement in a fight—the best thresholds were two to three drinks higher than that (Labhart, Livingston, Engels, & Kuntsche, 2018). If such levels of drinking are taken as likely thresholds of what is viewed as "intoxication", these patterns of occurrence of harms give some empirical weight to popular concerns about intoxication as a source of harm in the community, and a precipitator of assault or injury (see below).

Although there is a large ethnographic literature on subcultures and social worlds where intoxication is normative (Savic et al., 2016), the survey findings on situational norms for drinking are a reminder that intoxication is not necessarily expected or welcomed in societies as a whole. At a societal level, responses to intoxication are likely to be tolerant at most, and even when tolerated, the responses will seek to channel and constrain it to particular situations, roles and times.

Societal Responses to Intoxication

Responses to intoxication are oriented in two main directions: towards minimising any immediate harm from intoxication, and towards preventing or discouraging intoxication as a recurrent pattern of behaviour. There are a variety of potential immediate harms from intoxication. One is the danger of poisoning or other acute overdose effects, which may require medical assistance or at least watch and care for some hours afterwards. A second is the risk of self-harm or violence or injury to others while under the influence of alcohol or another drug. A third set of harms is threats to amenity, to use a community-planning term. The presence of intoxicated persons—threatening, unpredictable or uncouth in their demeanour and behaviour—may discourage others from using public transport or a park or coming into a restaurant or store.

Intoxication in Public Places

Societal responses to intoxication thus reflect a mixture of concerns and motivations. A primary political concern is with protecting people in public places from harm from others' intoxication; thus, criminal laws against public drunkenness have a long history. With the ready availability of cheap alcohol as an early product of the industrial revolution, European nations and their settler societies found they had to redouble their efforts to hold down the extent of public drunkenness. The main expedient was active street policing, with those arrested for public intoxication becoming a large part of the population of city jails and lockups. Thus, the Comptroller-General of Prisons in New South Wales, Australia, complained in 1896 that "men and women afflicted with the disease of habitual drunkenness are ignorantly dealt with as criminals.... Scores of these poor creatures spend years of their unhappy lives in moving backwards and forwards between the public-house and the prison" (Room, 1976, pp. 113–114).

For those staffing the criminal justice system, it was readily apparent that many of the drunkards were repeat offenders. By the late nineteenth century, there were substantial efforts to look beyond the intoxication episode and deal with the repeated pattern of behaviour, labelled "inebriety" (Baumohl & Room, 1987). The connection between chronic intoxication and serious mental deficiency or diseases was increasingly recognised, and as state mental hospitals grew in number, it was increasingly recognised that "chronic inebriates" were a large proportion of their patients. Specialist doctors pushed, with mixed success, for governments to fund "inebriate asylums" to provide treatment for inebriates and hopefully cure their habit of intoxication (Clark, 2014; Edman & Stenius, 2007; Tracy, 2004). The combined effects of the First World War (with its privations for all and military discipline for men), and of the prohibitionist phase of the temperance movement, substantially reduced public drunkenness and thus undercut support for state-supported inebriate treatment. In the 1940s and 1950s, inebriety was primarily handled in the health system in mental and general hospitals, and in the criminal justice system with local lockups, backed up by "prison farms" where those with multiple arrests for chronic drunkenness were sent to spend substantial periods as farm labourers (for the US, see Corwin & Cunningham, 1944; Spradley, 1970; for Australia, see Room, 1988).

In the post-Second World War period, the alcoholism movement, pushing forward a disease concept of alcoholism as a conceptual frame for understanding habitual drunkenness (Room, 1983), sought to replace criminal justice system handling of chronic intoxication with alcoholism or addiction treatment institutions in the health system, or halfway houses and other social housing in the welfare system. From a civil liberties perspective, it was also argued that public intoxication was a "status offence", used primarily as a way of getting poor and dishevelled men off the street and out of sight. Efforts were made in the US to get repeated arrests for public drunkenness declared unconstitutional, with the argument that this constituted punishment for acts (drunkenness in public) which were symptoms of a disease (alcoholism). Though in the end, the Supreme Court did not accept this argument, public drunkenness was decriminalised in many places in the 1960s and after, both in the US and elsewhere (Pennay & Room, 2012; Room, 1976).

However, the view of public intoxication as a blight on the amenity of public spaces remained. Local merchants, in particular, did not appreciate drunks on the doorstep of their shop, and often local residents' associations have felt the same way about intoxication in public spaces. Where public intoxication has been decriminalised, other measures for discouraging or deterring it have often been adopted. Such measures have included "detoxification centres", where an intoxicated person can be taken to sober up for a couple of days, and provisions under civil law for police to take someone found intoxicated in a public place to a shelter or other *proclaimed place* where they can be held until sober (Room, 1976, 1988). The growth of alcoholism treatment centres and sober housing in the US in the postwar period was in part funded by "urban renewal" programmes. Sociologists involved in such programmes remarked that "urban renewal" should be called "Skid Row removal", since a primary local motivation was often to get those publicly and chronically intoxicated off the streets and doorsteps (Hoch, 1991; Wittman & Polcin, 2014).

A more recent measure, now widely spread, for instance, in Australia (Pennay & Room, 2012), is to criminalise public drinking, so that it is illegal to be drinking, and often to have an open container, in public spaces. These provisions are likely to be at least as selectively applicable or enforced as public intoxication provisions were: in many places in Australia, for instance, it is legal for a restaurant customer to be drinking in the space on the public footpath where the restaurant is allowed to set tables, while it is illegal for someone to be drinking from a bottle on the footpath across the street. The prohibition has been pushed one step further back, to forbid any drinking rather than intoxication, but the primary object remains the elimination of intoxication in public spaces.

The Social Handling of Intoxication

Intoxication in Systems of Law

How intoxication is handled by societal response agencies is commonly governed or influenced by laws and regulations, whether criminal or civil. In different areas of law, the assumptions about how intoxication should affect the decision in a particular case can be very different. In the US, for instance, in civil cases under tort law on compensation for harm from negligence, the basic question is whether the party acted as a *reasonable person* would have acted; whether or not the person was intoxicated is seen as irrelevant. In general criminal law, intoxication can serve as a legal excuse for a crime for a limited range of offenses where *specific intent* to have committed the offense is required. Otherwise, bringing up the defendant's intoxication during the trial is usually not in the defendant's interest. In *per se* crimes such as driving while intoxicated, the intoxication is an element of the offense (Mosher, 1983). Depending on the particular laws and regulations in a society, whether and how intoxication is responded to by law enforcement or other social response agencies may vary tremendously.

Intoxication and Coerced Treatment

Repeated intoxication can be problematic for others in the household, family or workplace, and many of those coming to alcohol treatment acknowledge that they were under pressure from others to do something about their drinking (Storbjörk, 2006). More formally, in many countries, there are provisions for coerced treatment of alcohol and other drug problems. These can be under criminal law, often as a sentencing option backed up with the threat of instead going to prison if the treatment is not undertaken. Other provisions in many countries provide for "civil commitment", often under adaptations of mental health commitment laws, where the person's alcohol or drug use is seen as a danger to him/herself or to others (Carter & Hall, 2018; Israelsson & Gerdner, 2010). For instance, Finnish law in this area is applied to persons who are "given to insobriety or otherwise repeatedly making improper use of alcoholic substances or other intoxicants", and who also meet one of seven statutory tests ranging from "are manifestly violent, abuse their spouses or children" to "are in need of social assistance" (Porter, Arif, & Curran, 1986, p. 42).

Intoxication in Private Spaces

In most legal systems, the focus in prohibiting intoxication has primarily been on public spaces. However, in some places, for instance, the Northern Territory in Australia, it is possible to get alcohol and drinking banned in one's home to preclude intoxication in private, with the decision by the licensing authority based on "the wishes of the majority" of residents in a particular space (Northern Territory Government, 2018). Measures such as this, and other civil controls applied at individual levels, have primarily been adopted with particular relevance to Indigenous drinking in settler societies such as Australia (Smith et al., 2013). Otherwise, individualised restrictions which affect drinking in private spaces, common in the restrictive systems of alcohol availability set up in the first half of the twentieth century as an alternative to general prohibition where temperance movements had been strong, were generally abandoned half a century ago as unacceptable restrictions of individual choice, though there has been some reinvention of them in recent years (Room, 2012). Renewed attention to the role of alcohol in domestic violence is focusing attention again on potential harms from intoxication in the home, and how alcohol availability restrictions may reduce this (Lippy & DeGue, 2016).

Intoxication in Criminal Law: Often Dichotomous and Ill-Defined

In clinical thinking, it is well recognised that intoxication is a matter of degree. A clinical textbook (Schuckit, 2000), for instance, includes a chart of the "rough correlation between blood alcohol and behavioural/motor impairment" in its discussion of the diagnosis of Acute Alcohol Intoxication. In popular culture, too, there is a wide recognition of gradations in degree of intoxication, as in such sayings as the listing of the *five stages of intoxication: jocose, verbose, bellicose, lachrymose, comatose* (Spear, 2018). However, in the legal world, intoxication tends to be seen dichotomously, as either there or not. There is thus a substantial mismatch between popular and medical thinking about intoxication as a dimension with gradation in terms of degree, and the law's tendency to think of intoxication as either present or absent. Legislatures do not help with this: frequently intoxication is defined in law only in circular terms. A study of intoxication in Australian laws found that *"41% of* the criminal law provisions that attach significance to intoxication contain *no definition* of intoxication or a *very limited definition* (typically, simply to include the effects of other drugs as well as alcohol") (Quilter, McNamara, Seear, & Room, 2018, p. 38, emphases in original). Where definitions were offered in legislation, there was considerable variation in the concepts and wording, and in specifications on how the determination of intoxication is to be made. With respect to illicit drugs, intoxication was often defined in terms "of the mere *presence*" of the drug "in a person's system—no matter how much was consumed" (Quilter et al., 2018, p. 45, emphasis in original).

In the absence of any specification in the law, what counts as "intoxicated" is left to the individual judgement of police or others implementing the law, and then of those involved in the judicial process. This opens a wide door for prejudice and discrimination, whether conscious or not, in law enforcement and other social handling, by such factors as race and ethnicity, socioeconomic status, age and gender (e.g., Mazerolle, Marchetti, & Lindsay, 2003; Zemore et al., 2016).

The Diverse Relevance of Intoxication in Criminal Cases

The study of intoxication in Australian criminal law examined when and how it entered into the evidence and proceedings in the 327 cases involving intoxication (two-thirds involving alcohol) which were decided between 2010 and 2014 by the highest appeals courts in Australian jurisdictions (McNamara, Quilter, Seear, & Room, 2017). Intoxication came up often in these mostly quite serious criminal cases, most commonly in consideration of sentencing after a finding of guilt (in 145 out of 327 cases). From the defendant's perspective, bringing up intoxication is a two-edged sword: it may figure either in mitigating or aggravating arguments. In the trial phase of the case, intoxication can be used to support a defence—most notably in terms of mens rea, the argument that the defendant cannot be guilty because she/he was too intoxicated to form an intent to commit the crime. On the other hand, it can also contribute to or form an element of the offence. Particularly in sexual assault cases, the intoxication of the victim is also an issue, which depending on the circumstances can cast doubt on evidence or contribute to a finding of guilt, since an intoxicated person is considered incapable of consenting to a sexual act, although a victim's intoxication is often used to discredit female victims of sexual assault and rape.

Intoxication as an Excuse or as Increasing Blame: A Contested Issue

Particularly in countries such as Canada and Australia with legal traditions derived from British common law, the role of intoxication in findings of serious crime has periodically been in substantial political contention in recent decades (Stoduto, Bondy, & Room, 2006). Public attitudes tend to view intoxication as increasing the blame for a criminal act, while courts have wrestled with the issue of intoxication as an excuse—how intoxication relates to the legal tradition that a "guilty mind" intending the crime is required for conviction. A US study of attitudes concerning blame in an event ending in violence found that

American college students assigned more blame to a participant who is drunk, regardless of gender or whether the participant was the perpetrator or the recipient of the violence (Aramburu & Critchlow Leigh, 1991). In the same vein, a Canadian population study found that 92% agreed that a drunk person is responsible for his/her actions, and that this attitude was positively associated with believing that intoxication plays a causal role in violence (Paglia & Room, 1998). Against these attitudes, courts in common-law countries have tended to move in recent decades to a wider acceptance of an intoxication defence. Thus, the Canadian Supreme Court decided in 1994 that an intoxicated 72-year-old man who sexually assaulted a wheelchair-bound 65-year-old woman could not be convicted if he could show that he was in a state of extreme intoxication "akin to automatism or insanity". There was an immediate public furore: the *Toronto Star* reported that "judges across Canada admit to being under fire because of the perception that [the Court] has given drunk men an excuse to rape women…. 'Everywhere you go, you get it', said a British Columbia judge. 'You can't go to coffee or a lunch or a party without being attacked'" (Room, 1996; Vienneau, 1994). In June 1995, the Canadian parliament passed a bill designed to overturn the court's decision, stating that "self-induced intoxication" is not a defence with respect to any offence involving "assault or any other threat or interference by a person with the bodily integrity of another person" (Bondy, 1996). However, a 2018 court decision that this law is unconstitutional has again put the issue on the Canadian political agenda (DiManno, 2018; McQuigge, 2018; Star Editorial Board, 2018). Also reflecting a popular furore, in this case about "one-punch" deaths from assaults while intoxicated, the New South Wales parliament passed a law in 2014 which specifies a double penalty for assault causing death if the assailant was intoxicated at the time (Quilter, 2014).

Other systems of law have found solutions which steer around the issue of intoxication as a potential excuse for crime. In Germany, for instance, there is a separate *per se* crime of severe intoxication with harmful consequences, which is regularly invoked where a violent crime has occurred, but the accused was so intoxicated that intention is in question. In the 1990s, there were some 7000 sentences a year under this provision (Fischer & Rehm, 1996).

Policies to Prevent Intoxication

There are a wide range of strategies, of varying effectiveness, for preventing or reducing rates of harm from drinking or other drug use (Babor et al., 2010, 2018). Whether or not the strategy is specifically aimed at intoxication, if a strategy reduces social harms and injuries related to an intoxicating substance, it will almost certainly have been reducing rates or levels of intoxication. The focus here is on strategies which are more directly aimed at alcohol intoxication, and consideration of the effects of general restrictions on availability on rates of alcohol intoxication. We are thus considering availability restrictions where the substance is legally available—a circumstance in which government has more control over the circumstances in which the substance is sold and used than where the substance is not legally available. The findings from alcohol on policies to prevent intoxication are thus potentially applicable with suitable adjustments where cannabis has become legally available, for instance, but are not particularly relevant where a substance remains illegal (Room, 2018).

Server Responsibility and Intoxication

State control of the conditions under which alcohol is sold and served has a long history in many societies, with public order a major concern. A common provision in regulations governing those licensed to sell alcohol is a prohibition on serving or selling alcohol to those who are already intoxicated. However, cutting off someone who is drunk is against the economic interest of the seller, and may provoke an angry reaction; the general evaluative finding is that the prohibition on service to the intoxicated is rarely applied, even if backed up with server intervention training. However, the prohibition is somewhat more effective if backed up with regulatory enforcement (Babor et al., 2010, pp. 150–152; Graham et al., 2014). In some parts of the US, a further legal rule, known as "dram shop liability", makes the provider potentially liable for damages that occur to a third party because someone was served while already intoxicated. Though these liability provisions have been found to be effective in changing server behaviour enough to reduce drink-driving crashes (Rammohan et al., 2011), in a neoliberal age, it has proved almost impossible to implement this provision outside the US.

Policies to Prevent Drink Driving

There has been considerable success in a number of high-income countries in reducing rates of traffic crashes, and preventing drinking and then driving has been an important element of this. In most countries (where the blood-alcohol limits are 0.05% or 0.08%), this has been a matter of preventing driving after having more than two or maybe three drinks, so that the policies are fairly specifically aimed at preventing drinking to intoxication before driving. (In a few countries, e.g., Sweden with a 0.02% limit, the goal is essentially no drinking before driving.) What has worked in the campaigns against drink driving is worth examining for its implications on preventing intoxication and intoxication-related harms more generally (Graham et al., 2014). A notable feature of successful government efforts in this regard, as in Victoria, Australia, has been the integrated and sustained approach, including sustained political commitment, collaboration across government departments and investment in evaluation (International Technology Scanning Program, 2006).

Intoxication and Regulation of Availability

For alcohol, the literature is very clear that limiting availability—whether fiscally through tax and price, physically through limiting the number of sales outlets, or temporally through limits on times and days of sale—is an effective strategy to reduce amount of drinking and the rates of alcohol-related problems (Babor et al., 2010). Such strategies are thus featured in the World Health Organization's SAFER alcohol control initiative to reduce harms from alcohol (WHO, 2018).

The evidence is strong that such measures have their effect in considerable part by reducing the prevalence or degree of intoxication in the population. Alcohol consumption, like many other forms of consumer behaviour, is highly concentrated in the population, with 20% of those who drink at all accounting for about 80% of the total consumption (Room & Livingston, 2017); typically, episodes of drinking to the level of intoxication will account for half or more of the total alcohol consumed in a population (Callinan, Livingston, Room, & Dietze, 2018). Since heavier drinkers are more likely to gravitate to the cheapest drinks, raising the minimum price for a given amount of alcohol is also likely to affect rates of intoxication, as suggested by findings that a raised minimum price reduces rates of alcohol-attributable deaths (Zhao et al., 2013).

Future Trends in Alcohol Intoxication and Associated Harms: Is the Tide Changing?

In population surveys, approval for intoxication tends to be scanty. Approval of the many social and health harms which intoxication contributes to causing would be even rarer. One might think that measures such as limiting availability, which are likely to reduce intoxication, and which cost governments relatively little or even gain resources for them, would be passed and implemented. However, that has not been the general pattern in the neoliberal era of the last half-century. Rather, much of our knowledge of the effects of alcohol availability restrictions comes from studies of liberalisations of alcohol availability during that era (Olsson, Ólafsdóttir, & Room, 2002).

In most high-income countries, and in many others, drinking alcohol is an accepted behaviour, associated particularly with conviviality and surrounded by many social customs. In most of the world, alcohol is a legally marketed psychoactive substance. Alcohol is commonly served at receptions and celebrations in political and media circles; alcohol is "our drug" for those most politically influential at national and international levels. Also in this era, most of the market for alcohol is run for private profit, and the market is highly concentrated, with the beer and spirits markets increasingly dominated by a few transnational companies, with wine markets also heading in that direction (WHO, 2018, p. 130). In country after country, those in the alcohol market are among the most active political lobbies, visiting government ministers regularly and contributing regularly to political party coffers (e.g., FARE, 2017; Hawkins, Holden, & McCambridge, 2012).

As this is written, it appears that neoliberalism may be in retreat. Legislation for more restrictive controls on the alcohol market has begun to pass (e.g., Miller et al., 2017; O'Halloran, 2018). In Europe, as in several other high-income countries, alcohol consumption levels are falling (WHO, 2018, p. 45), and the current youthful generation seems to be cutting down on drinking (Pennay, Holmes, Törrönen, Kraus, & Room, 2018). We may be heading into an era in which rates of alcohol intoxication and of related harms decline in Europe and other high-income societies.

For other intoxicating substances, the current picture is mixed. The decline in youthful drinking does not seem generally to have been accompanied by an increased use of other substances. As cannabis becomes legally available for recreational use in an increasing list of jurisdictions, issues of market regulation to prevent intoxication-related harm parallel to those for alcohol need to be addressed. Particularly, but not only in North America, heavy use of opioids—from the pharmaceutical as well as the illicit market—has been an increasing problem (Fischer & Rehm, 2018), though the policy emphasis seems more on overdose poisoning than on intoxication. As the world slowly moves away from a *war on drugs* approach to substance use issues, pragmatic approaches to reducing harms from drug intoxication become more possible.

References

Aramburu, B., & Critchlow Leigh, B. (1991). For better or worse: Attributions about drunken aggression toward male and female victims. *Violence and Victims, 6*(1), 31–41.

Babor, T., Caetano, R., Casswell, S., Edwards, G., Giesbrecht, N., Graham, K., … Rossow, I. (2010). *Alcohol: No ordinary commodity – Research and public policy* (2nd ed.). Oxford: Oxford University Press.

Babor, T., Caulkins, J., Fischer, B., Foxcroft, D., Humphreys, K., Medina-Mora, M. E., … Strang, J. (2018). *Drug policy and the public good* (2nd ed.). Oxford: Oxford University Press.

Baumohl, J., & Room, R. (1987). Inebriety, doctors and the state: Alcoholism treatment institutions before 1940. In M. Galanter (Ed.), *Recent developments in alcoholism* (Vol. 5, pp. 135–174). New York: Plenum.

Bondy, S. J. (1996). A summary of public consultation on reform of the Criminal Code of Canada as related to a defense of self-induced intoxication resulting in automatism. *Contemporary Drug Problems, 23*, 583–593.

Callinan, S., Livingston, M., Room, R., & Dietze, P. (2018). How much alcohol is consumed outside of the lifetime risk guidelines in Australia? *Drug and Alcohol Review, 37*(1), 42–47.

Carter, A., & Hall, W. (2018). From coerced to compulsory treatment of addiction in the patient's best interests: Is it supported by the evidence? In C. Spivakovsky, K. Seear, & A. Carter (Eds.), *Critical perspectives on coercive interventions: Law, medicine and society* (pp. 15–29). London: Routledge.

Cavan, S. (1966). *Liquor license: An ethnography of bar behavior*. Chicago: Aldine.

Clark, C. (2014). *Reformers, Doctors and the State: Dealing with chronic drunkenness in Victoria 1870–1930*. Ph.D. dissertation, Melbourne School of Population and Global Health, University of Melbourne.

Corwin, E. H. L., & Cunningham, E. V. (1944). Institutional facilities for the treatment of alcoholism. *Quarterly Journal of Studies on Alcohol, 5*, 9–85.

DiManno, R. (2018, August 31). Extreme intoxication is once again a valid defence for sexual assault in Ontario. *Toronto Star.*

Edman, J., & Stenius, K. (Eds.). (2007). *On the margins. Nordic alcohol and drug treatment 1885–2007*. Helsinki: Nordic Centre for Alcohol and Drug Research (NAD). Retrieved October 2, 2018, from https://www.researchgate.net/publication/236862332_On_the_Margins_Nordic_Alcohol_and_Drug_Treatment_1885-2007

FARE. (2017, October). *FARE submission to the Senate Select Committee into the political influence of donations*. Canberra: Foundation for Alcohol Research and Evaluation. Retrieved October 4, 2018, from http://fare.org.au/wp-content/uploads/FARE-Submission-to-Political-Donations-Inquiry-FINAL.pdf

Fischer, B., & Rehm, J. (1996). Alcohol consumption and the liability of offenders in the German criminal system. *Contemporary Drug Problems, 23*, 707–729.

Fischer, B., & Rehm, J. (2018). Revisiting the 'paradigm shift' in opioid use: Developments and implications 10 years later. *Drug and Alcohol Review, 37*, S199–S202.

Graham, K., Miller, P., Chikritzhs, T., Bellis, M. A., Clapp, J. D., Hughes, K., … Wells, S. (2014). Reducing intoxication among bar patrons: Some lessons from prevention of drinking and driving. *Addiction, 109*(5), 693–698.

Hawkins, B., Holden, C., & McCambridge, J. (2012). Alcohol industry influence on UK alcohol policy: A new research agenda for public health. *Critical Public Health, 22*(3), 297–305.
Hoch, C. (1991). The spatial organization of the urban homeless: A case study of Chicago. *Urban Geography, 12*(2), 137–154.
International Technology Scanning Program. (2006). *Halving roadway fatalities: A case study from Victoria, Australia 1989–2004*. Washington, DC: Office of International Programs, Federal Highway Administration. US Department of Transportation. Retrieved October 3, 2018, from https://international.fhwa.dot.gov/halving_fatalities/halving_fatalities.pdf
Israelsson, M., & Gerdner, A. (2010). Compulsory commitment to care of substance misusers – A worldwide comparative analysis of legislation. *The Open Addiction Journal, 3*, 117–130.
Labhart, F., Livingston, M., Engels, R., & Kuntsche, E. (2018). After how many drinks does someone experience acute consequences – Determining thresholds for drinking based on two event-level studies. *Addiction* (early view). https://doi.org/10.1111/add.14370
Lippy, C., & DeGue, S. (2016). Exploring alcohol policy approaches to prevent sexual violence perpetration. *Trauma, Violence & Abuse, 17*(1), 26–42.
MacAndrew, C., & Edgerton, R. (1969). *Drunken comportment: A social explanation*. Chicago: Aldine.
Mazerolle, L., Marchetti, E., & Lindsay, A. (2003). Policing the plight of indigenous Australians: Past conflicts and present challenges. *Police and Society, 7*, 77–104.
McNamara, L., Quilter, J., Seear, K., & Room, R. (2017). Evidence of intoxication in Australian criminal courts: A complex variable with multiple effects. *Monash University Law Review, 43*(1), 148–194.
McQuigge, M. (2018, August 29). Excessive intoxication defence allowed against sex-assault charges, judge rules. *Toronto Star*.
Miller, P. G., Ferris, J., Coomber, K., Zahnow, R., Carah, N., Jiang, H., … Crane, M. (2017). Queensland Alcohol-related violence and Night Time Economy Monitoring project (QUANTEM): A study protocol. *BMC Public Health, 17*(1), 789. https://doi.org/10.1186/s12889-017-4811-9
Mosher, J. F. (1983). Alcohol: Both blame and excuse for criminal behaviour, and Presenter's comments. In R. Room & G. Collins (Eds.), *Alcohol and disinhibition: The nature and meaning of the link* (pp. 437–470). Washington, DC: USGPO, DHHS Publication No. (ADM) 83-1246.

Northern Territory Government. (2018). Get alcohol banned in a private premises. Retrieved October 2, 2018, from https://nt.gov.au/law/alcohol/get-alcohol-banned-in-a-private-premises

O'Halloran, M. (2018, October 4). Cancer warnings on labels as Dáil finally passes alcohol bill. *Irish Times*. Retrieved October 4, 2018, from https://www.irishtimes.com/news/politics/oireachtas/cancer-warnings-on-labels-as-d%C3%A1il-finally-passes-alcohol-bill-1.3650721

Olsson, B., Ólafsdóttir, H., & Room, R. (2002). Introduction: Nordic traditions of studying the impact of alcohol policies. In R. Room (Ed.), *The effects of nordic alcohol policies: What happens to drinking when alcohol controls change?* (pp. 5–16). Helsinki: Nordic Council for Alcohol and Drug Research, NAD Publication 42, 2002. Retrieved October 4, 2018, from http://www.dldocs.stir.ac.uk/documents/nad42.pdf

Paglia, A., & Room, R. (1998). Alcohol and aggression: General population views about causation and responsibility. *Journal of Substance Abuse, 10*, 199–216.

Paton-Simpson, G. (1996). The varied meanings of drinking and intoxication – A review. *Contemporary Drug Problems, 23*, 221–258.

Pennay, A., Holmes, J., Törrönen, J., Kraus, L., & Room, R. (2018). Researching the decline in adolescent drinking: The need for a global and generational approach. *Drug and Alcohol Review, 37*(Suppl. 1), S115–S119.

Pennay, A., & Room, R. (2012). Prohibiting public drinking in urban public spaces: A review of the evidence. *Drugs: Education, Prevention and Policy, 19*(2), 91–101.

Porter, L., Arif, A. E., & Curran, W. J. (1986). *The law and the treatment of drug- and alcohol-dependent persons: A comparative study of existing legislation.* Geneva: World Health Organization.

Quilter, J. (2014). One-punch laws, mandatory minimums and 'alcohol-fuelled' as an aggravating factor: Implications for NSW criminal law. *International Journal for Crime, Justice and Social Democracy, 3*(1), 81–106.

Quilter, J., McNamara, L., Seear, K., & Room, R. (2016). Criminal law and the effects of alcohol and other drugs: A national study of the significance of 'intoxication' under Australian legislation. *UNSW Law Journal, 39*(3), 913–949.

Quilter, J., McNamara, L., Seear, K., & Room, R. (2018). *'Intoxication' and Australian criminal law: Implications for addressing alcohol and other drug-related harms and risks. Canberra: Australian Institute of Criminology. Final Report.* Criminology Research Grant: CRG 20/14-15. Canberra: Australia

Institute of Criminology. Retrieved October 2, 2018, from http://www.crg.aic.gov.au/reports/1718/20-1415-FinalReport.pdf
Rammohan, V., Hahn, R. A., Elder, R., Brewer, R., Fielding, J., Naimi, T. S., … Task Force on Community Preventive Services. (2011). Effects of dram shop liability and enhanced overservice law enforcement initiatives on excessive alcohol consumption and related harms: Two Community Guide systematic reviews. *American Journal of Preventive Medicine, 41*(3), 334–343.
Room, R. (1976). Drunkenness and the law: Comment on 'The Uniform Alcoholism and Intoxication Treatment Act'. *Journal of Studies on Alcohol, 37*, 113–144.
Room, R. (1983). Sociological aspects of the disease concept of alcoholism. In R. Smart et al. (Eds.), *Research advances in alcohol and drug problems* (Vol. 7, pp. 47–91). New York and London: Plenum.
Room, R. (1988). The dialectic of drinking in Australian life: From the Rum Corps to the wine column. *Australian Drug and Alcohol Review, 7*, 413–437.
Room, R. (1996). Drinking, violence, gender and causal attribution: A Canadian case study in science, law and policy. *Contemporary Drug Problems, 23*, 649–686.
Room, R. (2005). Multicultural contexts and alcohol and drug use as symbolic behaviour. *Addiction Research and Theory, 13*, 321–331.
Room, R. (2007). Understanding cultural differences in young people's drinking. In M. Järvinen & R. Room (Eds.), *Youth drinking cultures: European experiences* (pp. 17–40). Aldershot, Hampshire and Burlington, Vermont: Ashgate.
Room, R. (2012). Individualised control of drinkers: Back to the future? *Contemporary Drug Problems, 39*(2), 311–343.
Room, R. (2018). Drug legalization and public health: General issues, and the case of cannabis. In H. Pickard & S. Ahmed (Eds.), *The Routledge handbook of philosophy and science of addiction* (pp. 518–530). New York: Routledge.
Room, R. & Collins, G. (Eds.). (1983). *Alcohol and disinhibition: The nature and meaning of the link.* National Institute on Alcohol Abuse and Alcoholism Research Monograph No. 12. Washington, DC: USGPO, DHHS Publication No. (ADM) 83-1246.
Room, R., & Livingston, M. (2017). The distribution of customary behavior in a population: The total consumption model and alcohol policy. *Sociological Perspectives, 60*(1), 10–22.
Room, R., Kuntsche, S., Dietze, P., Munné, M., Monteiro, M., & Greenfield, T. (2019). Testing consensus about situational norms on drinking: A cross-national comparision. *Journal of Studies on Alcohol and Drugs, 80*(6), 651–659

Savic, M., Room, R., Mugavin, J., Pennay, A., & Livingston, M. (2016). Defining "drinking culture": A critical review of its meaning and connotation in social research on alcohol problems. *Drugs: Education, Prevention and Policy, 23*(4), 270–282.

Schuckit, M. (2000). Alcoholism: An introduction. In M. A. Schuckit (Ed.), *Drug and alcohol abuse: A clinical guide to diagnosis and treatment* (pp. 68–111). New York: Springer Scientific and Business Media.

Smith, K., Langton, M., d'Abbs, P., Room, R., Chenhall, R. & Brown, A. (2013, October). *Alcohol management plans and other reforms.* Sydney: Indigenous Justice Clearinghouse. Retrieved October 2, 2018, from http://www.indigenousjustice.gov.au/briefs/brief016.pdf

Spear, D. (2018). The 5 stages of intoxication. Retrieved October 1, 2018, from https://www.dianespeartherapy.com/the-5-stages-of-intoxication/

Spradley, J. (1970). *You owe yourself a drunk.* Boston: Little, Brown.

Star Editorial Board. (2018, September 10). Let's be clear about the law about drinking and assault. *Toronto Star.*

Stoduto, G., Bondy, S., & Room, R. (2006). Self-induced intoxication as a defence. In N. Giesbrecht, A. Demers, A. Ogborne, R. Room, G. Stoduto, & E. Lindquist (Eds.), *Sober reflections: Commerce, public health, and the evolution of alcohol policy in Canada, 1980–2000* (pp. 265–288). Montreal and Kingston: McGill-Queen's University Press.

Storbjörk, J. (2006). The interplay between perceived self-choice and reported informal, formal and legal pressures in treatment entry. *Contemporary Drug Problems, 33*(4), 611–643.

Tracy, S. (2004). Building a boozatorium: State medical reform for Iowa's inebriates 1902–1920. In S. W. Tracy & C. J. Acker (Eds.), *Altering American consciousness: The history of alcohol and drug use in the United States, 1800–2000.* Amherst and Boston: University of Massachusetts Press.

Trygvesson, K. (2005). *Freedom in a bottle: Young swedes on rationales and norms for drunken behaviour.* Ph.D. dissertation. Stockholm: Stockholm University, Criminology Department and Centre for Social Research on Alcohol and Drugs. Retrieved December 9, 2018, from http://www.diva-portal.org/smash/get/diva2:198602/FULLTEXT01.pdf

Vienneau, D. (1994, November 9). Judges under fire for drunkenness defence. *Toronto Star.*

WHO. (2018, September 28). *WHO launches SAFER alcohol control initiative to prevent and reduce alcohol-related death and disability.* Geneva: World Health Organization. Retrieved October 3, 2018, from https://www.who.int/substance_abuse/safer/launch/en/

Wilsnack, R. W., Wilsnack, S. C., Kristjanson, A. F., Vogeltanz-Holm, N. D., & Gmel, G. (2009). Gender and alcohol consumption: Patterns from the multinational GENACIS project. *Addiction, 104*(9), 1487–1500.

Wittman, F. D., & Polcin, D. (2014). The evolution of peer run sober housing as a recovery resource for California communities. *International Journal of Self Help & Self Care, 8*(2), 157–187.

Zemore, S. E., Ye, Y., Mulia, N., Martinez, P., Jones-Webb, R., & Karriker-Jaffe, K. (2016). Poor, persecuted, young, and alone: Toward explaining the elevated risk of alcohol problems among Black and Latino men who drink. *Drug and Alcohol Dependence, 163*, 31–39.

Zhao, J., Stockwell, T., Martin, G., Macdonald, S., Vallance, K., Treno, A., … Buxton, J. (2013). The relationship between minimum alcohol prices, outlet densities and alcohol-attributable deaths in British Columbia, 2002–09. *Addiction, 108*(6), 1059–1069.

14

Intoxication and Harm Reduction

Adrian Barton

Introduction

It is generally acknowledged that for most people, at most times, the use of mind-altering substances are pleasurable experiences. We use such substances for all types of social occasions: celebrations, commiserations, ice-breakers when meeting new people, initiation ceremonies to university or new jobs and so on. Equally, most people who use such substances will overuse and become intoxicated on occasion. This is a recognised and generally accepted part of drinking alcohol and taking drugs: indeed, some research works show that it is often the case that users *seek* intoxication (Griffin, Bengry-Howell, Hackley, Mistral, & Szmigin, 2009; Measham & Brain, 2005). However, the reaction to intoxication varies due to several related factors which include the level of intoxication in relation to others, the social context and social space in which intoxication occurs, the time of day it happens, the frequency with which it

A. Barton (✉)
University of St Mark and St John, Plymouth, UK
e-mail: ABarton@marjon.ac.uk

F. Hutton (ed.), *Cultures of Intoxication*,
https://doi.org/10.1007/978-3-030-35284-4_14

occurs and the intoxicated behaviour in relation to cultural norms. In short, intoxication can be encouraged, tolerated, disapproved of and can on occasion lead to professional intervention. What is fascinating and is at the core of this chapter is the changing nature of social and political processes which are at work around reactions to intoxication.

This chapter revolves around the premise that drinking alcohol or taking drugs (from here in referred to simply as substance use) is generally a pleasurable activity that most people do throughout their lives without sustaining much in the way of personal harm, inflicting harm on those around them or harming society at large. However, it also recognises that *any* form of intoxication potentially carries with it harms and costs, and that in some cases harms and costs are directly attributable to substance use. 'Dealing with' the negatives of intoxication, especially in a policy sense, requires state interventions. Accordingly, this requires political decisions around what aspects of substance use the state needs to focus on, how and by whom that is measured and defined, who is best placed to address and reduce harms and costs and how this is achieved. As such, policy-based reaction to intoxication and substance use is as much about politics as it is about legal, scientific, therapeutic or medical interventions (Barton & Johns, 2013). For policy change to happen, politicians need to be aware of scientific and medical advances but often weigh these with changes in public attitude. It would appear that this is happening at the moment, as globally, at times, the strict prohibitionist approach towards illicit drug use is being abandoned for a more nuanced model which recognises the potential and actual harms of substance use, but equally recognises that intoxication is an embedded and pleasurable part of life for many people. This approach is referred to generically as 'harm reduction'.

At its core, harm reduction accepts that substance use will take place and that people will over-consume to the point of creating the potential for multiple problems to occur. In effect, by adopting and accepting the need for a harm reduction policy, politicians are implicitly recognising that prohibiting, proscribing and criminalising the use of some substances cannot prevent people from using them (Coomber, Moyle, & South, 2016). The logical consequence of accepting this is to question policies which are based on banning and criminalising substance use and intoxication. This is reflected in debates around harm reduction. To some, there is a common-sense simplicity to harm reduction making it a given, and something we should simply get on with delivering; to others the philosophy, policy and practice of 'doing' harm reduction is both a practical and political battleground, full of competing ideologies, mechanisms and cultures of blame. Central in this dichotomy is the debate about what constitutes 'harm', where harm is located and whether we adopt an individualised or community-based approach to 'dealing with' substance use.

This creates an interesting debate around the tension between individual pleasure, any potential harm this carries and the role of the state in curbing, controlling or protecting individuals in their choice about what is pleasurable but potentially harmful to the individual and communities they occupy (this is not unique to substance use: there are the same debates in a number of diverse areas including food, adventure sports, pornography and sexual practices). This debate has a long history: the line between individual pleasure, pain and harm and the role of the state in intervening has its roots in the work of eighteenth-century philosopher J.S. Mill (Vernon, 1996). Mill's key contribution to this is his contention that: 'the only purpose for which power can be rightfully exercised over any member of a civilised community, against his (*sic*) will, is to prevent harm to others' (Mill, 1962). Thus, according to Mill, the only time the state needs to intervene in individual actions is when those individual actions spill into community harm. On this basis, substance use which does no harm to others ought to be outside the remit of state control. Of course, this is open to all sorts of subjective, philosophical and political interpretations. These are often played out in terms of definitions and it is to this we now turn.

There are any number of harm reduction definitions which could have been used for illustrative purpose, but two have been chosen to make the point that organisations make subtle but politically important variations in their definitions. The two organisations are both international players with links to global politics: The World Health Organisation (WHO) and Harm Reduction International (HRI) which is an NGO in special consultative status with the Economic and Social Council of the United Nations. Whilst these two share key themes, HRI make telling and arguably more honest refinements to their definition of harm reduction. For example, the definition used by the World Health Organisation is:

> Harm reduction is a set of policies, programmes, services and actions that aim to reduce the harm to individuals, communities and society related to drugs, including HIV infection. (WHO, 2018)

In and of itself this is a good definition, but if it is looked at in terms of what it does not say, rather than what it does, this raises certain questions. For example, the WHO (2018) definition uses the word 'drugs' which to the lay reader implies only illicit substances, which may impact the range of activity included, as well as the political acceptability of the approach. What about alcohol or tobacco intoxication? They are 'drugs' but socially acceptable to most of the world although they cause as much harm as their illicit counterparts (Nutt, King, Saulsbury, & Blakemore, 2007). Equally, whilst there is a recognition in the WHO definition that harm reduction moves beyond the individual, it does not specify which areas of community or society it aims to deal with. Finally, it omits to mention that harm reduction does not mean cessation of use or even reduction of use. Thus, arguably whilst it is correct, the wording renders it politically acceptable to those who may not be fully informed about harm reduction, or who are philosophically opposed to it, yet pragmatically aware of its need.

The WHO definition can be compared to that of Harm Reduction International (HRI) (2018):

> 'Harm Reduction' refers to policies, programmes and practices that aim primarily to reduce the adverse health, social and economic consequences of the use of legal and illegal psychoactive drugs without necessarily reducing drug consumption. Harm reduction benefits people who use drugs, their families and the community.

Arguably, this is a more comprehensive definition as it recognises harm from intoxication is caused by legal and illicit substances, that harm can be reduced simply by changing the method of how the substance is used, and that harm reduction does not necessitate the cessation or reduction of use. However, politically this is 'risky', as it accepts use and intoxication, both present and continued. It also includes those legal psychoactive substances which are used by 'normal' people, thus ending the 'them and us' distinction that politicians often imply in debates about drugs risk and harm (Wheeler, 2019).

For the purposes of this chapter, it is the latter definition which is preferred. This is not to question WHO or to suggest that the organisation is not committed to harm reduction: rather it is simply the case that the HRI definition better reflects the lived reality of both the clients of harm reduction interventions and substance users overall and, in the main, the philosophy and approach of most of those charged with devising and delivering harm reduction policy and practice.

Constructions of Intoxication and Harm Reduction

As noted above, substance use and intoxication are a feature of most adults' life at some stage. However, whilst we recognise the embedded nature of substance use, we often fail to pause to consider the nature of intoxication, especially when intoxication becomes a 'problem'. Edwards (2005, p. 2) describes the state of the debates around intoxication and substance use thus:

> Posturing, fixed positions, monotonous repetition of untested assertions, and all of this with the facts of the matter ignored or trashed…[T]he public is not offered a debate of the quality, rationality or subtlety which the subject deserves.

Edwards (2005) is clearly referring to the often lazy and stereotypical clichés which are used especially amongst the media and lay audiences. Where intoxication is discussed, it is often located in binary divisions around 'good' intoxication and 'bad' intoxication as well as having a heavily gendered subtext depending on whether males or females are intoxicated (Greenfield, Pettianti, O'Malley, Randall, & Randall, 2010). Equally, there is tendency to ignore the science of intoxication and its chemical and biological materiality and simply focus on the actions of and social reactions towards substance users and the intoxicated. Harm reduction is treated in the same way, with a binary division between the 'deserving' and the 'underserving' recipient of interventions.

This tendency risks missing and downplaying some important aspects of how we understand and react to intoxication. For example, many writers are critical of the hegemonic social construction of intoxication, pointing to double standards around gender, age, class, ethnicity and the type of substance being used. Bancroft (2009, p. 10) eloquently illustrates this, citing the work of Scruton (2007) where the latter author argues intoxication via 'good' wine is 'markedly different' from that of other drugs. This is clearly a class-based perspective: intoxication, like disease, does not discriminate between class, ethnicity, sexuality or any other type of division—if you are drunk you are drunk, yet Scruton (2007) implies that it is somehow more acceptable to be drunk on 'fine wine' rather than to be drunk on cheap lager.

Arguably, it is the social class or wealth of the intoxicated being measured here rather than the level of intoxication, with severe moral and cultural overtones around the consequences of intoxication. As Becker (1967, p. 537) noted '…the aim of artificially inducing a change in one's consciousness is considered by many to be immoral' and this is seen as markedly different depending on the class, age, gender and ethnicity of the intoxicated. Thus, rather than intoxication being about the chemical properties of the substance being used and its biological effect on the body, it has become almost entirely about the morality of the user and their place in social and cultural hierarchy. In turn, this will impact on how we view intoxication and by extension how we view any measure to reduce the harms associated with substance use and intoxication.

The works of Barad (2003, 2012) become important here, especially in understanding the political and social acceptability of harm reduction practice. Essentially, Barad's argument is that whilst there may be a material existence, in this case intoxication, such materiality only becomes 'real' once we start to measure and observe it, that is, a phenomenon may be materially present—intoxication and substance-related harms—but it has no social or cultural meaning until we begin to measure it against prevalent norms and scientific and cultural conventions. Moreover, the meaning we attribute to that material phenomenon (and in policy terms the way we subsequently address it) is dependent upon how we measure it. Finally, Barad (2003) posits that once these determinate meanings have been produced, they act to exclude the production of other meanings. Thus, if we define, as Scruton (2007) does, intoxication via 'fine wine' to be morally and socially acceptable but intoxication via heroin unacceptable, we are not denying intoxication per se, but we are creating a reality based on cultural and moral measures. Put simply, we are basing our reaction on the morality (and in Scruton's case, the social class) of the user rather than the chemical impact of the substance on the biology of the intoxicated. This potentially carries over into harm reduction with some forms of intoxication being 'deserving' and 'acceptable' and others not.

This stance informs much of what follows. From here, the chapter provides an overview of the development of harm reduction, noting the political and social pressures on the genesis and development of modern harm reduction, but also looking at how measurement has impacted on what we now see as legitimate targets for harm reduction inputs.

Harm Reduction: Contemporary Developments

There is a well-rehearsed body of literature surrounding the genesis of contemporary harm reduction. Indeed Roe (2005, p. 244) argues that the genesis of harm reduction is based upon:

> an historic tension between those who see harm reduction primarily as a medical means of promoting health and mitigating the harm to individual, and a more activist group who see it as a platform for broader and more structural social change. (see also amongst many others Inciardi, 1999; Stimpson, 2010)

As noted above, the practice of harm reduction has a longer history than many would suggest (Roe, 2005; Winnifrith, 1994). Equally, there is a misunderstanding that our current approaches stem from the emergence of HIV/AIDs in the 1980s. Whilst it is undoubtedly true that we owe much of our current policy to that era, it needs to be noted that the beginnings of contemporary harm reduction policy and practice predate this. Arguably, the 'British system' (Barton, 2011) which emerged post-Rolleston (1926) and recognised that in some cases the prescription of a maintenance dose to a user was a better option than seeking abstinence is a case in point, but it is equally possible to suggest that harm reduction's genesis was in the Contagious Diseases Acts of the late 1800s (Smith, 1990). The recognition that abstinence was not always possible laid the foundations of contemporary harm reduction-based approaches to substance use and intoxication, mainly because the philosophy enshrined in the British model encouraged researchers, policymakers and practitioners across the globe to look beyond the abstinence model, despite social and political pressures to adhere to an 'intoxication to excess is bad' approach to dealing with substance use. Returning to the work of Barad (2003), it also calls for a different form of measurement: one where we accept intoxication will take place because of the material properties of the substance but where our measurement places no moral judgements on either the substance or the user. However, with reference to the work of Roe (2005), this further enhances the tensions between those who see harm reduction as a pragmatic objective response to substance use and those who see its potential to address deeper, embedded social inequality.

For example, around the same time as the HIV/AIDs panics, developments in public health were taking place, leading to the launch of 'new' public health models exemplified by the WHO's 1986 Ottawa Charter for Health Promotion. This document argued for the adoption of policies around public health and health promotion, noting that for it to be effective, health promotion needs supportive environments, strengthening of community actions, developing personal skills and reorienting health services (WHO, 1986). Arguably, it was on these developments that current approaches were founded. What was needed for a full-scale adoption of this approach to reducing harm from substance use was some form of catalyst. Undoubtably, the catalyst in moving a public health-based approach using methods embedded in harm reduction into the mainstream of policy and practice was the onset of HIV and AIDS in the 1980s, and the response of various governments to that crisis.

To set one such government-led response in context, Britain was undergoing a transformation in terms of its economic and social basis (see McSmith, 2010). As a result, high levels of structural unemployment and the accompanying urban decay were creating a number of social problems, amongst which were rising rates of acquisitive crime and rising levels of heroin use. It was soon apparent that there was a relationship between heroin use and crime (Bennett & Holloway, 2005). This led to heroin users being seen as a key driver of the 'crime problem' and being seen only as deserving of punishment. Yet crime was not the only problem associated with heroin use. Within those heroin users, there were high levels of injecting drug users (IDUs) often taking part in unsafe injecting practices, leading to a rise in certain types of diseases, mainly hepatitis (Drucker, Alcabes, & Marx, 2001). In some instances, these diseases were transmitted to the non-drug using population, generally through unprotected sex with an infected drug user, many of whom were turning to sex work to fund their substance use (Silbert, Pines, & Lynch, 1982).

In practice, the mainstay of many governments' initial foray into harm reduction took the form of needle exchanges and syringe exchange programmes (SEPs). Whilst technically people who inject drugs (PWID) could purchase clean needles, the 'heroin epidemic' led to the Royal College of Pharmacists advising their members to reduce or cease the sales of needles between 1982 and 1986 (Wright, 2006, p. 47). Wright notes:

> From 1982 to 1986 the Society had taken a firm stance that needles were not to be given to drug misusers, on the grounds that this would help to curb the increase in numbers of people injecting. A statement by the Council required pharmacists to "restrict the sale of syringes and needles to bona fide patients for therapeutic purposes".

This decision was largely based on the growing number of PWID and was arguably based on moral judgements about the nature of the customer rather than their pharmaceutical need. Whilst some PWID would have used risky injecting practices anyway, it is highly possible that during this period many IDUs shared needles through expediency rather than choice. There are implications here about how intoxication was seen at that time. The act of denying clean needles to PWID at least implies that the nature of intoxication caused by injecting heroin to a degree where all manner of unsafe practices were taking place was beyond what was acceptable and placed the IDUs as social and medical outcasts.

However, when evidence began to emerge about the transmission of diseases through infected blood (Robertson, Bucknall, Welsby, & Roberts, 1986), this practice ceased. The UK's first needle exchange opened in Peterborough in 1986 with myriad others following closely in its wake. The UK were following the Netherland's approach where the first needle exchange was opened in 1984 and New Zealand quickly followed the UK with the opening of an SEP in 1987 (Cahill & Schaefer, 2009). As a response to the HIV epidemic, a 1988 report on Aids and Drug Misuse from the Advisory Council on the Misuse of Drugs (ACMD) declared 'the spread of HIV is a greater danger to individual and public health than drug misuse'. In turn, Margaret Thatcher introduced harm reduction as a policy in 1988 (Stimpson, 2010), and since then, harm reduction programmes for HIV prevention have been adopted in more than half of the 158 countries where people inject drugs (https://www.who.int/hiv/topics/idu/en/). Importantly, it must be noted that the political and moral rationale for introducing harm reduction was not the helping of substance users, rather it was couched in terms of fighting HIV for the benefit of the general population. For whatever reason, a specific version of harm reduction practice and policy had become mainstream and accepted. But, and importantly, the focus was to be on the individual rather than any underlying social, environmental or structural factors.

Whilst the initial focus was on PWID and halting the spread of HIV, harm reduction for recreational substance users soon became established, partly because of the growth of 'rave culture' and the accompanying use of substances such as lysergic acid diethylamide (LSD), ecstasy and amphetamines (Manning, 2007). The nature of the harm reduction messages promoted during this period is interesting. Agencies working with recreational substance users during this period clearly felt that their messages needed to be relevant to the user and perhaps not follow the political line that intoxication via illicit substances is bad and that substance users should 'just say no'. Rather than adopt this latter abstinence-based approach, harm reduction messages accepted substance use and were aimed at directly informing users on how to use substances safely to gain the maximum enjoyment (for a good example of this see the Peanut Pete[1] website here: http://michaellinnell.org.uk/michael_linnell_archive/peanut_pete/peanut_pete.html). This recognition that substance use was an integral part of many people's lives went against the dominant messages coming out of central governments such as the '*Just Say No*' message led by Nancy Reagan in the US and the *Heroin Screws You Up* message promoted by the British government.

In effect, substance workers were challenging political rhetoric and criminal justice policy by acknowledging the regular use of illicit substances and the changing social attitudes to substance use and intoxication. The normalisation of drug use was being recognised, thanks in no small part to the work of Parker and colleagues (Parker, Aldridge, & Measham, 1997), and even amongst the most committed abstinence supporters, there was a realisation that banning substances by using the criminal justice system to prevent use was failing. This is important as it endorses the work of Barad cited above (2003) because we see a different form of measurement taking hold and a different form of reality emerging. Instead of measuring and 'dealing with' substance use as a crime problem, this emerging form of measurement began to create a new reality where substance use was seen more as a health and welfare problem.

However, the political reluctance to accept recreational use and intoxication, as well as the accompanying fear that accepting recreational use can be construed as condoning substance taking, led to a failure to provide meaningful messages about how to take substances and manage intoxication in a safer way. In turn, this put the health and well-being of recreational substance users at risk. Again, this led to the British government being forced into facing the dilemma of how to help recreational substance users reduce the risk associated with their intoxications, whilst still maintaining a 'substances are bad' rhetoric. This was not a problem unique to the UK—most other nations were facing the same challenge. The next section examines how governments reacted and how emerging expertise and activist groups were instrumental in expanding the concept and practice of harm reduction.

Harm Reduction: A Different Approach to Measurement and Understanding

To summarise, harm reduction had been allowed a foothold into the 'war on drugs' due to the emergence of HIV/AIDS and an accompanying emergence of a 'new' public health approach to social problems. One possible unintended side effect of government forays into the world of substance use was a recognition that whist being marginal, relatively large proportions of the population were using some form of illicit substance, and as opposed to being seen as deviant, substance use was a normalised and accepted part of everyday culture (Parker et al., 1997). Due to this many governments were forced to rethink policy: whilst it might be fine to have a normative, long-term vision of a 'drug free society', the lived reality was clear—substance use at all levels of intoxication was widespread, and as a result some form of harm reduction input was in order to address a range of needs and problems. This led to significant policy changes throughout many nation states. Kubler (2001, p. 623) neatly makes this point. Although he specifically mentions Western Europe, this could equally be applied worldwide, as Kubler argues:

> Public policies…related to the use of illegal drugs have recently undergone important change throughout Western Europe. Originally based on the prohibitionist regime established by a series of international conventions in the early twentieth century, many national drug policies have moved, in the 1980s and 1990s, toward strategies aimed at drug users unwilling or unable to end consumption.

Yet, whilst this widening of the reach and scope of harm reduction is to be applauded, the underlying assumption was that harm reduction was still very much the preserve of work which social intervention organisations (health, welfare, social work, schools) did when 'dealing with' the intoxication practices of individual substance users. Thus, the individual became both the cause and solution to harmful practices related to drug intoxication, and success could only be seen as an individual achievement. This was (and is) true to a point, but it was also unrealistic, if, sadly, to be expected given the way governments often address a range of social problems. This also illustrates one of the key challenges facing harm reduction practice in as much that whilst there is a whole range of intoxications and an accompanying plethora of harm reduction approaches, it is often politically and culturally 'safe' to focus on PWID and treatment rather than accept and embrace the reality and potential that harm reduction practices have on addressing all forms of intoxications.

Many other social problems which manifest in individual behaviours have their roots in deeper more entrenched social structures and environments (Akers, 2009). There is a long-recognised school of thought that argues by focusing on the individual rather than the structural; governments can downplay their roles in allowing structural inequalities to exist and foreground the moral irresponsibility of the individual (Box, 1987). This was recognised by Moore and Dietze (2008) where, looking at the Australian context, they acknowledged and celebrated the rise of harm reduction as the primary policy option in Australia, but lamented the 'piecemeal and fragmented' nature of policies which aimed to address those structural barriers which existed such as drug laws, poverty, social class and marginalisation.

However, as with many policy areas, harm reduction is not static and fixed. It began to develop in a manner which saw the individualised pathology of the original harm reduction interventions being bolstered by movements promoting harm reduction policies aimed at addressing the harms related to intoxication created by environmental (Rhodes, 2009) and structural (Moore & Dietze, 2005) factors. Kubler's (2001) work provided a theoretical review of why this may have been the case. He draws on advocacy coalition framework theory (ACF) and social movement theory, and then applies these approaches to Swiss drug policy. Space precludes a detailed analysis, but what is important for our purposes here is Kubler's (2001, p. 630) argument that harm reduction was allowed to grow as a result of changes in deep core levels of understanding about substances, noting a shift from a belief that 'deviant' individuals need to 'get back on track' to an emerging belief that individual autonomy and integrity is more important than slavish devotion to sociocultural norms: in short, substance users deserved help as much as anyone else, but they needed to be free to refuse help when offered.

Secondly, Kubler (2001, pp. 630–631) noted a change in policy core beliefs. Under the prohibitionist model, core policy favoured the 'just say no' approach where abstinence was key and coercive pressure was used to force substance users into treatment. In what was then the emergent harm reduction paradigm, core policy beliefs moved towards the stance that treatment must be voluntary, with the decision to enter treatment made by the substance user. Moreover, if the user was unwilling or unable to enter treatment, then help should be offered until the user is ready to seek treatment. Finally, Kubler (2001, p. 630–632) explored how changes translated into instrumental policy beliefs. For example, the changing approach towards a harm reduction paradigm advocated a loosening of repression, a reduction of environmental and structural strains and de-stigmatisation of substance users and their intoxication practices.

Since Kubler wrote his paper, what were new core beliefs and instrumental policy approaches have matured and blossomed. McCann (2008, p. 8) argues that in less than a decade, harm reduction had become so powerful that we reached a position within some countries where:

> The character of policy making was changed as were its politics, the activists involved, and the object of policy—the IDUs themselves. The IDUs were now officially regarded as primarily sick, rather than a primarily criminal, population whose lives must be stabilised so that they stay healthy and alive, if they are eventually to overcome their addiction.

Indeed, such was the strength and confidence of harm reduction protagonists that authors such as Rhodes (2009, p. 193) were able to draw on a range of academic, policy and theoretical sources (including social epidemiology, political economy and the sociology of health) to champion a holistic approach to harm reduction, built on the concept and practice of 'risk environments'. This notion of temporal and spatial risk was not confined to harm reduction—the same criterion has been applied to intoxication in the Night Time Economy (Bancroft, 2009). Rhodes (2009), focusing on harm reduction, argued that substance use harms related to intoxication were products of the social situations and environments in which individuals participate. Thus, rather than see the locus of responsibility at the individual level, a better and more realistic approach was to see intoxication and its related harms as being just as much the responsibility of those organisations and social institutions that have a role in producing harms. So, for example, police enforcement which creates conditions where unsafe injection practice take place can be seen as a harm producer. That said, Rhodes (2009, p. 199) recognised the practical and political difficulties in introducing such an approach, and drawing on the work of Glass and McAtee (2006), he noted:

> Interventions which target social conditions producing drug harms may be more effective than interventions targeting specific behaviours, *even if* these social conditions are not easily translated into specific epidemiological causes or risk factors.

Nevertheless, champions of this holistic approach promoted the benefits of sharing responsibility for drug harms between individuals and socio-economic structures largely because it shifts notions of blame from individual substance users by recognising the complex relationship between socio-economic structures and individuals. This combination of society taking responsibility as promoted by Rhodes (2009) and the shifts in core beliefs and practices identified by Kubler (2001) clearly had some purchase. However, the next logical step in the development of harm reduction would require some brave political decision making. The next section moves to examine recent developments governments have taken in reducing structural harms.

Contemporary Developments: Measuring a New Reality?

It is safe to say that harm reduction is an entrenched and established approach to substance use and intoxication in a large number of countries. Moreover, it is increasingly the case that many jurisdictions have begun to embrace the notion of shared responsibility: equally some large jurisdictions are still wedded to the 'war on drugs' and a prohibition model. This final section takes a brief look at where harm reduction in relation to diverse intoxication practices is potentially taking us.

One of the key harms that the prohibition model carries in its wake is the criminalisation of some substances and self-evidently the subsequent criminalisation of substance users. Carrying a criminal record for a drug offence can have a significant impact on career development and does mitigate against certain types of employment in most countries across the globe with a variety of consequences almost all of which are negative. For example, in a US context, a convicted 'drug felon' cannot get welfare payments, public housing student loans, or a mortgage, so the effects are punitive and far reaching, and in some cases based on little more than a youthful indiscretion. Also, detecting, prosecuting and punishing some types of substances and substance users places a strain on overstretched criminal justice systems, where, arguably, resources could be better used to address more serious and harmful types of offending. Many governments are now realising this, especially in relation to cannabis, which is, after alcohol, the world's favourite recreational intoxicant. As a result, significant legal changes have already taken place. For example, in the USA, nine states have now legalised the possession, production and use of cannabis for personal use. Further developments include Canada's legalisation of cannabis in October 2018, following Uruguay who introduced a legal, regulated cannabis market in 2017. A growing number of governments have also either formally decriminalised cannabis use or possession such as the Czech Republic in 2010, and Portugal in 2001, or have a de facto informal decriminalisation policy in place. There is also evidence that some jurisdictions are moving beyond cannabis: Colorado became the first state to decriminalise the personal possession and use of 'magic mushrooms' in May 2019.

Alongside this, many governments are moving rapidly towards ensuring substance use is taking place in safe conditions. Safe injecting facilities are now becoming common place across many countries, aimed at making sure users are safe and can access advice and care if required (Mitchell, 2017). For recreational users, substance testing units are becoming an established feature of festival landscapes. For example, in the UK, drug testing units were available at around ten festivals in 2018, often with the support of the local police (Wilding, 2017). The harm reduction impact of this approach is tried and tested: Switzerland, where some substances are illegal, adopted this practice and there have been no deaths attributed to so-called party drugs (which would include MDMA, cocaine, amphetamine and LSD) in the past seven years (Wilding, 2017). Measham (2019) provides research evidence for the impact of drug testing, and grass-roots organisations like 'knowyourstuff' (https://knowyourstuff.nz/) in New Zealand have pioneered this important harm reduction approach to substance use. Elsewhere in the Southern Hemisphere, authors such as Camilleri and Caldicott (2005) have long been champions of drug testing.

Equally, the prohibition model is based on seeing the 'blame' for substance use firmly in the hands of the user. Harm reduction, as noted above, seeks to change this perspective and move debate and practice into accepting that socio-economic conditions need to be factored into any policies aimed at reducing substance-related harm. Again, just as with the criminalisation of substances, governments across the globe are beginning to enshrine harm reduction's approach in policy. One example amongst many is the approach adopted by New Zealand where:

> Alcohol and other drug issues are closely intertwined with social factors such as income, employment, housing and education. This means that effective government intervention requires a cross-agency response. (New Zealand Ministry of Health on-line, 2018)

Although as with many government's policies across the globe, this is not necessarily the case in practice; it often being that the rhetoric of governments does not match up to proffered practice or the lived realities of the receivers of policy (Barton & Johns, 2013).

That notwithstanding, taken together these moves mark a significant and often brave move on the part of national governments. In effect, what governments are acknowledging is that criminalising intoxication, defining and then measuring it as a 'crime' or as 'deviant' behaviour are counterproductive in terms of reducing intoxication-related harms. Accompanying this is a tacit recognition that prohibition will not, and arguably cannot, stop use.

However, despite this, some jurisdictions are still wedded to the prohibition model and seek to restrict harm reduction approaches. For example, Davidson, Lopez, and Kral (2018) report on their findings regarding the use of 'underground' supervised injecting facilities in the USA and the difficulties this poses for workers and users alike; Russia's hard-line drug policy has been questioned on a number of grounds including global public good and as a violation of human rights (Arps & Golichenko, 2014; Babor et al., 2010); Singapore and the continuation of the death penalty for drug law violations generates much debate (Leechaianan & Longmire, 2013); and the unlawful killing of over 8000 drug users in the Philippines continues to raise serious questions about human rights violations in that jurisdiction (Muggah, 2017). Even in countries where harm reduction is established, the lack of open commitment, combined with political intransigence and expediency, creates a confusing and complex environment. Nutt (2015, p. 2), looking at British drug policy, argues:

> The government has been resisting evidence because they think there's political advantage in pretending that the old policy will work. And they're scared of being shown to have got it wrong. The Home Office is resisting it because it's not independent; it's actually working to the politicians rather than to the people and advisory experts. It's a peculiar collusion between the civil service and politicians, to the detriment of everyone.

Concluding Thoughts

Intoxication and harm go hand in hand and range from a mild alcohol-induced hangover all the way through to premature death. We know this because materially, it has been forever the case. As demonstrated above, how we view and measure intoxication (Barad, 2003), how we reduce harms and where we place blame for the negative consequences of substance use varies, and is as much to do with politics, protecting 'good citizens' from 'deviant populations', mobilising pressure and practice development as it is to do with compassion for the harmed. That said, since harm reduction made a foothold into the dominant prohibition paradigm, the evolution of both the concept and practice of harm reduction has seen it become the dominant model in approaching the harms related to intoxication. Accompanying that, or indeed arguably leading the way, is the change in how we measure and therefore understand intoxication and harm reduction. We have now reached a stage where governments of all persuasions are moving towards accepting intoxication as a norm and putting policies in place to address intoxication-related harms. Moreover, there are the beginnings of a movement where some jurisdictions are looking at structural and environmental causation of harm and in some instances seeing access to harm reduction as a basic human right. These are significant changes in a prohibition approach to substance use and intoxication that had its roots in the invasive, punitive and morally repugnant Contagious Diseases Acts of the 1800s. It will be illuminating to see how much further harm reduction, as a response to multiple ways of becoming intoxicated, develops in the next decade.

Note

1. Peanut Pete was a cartoon character created by the Manchester Lifeline Project. He was a recreational drug user who often pushed his use of the drug little bit too far. The cartoons were amusing but had a serious message, aimed specifically at a certain type of substance user.

References

Advisory Council on the Misuse of Drugs. (1988). *Aids and drugs misuse.* London: ACMD.

Akers, R. (2009). *Social learning and social structure: A general theory of crime and deviance.* New York: Routledge.

Arps, F. S. E., & Golichenko, M. (2014). Sex workers unite! Litigating for sex worker's freedom of association in Russia. *Health and Human Rights Journal, 16*, 2.

Babor, T. F., Caulkins, J. P., Edwards, G., Fischer, B., Foxcroft, D. R., Humphreys, K., …, Reuter, P. (2010). *Drug policy and the public good.* New York: Oxford University Press.

Bancroft, A. (2009). *Drugs, intoxication and society.* Cambridge: Polity Press.

Barad, K. (2003). Posthumanist performativity: Toward an understanding of how matter comes to matter. *Signs: Journal of Women in Culture and Society, 28*(3), 801–831.
Barad, K. (2012). On touching – The inhuman therefore I am. *Differences: A Journal of Feminist Cultural Studies, 23*(3), 801–831.
Barton, A. (2011). *Illicit drugs: Use and control* (2nd ed.). Routledge: London.
Barton, A., & Johns, N. (2013). *The policy making process in the criminal justice system.* London: Routledge.
Becker, H. (1967). History, Culture and Subjective Experience: An exploration of the social bases of drug-induced experiences. *Journal of Health and Social Behaviour, 8*(3), 163–176.
Bennett, T., & Holloway, K. (2005). *Understanding drugs, alcohol and crime.* Maidenhead: Open University Press.
Box, S. (1987). *Recession, crime and punishment.* London: Macmillan.
Cahill, S., & Schaefer, N. (Eds.). (2009). *Syringe exchange programs around the world: The global context.* Gay Men's Health Crisis. Retrieved from September 9, 2018, from http://www.gmhc.org/files/editor/file/gmhc_intl_seps.pdf
Camilleri, A. M., & Caldicott, D. (2005). Underground pill testing, down under. *Forensic Science International, 151*(1), 53–58.
Coomber, R., Moyle, L., & South, N. (2016). The normalisation of drug supply: The social supply of drugs as the "other side" of the history of normalisation. *Drugs: Education, Prevention and Policy, 23*(3), 255–263.
Davidson, P. J., Lopez, A. M., & Kral, A. H. (2018). Using drugs in un/safe spaces: Impact of perceived illegality on and underground supervised injecting facility in the USA. *International Journal of Drug Policy, 53*, 47–54.
Drucker, E., Alcabes, P. G., & Marx, P. A. (2001). The injection century: Massive unsterile injections and the rise of human pathogens. *The Lancet, 358*(9297), 1989–1992.
Edwards, G. (2005). *Matters of substance: Drugs: Is legalization the right answer – Or the wrong question?* Harmondsworth: Penguin.
Glass, T. A., & McAtee, M. J. (2006). Behavioral science at the crossroads in public health: Extending horizons, envisioning the future. *Social Science and Medicine, 62*, 1650–1671.
Greenfield, S. F., Pettianti, H. M., O'Malley, S., Randall, P. K., & Randall, C. L. (2010). Gender differences in alcohol treatment: An analysis of outcome from the COMBINE Study. *Alcoholism: Clinical and Experimental Research, 34*(10), 1803–1812.

Griffin, C., Bengry-Howell, A., Hackley, C., Mistral, W., & Szmigin, I. (2009). "Every time I do it I absolutely annihilate myself": Loss of (self)consciousness and loss of memory in young people's drinking narratives. *Sociology, 43*(3), 457–476.

Harm Reduction International. (2018). Home Page. Retrieved September 12, 2018, from www.hri.global

Inciardi, J. A. (1999). *Harm reduction: National and international perspectives.* Thousand Oaks: Sage.

Kubler, D. (2001). Understanding policy change with the advocacy coalition framework: An application to Swiss drug policy, in. *Journal of European Public Policy, 8*(4), 623–641.

Leechaianan, Y., & Longmire, D. (2013). The use of the death penalty for drug trafficking in the United States, Singapore, Malaysia, Indonesia and Thailand: A comparative legal analysis. *Laws, 2*(2), 115–149.

Manning, P. (Ed.). (2007). *Drugs and popular culture.* Cullompton: Willan.

McCann, E. (2008). Expertise, truth and urban policy mobilities: Global circuits of knowledge in the development of Vancouver, Canada's 'four pillars' drug strategy. *Environment and Planning, 40*, 885–904.

McSmith, A. (2010). *No such thing as society.* London: Constable.

Measham, F., & Brain, K. (2005). 'Binge' drinking, British alcohol policy and the new culture of intoxication. *Crime, Media, Culture: An international journal, 1*(3), 263–284.

Measham, F. C. (2019). Drug safety testing, disposals and dealing in an English field: Exploring the operational and behavioural outcomes of the UK's first onsite 'drug checking' service. *International Journal of Drug Policy, 67*, 102–107.

Mill, J. S., in Warnock, M. (1962). *Utilitarianism and on liberty.* London: Fontana Library.

Mitchell, F. (2017). Glasgow, Scotland tackling injection of drugs in public spaces through the introduction of safer facilities. *The Lancet, 4*, 4.

Moore, D., & Dietze, P. (2005). Enabling environments and the reduction of drug-related harm: Re-framing Australian policy and practice. *Drug and Alcohol Review, 24*(3), 275–284.

Moore, D., & Dietze, P. (2008). Drugs and public health: Australian perspectives on policy. South Melbourne: Oxford University Press.

Muggah, R. (2017). Duterte's drug war in the Philippines is out of control, he needs to be stopped, *The Guardian.* Retrieved June 18, 2019, from https://www.theguardian.com/global-development-professionals-network/2017/

jan/05/rodrigo-dutertes-drug-war-in-the-philippines-is-out-of-control-he-needs-to-be-stopped
New Zealand Ministry of Health. (2018). *National drug policy 2015–2020*. Retrieved August 23, 2018, from https://www.health.govt.nz/publication/national-drug-policy-2015-2020
Nutt, D. (2015). quoted in an interview with PI Media (UCL student media). Retrieved September 26, 2018, from https://pimediaonline.co.uk/investigation/legalise-it-an-interview-with-professor-david-nutt-on-uk-drug-policy/
Nutt, D., King, L. A., Saulsbury, W., & Blakemore, C. (2007). The development of a rational scale to assess the harms of drugs of potential misuse. *Health Policy, 369*(9566), 1047–1053.
Parker, H., Aldridge, J., & Measham, F. (1997). *Illegal leisure*. London: Routledge.
Rhodes, T. (2009). Risk environments and drug harms: A social science for harm. In *International Journal of Drug Policy* (Vol. 20, pp. 193–201).
Robertson, J. R., Bucknall, A. B. V., Welsby, P. D., & Roberts, J. J. K. (1986). Epidemic of AIDS related virus (HLTV 3/LAZ) infection among intravenous drug users. *British Medical Journal*. (Clinical research ed.), *292*(6519), 527–529.
Roe, G. (2005). Harm reduction as paradigm: Is better than bad good enough? The origins of harm reduction. *Critical Public Health, 15*(3), 243–250.
Scruton, R. (2007). The philosophy of wine. In J. Robinson & B. C. Smith (Eds.), *Questions of taste: The philosophy of wine*. Oxford: Signal Books.
Silbert, M. H., Pines, A. M., & Lynch, T. (1982). Substance abuse and prostitution. *Journal of Psychoactive Drugs, 14*(3), 193–197.
Smith, F. B. (1990). The contagious diseases acts reconsidered. *Social History of Medicine, 3*(2), 197–215.
Stimpson, G. V. (2010). Harm reduction: Moving through the third decade. *The International Journal on Drug Policy, 21*(2), 91–93.
Vernon, R. (1996). John Stuart Mill and pornography: Beyond the harm principle. *Ethics, 106*(3), 621–632.
Wheeler, C. (2019). Michael Gove: A cocaine party – Then an anti-drugs article. *The Times*. Retrieved June 14, 2019, from https://www.thetimes.co.uk/article/backers-rally-around-contrite-michael-gove-after-cocaine-confession-l873hqzp8
Wilding, M. (2017). How the UK's music festivals changed their tune on drugs. *The Vice*. Retrieved August 14, 2018, from https://www.vice.com/en_uk/article/gybgeb/how-the-uks-music-festivals-changed-their-tune-on-drugs-safe-sesh

Winnifrith, T. (1994). *Fallen women in the nineteenth-century novel.* London: St. Martin's Press.

World Health Organisation. (1986). *Ottawa charter for health promotion.* Retrieved August 8, 2018, from http://www.who.int/healthpromotion/conferences/previous/ottawa/en/

World Health Organisation. (2018). *People who inject drugs.* Retrieved September 12, 2018, from www.who.int

Wright, M. (2006, August 11). Exchanging views of needle exchange. *The Pharmaceutical Journal.* Retrieved August 11, 2006, from https://www.pharmaceutical-journal.com/PJ,-August-2006/315.issue

Index[1]

[1] Note: Page numbers followed by 'n' refer to notes.

F. Hutton (ed.), *Cultures of Intoxication*,
https://doi.org/10.1007/978-3-030-35284-4

CPSIA information can be obtained
at www.ICGtesting.com
Printed in the USA
LVHW011645191220
674620LV00004B/169

9 783030 352837